WIND IN THE BLOOD

WIND IN THE BLOOD

Mayan Healing and Chinese Medicine

HERNÁN GARCÍA
ANTONIO SIERRA
GILBERTO BALÁM
Translated by Jeff Conant

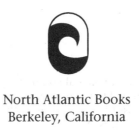

North Atlantic Books
Berkeley, California

Published by
North Atlantic Books
Berkeley, California

Original publishers:
Educación, Cultura y Ecología, A.C. (EDUCE), Foro de Apoyo Mutuo (FAM) México, Venta de Medicamentos y Materiales Educativos en Servicios de Salud, S.A. (VEMMESS), Promición de Servicios de Salud y Educación Popular, A.C. (PRODUSSEP), Guadelupe Huelsz

Cover photo by Ignacio Alcantara and Reynaldo Izquierdo
Cover and book design by Treehouse Graphics
Original art by María Teresa Munguía. Additional drawings by Preet Srivastava.
Drawing on page 20 from *Healing With Whole Foods: Oriental Traditions and Modern Nutrition,* by Paul Pitchford (Berkeley: North Atlantic Books, © 1993). Reprinted by permission of the publisher.

Printed in Canada

Wind in the Blood: Mayan Healing and Chinese Medicine is sponsored and published by the Society for the Study of Native Arts and Sciences (dba North Atlantic Books), an educational nonprofit based in Berkeley, California, that collaborates with partners to develop cross-cultural perspectives, nurture holistic views of art, science, the humanities, and healing, and seed personal and global transformation by publishing work on the relationship of body, spirit, and nature.

North Atlantic Books' publications are available through most bookstores. For further information, visit our website at www.northatlanticbooks.com or call 800-733-3000.

Library of Congress Cataloging-in-Publication Data
García, Hernán.
    [Medicina maya tradicional. English]
    Wind in the blood : Mayan healing and Chinese medicine / by Hernán García, Antonio Sierra, and Gilberto Balám; translated by Jeff Conant.
        p.   cm.
    Includes bibliographical references and index.
    ISBN-13: 978-1-55643-304-7
    ISBN-10: 1-55643-304-2 (alk.paper)
    1. Mayas—Medicine. 2. Medicine, Chinese. I. Title. II. Sierra, Antonio.
III. Balam Pereira, Gilberto.
F1435.3.M4 G3713 1999
610'.89'974152 21—dc21   99-045353

5 6 7 8 9 MQ 23 22 21 20

This book includes recycled material and material from well-managed forests. North Atlantic Books is committed to the protection of our environment. We print on recycled paper whenever possible and partner with printers who strive to use environmentally responsible practices.

HEALING SONG

This is to cool burning fever and to cool fire, the ailment fire.

My foot's coolness, my hand's coolness,
      as I cooled this fire.
Fivefold my white hail, my black hail, yellow hail,
      as I cool the fire.
Thirteenfold my red cloth, my white cloth, my black cloth, yellow
      cloth, when I answered the strength of this fire.
A black fan my emblem,
      as I answered the strength of this fire.
With me comes the white water-maize,
      and I answered the strength of this fire.
With me comes the water-lily,
      and I have answered the strength of this fire.
Just now I settled my foot's coolness, my hand's coolness.
      Amen.

      —from *Ritual of the Bacabs,* in *The Sun Unwound:*
        Original Texts from Occupied America

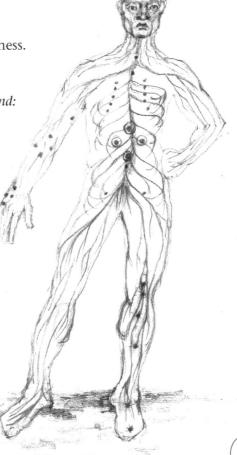

HEALING SONG

This is not of bathing ... cool fire, the diligent fire.

My roots coolness, my hand's coolness,
as I cooled this fire.
Even in my white hail, my black hail, yellow hail,
as I cool the fire.
Threefold my red cloth, my white cloth, my black cloth, yellow
cloth, when I answered the strength of this fire
As I bear out my emblem?
as I answered the strength of this fire.
With me comes the white water-maker,
and I answered the strength of this fire.
With me comes the water-lily,
and I have answered the strength of this fire,
just now I cooled my root's coolness, my hand's coolness.
Amen.

—from Ritual of the Bacabs, in The Sun Unwound:
Original Texts from Occupied America

TABLE OF CONTENTS

AUTHORS' ACKNOWLEDGEMENTS

THIS WORK IS A COLLECTIVE fruit whose principal protagonists are the *curanderos* of Campeche and Yucatán with whom we have worked for several years. With them we realized a series of encounters, workshops, monthly meetings, individual interviews, and observations of their practice. Several of them worked collectively with us in the preparation of this book. Unfortunately, for reasons of space, we have not included the numerous anecdotes and personal narratives of the *curanderos*.

From the region of Camino Real in the state of Campeche a great number of *curanderos* participated: they were shamans, herbalists, masseuses, bone setters and midwives from the communities of Santa Cruz Ex Hacienda, San Nicolás, Tankuché, Calkiní, Dzitbalché, Bacabchén, Poc Boc, Hecelchakán, Dzotchén, Cumpich, Santa Cruz Pueblo, Concepción, Sacabchén and Pucnanchén.

From these communities the *curanderos* who participated actively in the work brought together in this book are: Hipólito Naal Ke, Amelia Naal Tzuul, Pedro Tzulub, Fidelio Colli Mech, Eugenio Brito Che, Flora Ku Almeida, Aurelio Mech, Francisco Ak Canul, Nemencia Huchin Flores, María Socorro Herrera de Uk, Elena Falcón Herrera, María Noemí Quetz Tzec, Rosalía Pedroza Garduño, Felipe de Jesús Aguilar Pool, Guillermina Canul Chi, Florencia Sofía Pérez Más, Fortunato Cahuich Tum, Margarita Ortiz Camal, Matilde Chan Ake, Maximo Tun Chan, Ermilo Sima Pech, María Zenaida Ortiz Uh, José Dolores Ortiz Camal, Mariano Ortiz Uh, Ana María Cahuich Canul, Benita Mis Dzib, Catalina Tun Yan, Agustina Mis Dzib, Marcelina Yah Mis, María Jacinta Cohuo Naal, Eufracia Uk Naal, Isabel Mancilla Cohuo, Gilberto Sunza Dzul, Hilaria Tamay Mancilla, Juanito Cahuich, Ignacia Cocom Eguan, María Concepción Uk Chan,

María Leonida Chan Pech, Elena Josefina Ku Chan, Natalia Uk Chan, Eutalio Sunza Dzul, Alberto Queb Yak, Ursula Tamay Canche, Dionisia Ek Chi, Eusebia Ek Chi, Cristina Uk Ek, Antonia Chin Ek, and Hermenegilda Ku Ek.

We would like to acknowledge, as well, the support of workers at various regional centers of the National Indigenous Institute (INI) in the states of Yucatán and Campeche, especially the center in Calkiní.

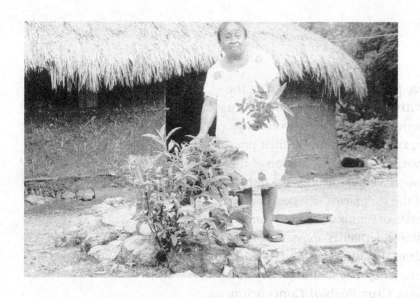

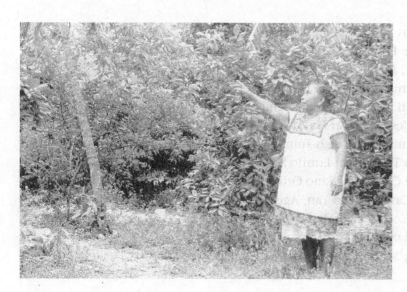

TRANSLATOR'S ACKNOWLEDGEMENTS

THE TRANSLATOR WOULD LIKE TO ACKNOWLEDGE the friendship and generosity of countless people in numerous villages in Chiapas and Guatemala who opened their houses and their lives to me during the course of this work. I thank, as well, those without whose kindness and support in a difficult moment this work of translation would be undone, or worse, lost. For original artwork I thank Preet Srivastava, and for invaluable help with both resources and refuge during the course of the work, I thank Matthew Graham, Thomas Doughty, Nicole Andersen, Annick Garcia, Alfonso Jaramillo, Darin De Stefano, Claudia Peniche, and Karla Quiñones. In encounters between different worlds there is always a shock; this work, like those who have supported it, is bound by the hope of minimizing the shock in order to facilitate understanding.

Finally, I would like to dedicate the work to all of those who, within and outside of the villages of the Mayan regions, have sacrificed everything to preserve and protect cultural knowledge and dignity.

TRANSLATOR'S FOREWORD

MY FIRST ENCOUNTER with Mayan medicine occurred in the Guatemalan highland village of Todos Santos Chuchumatan. For several days I took long walks in the mountains with the *comadrona*—the midwife and healer of that village—and she introduced me to the native medicinal plants and explained to me the rudiments of the local botanical medicine. An elderly Mam Maya woman, she spoke very little Spanish—and I spoke no Mam—which made the long cool mornings pass slowly; but her patient explanations, using signs, gestures, and the few words available to us both, seemed to me both detailed and complete. Beyond awe at her complete familiarity with the flora of those hills, I was impressed by two things: that the plants familiar to me from my home in California were put to similar uses here—bougainvillia for cough, plantain for infections of the mouth and throat, psyllium seed for cleaning the gut, cornsilk for infections of the urinary tract and bladder—and that the native medicine embraced concepts completely foreign to Western industrial medicine. She described to me unfamiliar illnesses such as fright, envy, and the evil eye—*susto, envidia,* and *mal de ojo* —and explained to me how she treated them. That these illnesses, described in *Wind in the Blood* as "spiritual illnesses," were treated with herbal remedies equal to the treatments for, say, headache, diarrhea, and diabetes, impressed me as interesting both from an anthropological and pragmatic perspective.

These non-Western diseases and their classification—central to the local medicine—are perhaps indicative of the values, the vision, and the historical situation of the culture, much as cancer, heart disease, AIDS, and the discourse surrounding them are indicative of the conditions and cultural underpinnings of Western post-industrial cultures at the current moment. With a slight shifting of terminologies and paradigms we might see that the illnesses defined by Mesoamerican peoples—fright, envy, desire—are quite common—even pandemic—in the so-called "first world" as well. Western medicine is beginning to deal on a vast scale with disorders that might be classified as types of fright and envy—attention deficit disorder, post-traumatic stress, depression, anorexia, and nervous anxiety, to name a handful—but has yet to learn the lesson integral to Mayan medicine: that dealing with these diseases must be done systemically, both by treating the body as an entity and by examining the causes of disease in the individual's relation with society as a whole.

Another class of diseases which came to my attention during those long mountain walks include illnesses involving cold, heat, and wind. This brought to mind Chinese medicine—of which I had a rudimentary knowledge—with its theory of the five elements and the thermal qualities of illness and treatment, its understanding of the seven emotions and the atmospheric influences. The comparison, simple as it was, never left me. I imagined that native Mesoamerican medicine had at one time been as "advanced"—that is, sophisticated in its concepts and integrated in its practice—as Chinese medicine. My assumption was, and still is, that the vastly different cultural histories of China and Mesoamerica—the one a highly literate monarchical beauracracy lasting thousands of years, the other a largely oral culture with a literate priest class whose foundations (and whose entire library of literature and histories) were systematically uprooted and destroyed by conquest and colonization—caused Chinese medicine to become widely known and highly respected throughout the world, while Mesoamerican medicine virtually disappeared.

Over the next few years my original impressions remained as I encountered Mayan medicine in practice in villages throughout Chiapas, Mexico. I found the ancient concepts still very much alive among the Mayan people, sometimes in forms difficult to distinguish, sometimes astonishingly clear. I once asked my friend Raphael, a Tzeltal Maya healer with Western training, to explain *susto,* fright. He answered: "fright is when something happens to scare you and your soul leaves your body. Without the soul, the body is weak and gets sick easily. The only way to cure it is to bring the soul back." When I asked him if any Western remedies could bring the soul back into the body, he said it was possible, but he'd never heard of them.

The first Mexican edition of this book, *Medicina Maya Tradicional,* was printed in May, 1996, in a modest edition of 1000. I discovered the book in San Cristóbal de las Casas, Chiapas, in the winter of 1997 in the office of PRODUSSEP, one of the popular health organizations that had a hand in publishing it. I immediately recognized in it the confirmation of my speculations. On reading the text I found that the similarities between Mayan and Chinese medicines were more profound than I could have imagined, down to the use of the very same pressure points.

The authors of the book—three doctors working in rural communities in the state of Campeche—were taking a bold new approach to popular healthcare in indigenous areas. The traditional post-conquest attitude towards this work is typical: Doctors arrive in a village and offer their expertise to a population which they consider backwards or ill-informed at best. The doctors bring their understandings of health and disease and attempt to train the people in the basics of health technology. But the people respond slowly, stubbornly, or not at all. Unbeknownst to the doctors, the rural indigenous population maintains its own ideas on the subject.

But these doctors—Balám, Sierra, and García—took the traditional cultural understanding of health as a point of departure for treating illness. They asked a lot of questions, and listened carefully to the answers. What is so radical in this approach is simply that it appreciates the indigenous culture in its own right, and perceives the validity of the ancient medicine, even in its currently fragmented form. Surprising as it may be to some, even at this late date, an attitude so free of culturally bound assumptions and stereoptypes—and so determined to respond to the culture on its own terms—is rare in the fields of development and popular health.

Traveling in the Mayan regions—particularly in war torn Guatemala and Chiapas—one cannot remain unaware of the violent upheaval which has overturned these cultures since the conquest, and which continues to the present moment. As national and global forces bare the earth in their search for resources to feed industry, one of the first victims, besides the land itself, is culture. When, in July of 1562, Friar Diego de Landa ordered the destruction of 5000 Mayan idols and 27 hieroglyphic scrolls, the damage to cultural memory was irreversible; this was merely the beginning of a process which continues with the imposition of occidental cultural notions—of the nature of knowledge, of medicine, of nature itself—on the Mayan people.

Visiting the ruins of Tikal in Guatemala, I met a practitioner of the traditional medicine, a *curandero*. My traveling partner was suffering from kidney stones, and we asked the *curandero* if he could do anything to alleviate her pain. He gladly agreed to help, and asked only that we respect his practice by *not* insisting to pay him. As he proceeded with the diagnosis his questions centered on the subject of fear and doubt; it seemed that, for him, kidney stones were a matter of residual fear inhabiting the kidneys. This struck me, again, as profoundly similar to a Chinese diagnosis, where the emotion associated with these organs is fright.

In the early hours of the morning, before the first light split the lowland mist, he performed a massage, with the intention of "breaking" the stones. He chanted softly as he worked, and when he finished he was visibly exhausted by the process. He said that he had only been able to break one of the two stones that he had detected, but that the other would dissolve in the coming weeks. He recommended pineapple juice and a tea of maidenhair fern to be taken daily.

A few hours after the treatment, my friend experienced severe pain and discovered blood in her urine. The pain passed and we continued our travels. A week later she came down with a high fever and a severe kidney infection. By the time she got to a hospital the infection was gone, and, as an ultrasound proved, so were the kidney stones.

This serves as an example, to my mind, of the effectiveness of traditional Mesoamerican medicine. But the great challenge comes in integrating this medicine with occidental understandings. Another example illustrates: in the village of Roberto Barrios, not far from Tikal but on the Mexican side of the border, I was asked to visit a man who was suffering from a severe infection in his foot, to give my opinion on the matter. Entering his hut, I saw the man lying on his side on a dirty straw mat on the mud floor of a house filled with cobwebs and the greasy black soot of a cooking fire. His right foot was swollen to twice its natural size and covered with open, festering sores. The foot was also completely filthy, covered with dirt, as if it hadn't been washed in days. My immediate suggestion was to wash the foot in water, wrap it in a clean bandage, and keep it dry. When I asked why the man had not visited the village clinic, I was given an unclear response. I suggested bringing the resident clinician but was asked not to. And the reaction to my advice of washing the foot was less than positive, for reasons which were equally unclear.

I went to the clinic and mentioned the situation to the health promoter on duty, who explained, "he won't come to the clinic because he doesn't believe in the medicine. He's seeing a *brujo* (witch) who tells him that clinic medicine is poison." I asked if they could at least get him to wash his foot, and was told that the *brujo* had advised against putting water on the foot. The heat of the infection, combined with the cold nature of water, would disrupt his spirit and complicate the illness.

The Mayan notion of cleanliness, as we'll see in the book, is very different from the Western notion, and has nothing to do with germ theory. This presents one of the most basic problems for health workers with Western training working in indigenous areas, a problem which the authors of this book are attempting to resolve. The man with the foot infection in Roberto Barrios may have ended up losing his foot due to the inability of the local medicine to stem the infection. In cases like this, one cannot simply privilege one cultural system over the other; we cannot expect Western medicine to work consistently for Mayan *campesinos* any more than we can expect Mayan medicine to work for stockbrokers on Wall Street. It is in the resolution of this challenge that this book offers hope.

The value of a comparison between Mayan medicine and Chinese medicine is in dispelling the stereotypes associated with indigenous healing, and in giving credence to terms like "evil eye," "fright," and other concepts central to the Mesoamerican concept of physical and social harmony. Euroamerican culture has begun to embrace traditional Chinese medicine—due, in large part, to detailed scientific studies which prove the effectiveness of Chinese acupuncture and explain it in terms comprehensible in the West. It is time to expand this acceptance to the realm of traditions born on our own continent. Though most readers will not apply this medicine in their own lives, by making this information available, and presenting it in a context which establishes its legitimacy and efficacy, I would hope to take one small step towards reversing the trend of domination and destruction which has characterized occidental relations with indigenous American cultures. As a journey of a thousand miles begins with a single step, so the reversal of the trend of marginalization begins with a simple gesture of understanding. If this book inspires the slightest rethinking of historical and conceptual relations on the continent, the step will have been well taken.

—Jeff Conant, April 1999

PREFACE

WE LIVE IN A TIME OF REEVALUATION. The global "new order" has not succeeded in erasing all of the ancient practices of rural peoples, nor has it removed their need to sustain these practices. Knowledge continues being exercised in many parts of the world which remains largely obscure to an urban public who find illumination only in their television screens and computer monitors. Fortunately, people stubbornly continue seeking meaning in the places where it has always resided. Today, long enduring cultures are increasingly conscious of the importance of maintaining their traditional knowledge, their way of fighting off the darkness. Scholars and educators throughout the world have begun, painstakingly, to recognize a past rich in knowledge, and the trajectory—the cosmovision—that has made it cohere and endure. In our case we are talking about the vital history of Mesoamerica.

Today this body of knowledge is being rebuilt bit by bit. When the interests of one traditional community coincide with the curiosity of a group of respectful scholars, the result is illuminating; many paths suddenly open towards deeper discoveries and fissures in our common understanding. This book is the product of such an effort. The authors, doctors by trade, submerged themselves in rural health promotion in Campeche and began to glimpse patterns which, though fragmentary and disarticulated, suggested the existence of a local conceptual system for the treatment of disease and the location of its causes. This system only began to fully emerge when the doctors, with some effort of the imagination, put aside the conceptual instruments they had received from Western medical practice and began to use the Chinese theoretical system as a lens through which to study local tradition. This shift in viewpoint unleashed a surprising wave of successes, including the assembly of this book. Primarily, the authors began to lay bridges between the dispersed fragments using a system which was well suited to such an undertaking. This brought about a synthesis of accumulated traditions and conceptions of the human body, of the processes of health and disease, and the balance of opposing forces. Above all, the traditional Mayan healers involved in the project encountered that necessary mirror which allowed them to share their knowledge with ease and fluidity—knowledge which had previously been devalued and ignored by doctors and anthropologists alike. These Mayan healers, devoted practitioners, felt that their curiosity was shared, that they could reconsider and explain their world view, that there was now someone who could receive their knowledge respectfully and thoughtfully.

This book comes to light after years of communal and communitarian work. Many traditional healers from various communities in Campeche and Yucatán—principally the region of Camino Real in Campeche—have contributed to the work. These healers were not merely "informants," in the anthropological sense. The learning was vast and mutual—cross-cultural dialogue, they call it—and made it possible to understand the present state of a Mayan system of acupuncture which is inscribed in a wide body of medical knowledge rooted in the Mayan cosmovision, or world-view. It is a holistic vision which makes no attempt to isolate a symptom or establish a disease without recognizing the point of balance between human action and those qualities, forces, and phenomena in which it takes part.

The intent here is to produce some teachings; "local knowledge" has a value that would be worth our while to recognize. This knowledge will be accessible in the degree to which it is studied in close collaboration with its ancient and honorable bearers. This collaboration will be possible only if those who attempt it, from this side of the cultural border, eschew the custom of devaluing the evidence—a custom which the current Mexican educational system continues propagating. We must assume the shared responsibility of envisioning new ways to approach ancient knowledge without idealizing it, and be disposed to look closely and to amaze ourselves with the discovery. Only in this way will we find ourselves atop the cultural garbage that threatens to suffocate us.

—Ramón Vera Herrera, April 1996

INTRODUCTION

Once upon a time, three blind men ran into an elephant. The first one approached the elephant at the trunk, the second at one leg, and the third at the torso. The first said, "This animal is like a snake, only strong, and wrinkled." The second replied, "What are you talking about? It seems more like a tree trunk." The third man retorted, "You're both out of your minds! This animal is like a huge wall."
    —Indian Fable

AS DOCTORS, EACH ONE OF US is familiar, by different routes, with the health needs of *campesinos* and indigenous people. We began our work by interpreting, through our own conceptual framework, the society in which they live, the roots of their diseases and their medical practices. After many years of experience working in rural indigenous areas, we have come to appreciate the existence of ways of comprehending the world that are different from our own.

From the beginning we pronounced our respect for popular forms of culture and we occupied ourselves with recovering certain cultural elements, especially those elements which would be useful for educational and clinical work. But our knowledge of the culture was limited, and sometimes it seemed to us that elements of traditional culture actually obstructed the work of community health education. Because of the limited and partial vision with which we began, we saw the culture of the *campesinos* and indigenous people as if it were nothing more than the sum of disarticulated elements—some good, others bad.

In rural and urban populations throughout Mexico, little by little—according to the degree of trust we each established with members of the communities—we began to hear comments like the following:

- "My sister was struck by a wind and her face swelled up. It's not a sickness of doctors, so I didn't say anything to you, and I took her to a *curandero* who cured her in a few hours."
- "I tie a red bandanna to my son's wrist to protect him from the evil eye."
- "My wife is pregnant and can't eat the foods that the doctors recommend because they are cold foods."

- "I can't wash my hands because I just came from working and I am feeling hot."
- "This morning my two-year-old daughter was almost kidnapped by *aluxob*. I was out harvesting coffee, and who knows how she wandered off and fell forty meters downhill. When I reached her she was alright, and she spoke to me about the children who had carried her away."

Comments like these opened the door to a world with a different logic. We realized, slowly, that in indigenous and rural *mestizo* communities, as much as in urban and suburban centers, there exist patterns of thinking with prehispanic roots—an alternative logic by which the people interpret and act in the world. We came to understand then that the indigenous world obeys a different law, another knowing, a different structure of thought than does Western culture. This realization brought us closer to the field of traditional medicine where we could begin to obtain elements that would help us understand and decipher the culture as such.

In Campeche and Yucatán, we came into contact with the Mayan *curanderos* of the region, and worked with them in a process of investigation and action; we recognized their role as essential to the health of the community, as well as to our own understanding of—and interaction with—the culture. The indigenous healer is, in many cases, a traditional authority or community leader, and in general is recognized as a servant of the community. To the present day these healers are essential to their communities. The recognition they receive, despite changing social conditions, allows them to continue exercising their medical practice.

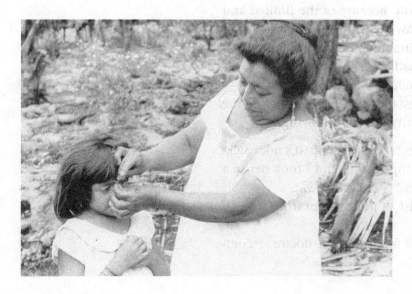

In the beginning of our work in the Mayan regions, the principal objective was to understand their conception of health, the contemporary state of Mayan traditional medicine, and the current world-view. As we deepened our understanding of this traditional medicine, we discovered a set of conceptual and practical elements which appeared to be integrated in a series of conceptual principals—indicating the presence of a system of great richness and depth. Catching glimpses of the system of traditional medicine, we found that the conceptual and practical elements were fragmented, unordered, disarticulated, and disperse; it became necessary to look to the roots of the system in order to understand its applications.

EXISTING INFORMATION ON TRADITIONAL MAYAN MEDICINE

Current knowledge about Mayan medicine springs from various sources. It has not been possible to reconstruct the most basic understanding of the ancient Mayan medical system, nor has it been possible to a large degree for the Mayan people themselves to recall traditional concepts of disease in order to combat it. The conceptual information that we have has been scattered and inconsistent. There remain no prehispanic Mayan medical texts that we can decipher, and thus no direct sources from the pre-conquest era that we can use to approach the subject.

Diego De Landa, the most important historian of Mayan culture from the early years of the conquest, makes mention of some illnesses suffered by the native peoples in the thirteenth and fourteenth centuries, and of the orations which were used to invoke gods of medicine such as *Ixchel, Itzamna, Citbolotun* and *Ahau Chamaez*.[1] During various moments of the conquest the well-known books of the *Chilam Balam* appeared, written by indigenous authors in the Mayan language with the Roman alphabet; each volume took the name of its place of origin: *Kaua, Ixil, Tekax, Nah, Teabo* and *Chumayel*. It is generally supposed that these texts were based upon ancient hieroglyphic texts.[2] Some of the originals are in libraries in the United States, while others have been lost. Nevertheless it has been possible to rescue some formulas and medical terms contained in these texts.[3]

The manuscripts *Sotuta* and *Mena*—although they date from the epoch of the conquest—were written by indigenous authors and make reference to prehispanic medical knowledge. Consulting these works, we can begin to hypothesize about the changes that Mayan medicine has undergone over the centuries; for example, we observe that many diseases mentioned in these manuscripts have disappeared or their names and etiologies have changed with the passage of time.

In the *Codex Pérez*, an original manuscript from Mani, Yucatán, the months or *"katunes"* are transliterated into the Gregorian calendar, and the dates and times corresponding to certain diseases are noted.

The Ritual of the Bacabes[4] is a fundamental text in the field of Mayan studies. It seems to have originated in Nunkiní, Campeche at the end of

Introduction

the sixteenth century, and is closely tied to the *Codex of Calkini* and *The Chilam Balam of Chumayel*. This work is presented with not only the clearest Mayan literary style, but with Mayan medical, magical, and religious concepts that show almost no European influence. The texts are mostly spells and formulas for the healing of diseases—a combination of medical, botanical, magical, and spiritual knowledge presented in an esoteric, literary, and occasionally obscure style.

Another volume, *Recetarios de indios en lengua maya* (*Formulas of the Indians in Mayan Language*), was written during the colonial epoch, as recorded by Barrera Vazquez.[5]

A volume of incantations in Mayan language, whose origin remains unknown, is in the Ayer Collection of the Newberry Library in Chicago.

A book known as *El judio (The Jew)*,[6] dated 1775, has had a controversial history in the area of Mayan studies. With the passage of time, the extant copies have undergone various modifications of their contents, which comprise indigenous medical knowledge.

In recent times there has been considerable research into the contemporary state of traditional medical knowledge. From the nineteenth and early twentieth century the outstanding investigators in the field have been Dondé (father and son),[7] Benjamin Cuevas,[8] and Rejón.[9] In terms of contemporary study the best known are Villa Rojas, Redfield, Thompson, Barrera Vázquez, Roys, and Souza (see bibliography).

What is known of prehispanic Mayan medicine, with some information currently lost or unavailable, can be briefly summed up as follows:

- Disease was caused by the gods and spirits. The majority of illnesses had "supernatural" causes and disease prevention and cure had a generally mystical character. Particular diseases bore relations with specific gods.
- The winds were responsible for causing many diseases.
- The ancient Maya represented fundamental illnesses with animal symbols.
- There were relations between factors such as the cardinal directions, the winds, animals, and disease.
- Time was conceived of as sacred. Personified periods such as years, months, and days had great influence over the world and human life.
- Diseases were categorized according to principles of hot or cold.
- As the cause of disease was attributed to divinity, the functions of priests and healers were combined. This function still survives, most notably in the role of the *j'meen*.

- Illnesses were diagnosed by palpation, divination, and discussion with the patient.
- Among the main resources used to cure disease were medicinal plants, the recitation of psalms, and the practice of bleeding.

THE CHINESE MEDICAL SYSTEM AS AN INSTRUMENT FOR BROACHING TRADITIONAL MAYAN MEDICINE

Given the degree of conceptual fragmentation existing in Mayan medicine, the path towards discovering the roots of the system was, of course, by way of other systems which would help us conceive of the puzzle as a whole. We came to the work first from the perspective of Western medicine and anthropology, but from this perspective we encountered many dead-ends. The conceptual categories that we were using were not sufficient to observe, understand, and integrate the fragmented elements at hand. If we were to consider Mayan traditional medicine systematically— that is, as a logically structured holistic field—we had to find its theoretical base. Our schematics, however, gave us no room to move in this direction.

Fortunately, two members of our group had been trained in acupuncture and elements of traditional Chinese medicine. Starting from 1984, we began to take note of the fact that many concepts and health practices found in the indigenous communities became accessible by way of conceptual groundwork from the Chinese system.

The Western anthropological/medical model, because of its vast differences from indigenous concepts and practices, often glossed over the traditional practices in a superficial way without a view to the depths of the system, or interpreted the traditional techniques in a distorted manner. An example illustrates: a Mayan midwife might use a "hot" plaster placed on the little toe to stimulate uterine contractions and facilitate birth; this practice would be interpreted differently by a Western doctor or anthropologist than it would by a doctor or anthropologist with training in the Chinese system. The Western practitioner might describe and interpret the phenomena in terms of its symbolic significance, if he were able to approach it at all. As likely as not he would find no medical explanation for a relation between a poultice on the toe and a uterine contraction. The Chinese practitioner, on the other hand, would recognize a technique from his own repertoire, recalling that in Chinese practice this area of the foot is stimulated to trigger uterine contractions. In this case the researcher or practitioner suddenly has a deep relation with the indigenous practice, and, starting from the practice, can work towards an understanding of the theoretical basis of Mayan medicine.

Chinese Traditional Medicine is a complex system derived from the synthesis of many medical and spiritual currents realized over thousands of years of discovery, invention, systematization, and discussion; it involves a world-view and understanding of the human body with attendant interpretations of the phenomena of health and disease. In its present form, Chinese Traditional Medicine comprises a wide array of practices which share a common philosophical base from which the practitioner sets out on her or his task of healing.

The philosophical and medical categories from Chinese medicine are available to us because these traditions were not persecuted and destroyed as was traditional Mexican medicine, and were, in fact, systematized and broadened over the course of thousands of years—most recently under the administration of the People's Republic of China, which has shown a great commitment to the preservation and exploration of traditional medicine.

The decision to use the Chinese system as a model to aid in our understanding of Mayan medicine brought us to an in-depth study of other conceptual relations—how the Maya conceived of etiological factors (the causes of disease), the importance given to emotional states (fear, anger, etc.), the role of climatic conditions (air, heat, cold), and certain diagnostic techniques in which we found coincidence, like the use of the radial pulse, massage, bleeding, cupping, the herbal pharmacopoeia, and the stimulation of specific points on the body. Using Chinese conceptual categories as an instrument for broaching Mayan traditional medicine permitted us to observe and study concepts and practices which normally pass by the Western practitioner or anthropologist, without excluding so much and without so much distortion in the interpretation.

It does not interest us to demonstrate the similarities between these two medical systems "per se." We are not trying to force comparisons between the two, nor to support current anthropological arguments. We were, and are, simply attempting to understand traditional Mayan medicine, in its fragmented state, and to do so by using the categories given us by the Chinese system.

Some social scientists suggest that cultural and technological systems (i.e. the field of health) develop according to patterns found in the natural world, suggesting that similar cultural patterns or structures develop among cultures with similar relations to the natural world. According to this theory, so-called hunting and gathering people the world over will develop common technologies, as will small-scale agricultural peoples, and so on.[10] Our understanding of the profound similarities between Chinese and Mayan medicine is based in this view of cultural development.

Our extensive reliance on our colleague Dr. Sierra, trained at the Institute of Traditional Chinese Medicine in Beijing, has allowed us to deepen the concepts, categories, and judgments between the two cultures, and has given us access to many books and documents written in Chinese.

CONTACT WITH MAYAN MEDICINE

At the outset of the investigation the principal objective was to understand the conception of health among the Maya. As we approached a deeper understanding of the medicine, we abandoned many of our previous judgments and began to accept that certain classifications with indigenous roots—like "fear" *(susto),* "the evil eye" *(ojo),* and *"empacho"*

(a type of indigestion)—exist in complex interrelationships and serve to explain cases that might be inexplicable from the standpoint of Western medicine. Some of these illnesses, we found, can be approached more readily from the Chinese medical perspective. Moreover, we have observed that the treatments used in these types of cases are effective to a great degree.

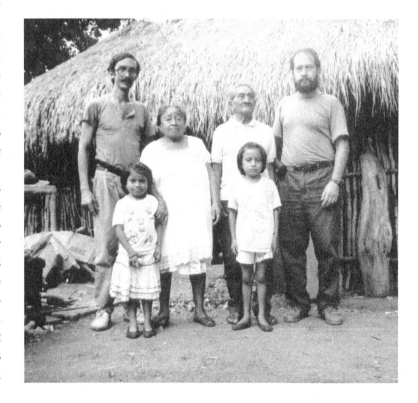

We take our information and facts from various sources. The primary source has been Gilberto Balám, a doctor who has worked with Mayan medicine for over 20 years, sustaining close relations with a number of *curanderos,* and who has organized several meetings of traditional medical practitioners in Yucatán and Campeche. This work has brought to light several publications. The doctors García and Sierra have worked in Mayan

Introduction

communities in Campeche since 1989, and have also enjoyed the opportunity of working in conjunction with various *curanderos*.

During 1991 and 1992 a conference was held in Calkiní in which about 40 *curanderos* participated, among them *j'meenob* (shamans), *yerberos* (herbalists), *hueseros* (bone setters) and *parteras* (midwives). The conference was arranged into four workshops designed to deepen familiarity with Mayan disease classification, both "organic" and "spiritual." We had participated in monthly meetings with some of the *curanderos* over the course of three years, undertaking a personal study of various medical therapies and techniques. The *curanderos* from several communities in the region of Camino Real in the state of Campeche have worked with us in the systematization of this work, and deserve the greater part of the credit.

From 1989, when we began to use Chinese medical concepts to approach Mayan medicine, we have seen increasing affinities between the two practices. In the village where we began our work in health education we used Chinese massage techniques and demonstrated the use of acupuncture needles. This aroused great interest among several community members, who began to participate more fully in our work. Only later did we discover that these were the *curanderos* of the community. They surprised us further by showing us their own collection of therapeutic needles, or "spines."

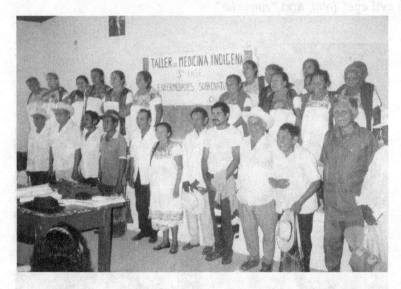

We discovered that from the moment we began to introduce Asian techniques like *Shiatsu* massage and acupuncture into our community health work, we were received differently than when we had presented ourselves as Western doctors. The people in general, but particularly the *curanderos*, identified with us more readily, and soon opened up and began sharing with us their own form of massage—*jet*—and the applications of Mayan acupuncture, known as *jup* and *tok*.

In some communities the *curanderos* and their apprentices invited us to teach them and to attend their consultations. The experience was enlightening, and was, in fact, the first occasion in our educational work in which we experienced a truly "horizontal" relationship: on both sides there was great respect and a deep desire to understand the other's perspective. For the *curanderos* this was a new experience. Up to this point doctors from the outside had generally developed a one-sided relationship with the *curanderos* and their medicine, considering it "primitive" and lacking in modern sanitary techniques. The doctor speaks and the *curandero* listens. Anthropologists, on the other hand, had simply reversed the relationship. They would visit the *curanderos* to get information (if the *curandero* was willing to share it), leaving nothing in return. The anthropologist asks questions and the *curandero* answers them.

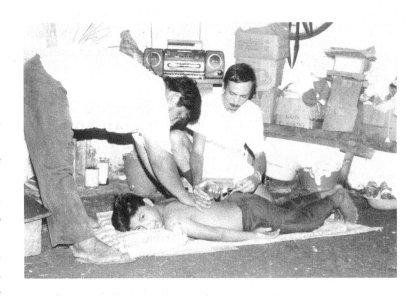

In the consultations we witnessed, the *curanderos* and patients opened themselves up, explaining and demonstrating concepts and medical practices, explaining their understanding of health and disease, their relation with "supernatural" forces, the use of prayer, and their knowledge of medicinal plants. This way of working—and watching them work—increased our contact and broadened our reputation with the *curanderos* of the area. During these consultations we deepened our understanding of the conceptual elements of the medicine, the forms of application of the spines, and the use of bleeding, cupping, massage, prayer, cleansings, and medicinal plants.

This of course gave us a broader field of comparison with Chinese medicine. And, again, the learning was mutual. For example, the use of moxibustion (applying heat to various points of the body by burning ground mugwort), previously unknown, has been well received. Today several *curanderos* have incorporated moxibustion into their practice, especially in treating cases of "cold," using the points already familiar to them. They have obtained good results.

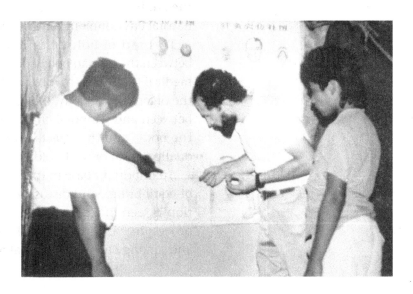

We have also had the opportunity to work with patients confronting traditional ailments such as *tipté, cirro, corrimiento* (to be explored further along), and other syndromes with no equivalent in Western medicine—but with some similarities to Chinese diagnostics with its notion of "energetics." In this way we have been able to systematize some of the information we have learned about the traditional techniques.

THE MAYAN CONCEPTUAL SYSTEM ON THE YUCATÁN PENINSULA

Currently, thanks to many years of study in Campeche and Yucatán, we are able to conceptualize traditional Mayan medicine in a holistic and dynamic way; and we can propose a different way of looking at the phenomena involved. The work we have done has brought us scarcely to the beginning of a constructive understanding of, and a way of reconstructing, the theoretical system. The model that we chose—Traditional Chinese Medicine—does not explain the entire system. The two systems are not equivalent, merely similar in their conceptions.

The Mayan system is based on a conception of the cosmos in which there is a profound relation between cosmic manifestations and human life. The human being is seen in an integral and interactive relation with the cosmos, which includes both nature and society. According to this system, individual actions have cosmic repercussions, and any change or action in nature, the family, or the community also affects the individual. Due to this understanding of the cosmos, Mayan medicine involves the study of these relationships and of the influence of the social and natural environment on the human body.

This sort of holistic thinking—a conception of profound relation between the human body and the cosmos which is lacking in the Western medical tradition—involves the study of the deep relation between all of the organs of the body, the relation of the body and the soul, the relation between and temporal characteristics of disease in the different areas of the body, and the effects on the body of the primary Mayan medical duality—that of heat/cold.

An important base in this system is the conception of health as a state of equilibrium, and disease as the rupture of this equilibrium. This relation is seen in a dynamic form: health and disease are understood as a process in which the individual searches for a state of balance between and among changing internal and external elements. These encompass factors of diet, climate, infection, constitution, emotions, and "energetics." Many of the qualities of foods and of environmental factors are seen in terms of heat and cold and thus are potential causes of illness.

Among the Maya the external vehicle primarily responsible for setting off a state of imbalance in the body is wind. This concept encompasses various influences including climate, infection, and "energy." The wind is the element which unites the "natural" world with the "supernatural," or "the world of the winds." It can be a physical phenomenon that sets the body out of balance, it can be a force generated by people, animals, or plants, or it can be a living emissary of "supernatural" forces *("dueños")*.

In this system it is understood that nature determines the course of human life—giving life and bringing death—and is seen to be animated, to have its own personality. The natural world is deified and venerated. The forces which set an individual out of balance can be produced by the organism itself, by the family and community, by nature, or by the gods. Showing a lack of respect for any of these elements, breaking the family or social balance, insulting the natural world, the cosmos or the gods, can bring negative effects to the individual, throwing her or him out of balance and producing disease. Health is the result of living in harmony with social and natural laws, and disease and disequilibrium are the results of transgressing these laws.

Preventive and curative methods cohere with this basic understanding of health and disease. These understandings possess a symbolic and mystical character, like all medicines, and they are based on a profound set of beliefs about the functioning of the world and the body. Although these beliefs do not incorporate the occidental understanding of microbiology, and though they possess a logic far different from Western logic, we can no longer simply label them "irrational" as was done by the Europeans who conquered and colonized the Mayan regions during the eras of enlightenment and reformation.

We consider therapeutic and pharmacological efficacy to be very important, but we also believe that symbolic efficacy is of primary importance, with its psychoneuroimmunological repercussions. This relates, as well, to the "energetic" element of the medicine, without which we lack a complete vision of the forces involved. In the Yucatec Maya conceptualization of the human body we find a life-force (the *ool*) which is the source of vital energy, and which differs from the soul (the *pixán*). These concepts were deformed by Spanish Christianity over the course of the conquest and colonial period, which gave them a suspicious and supernatural character. In therapeutic practice several distinct types of balancing energies work through the diagnostics of heat and cold, the acupuncture therapies, and the cleansings.

In the following chapters we give a description of the principles—conceptions of the body and the cosmos, causality, diagnostics, and therapeutics—of contemporary traditional Mayan medicine, followed by their Chinese counterparts. Though the comparisons may be rough at times, the reader will be able to look through the lens of Chinese elemental theory and other conceptualizations in order to better understand the fragmented and obscure aspects of Mayan medicine. To facilitate understanding we have chosen to put the elements of Chinese traditional medicine and culture after their Mayan equivalents without trying to force comparisons. If there is some element of Chinese or Mayan theory that has no counterpart, we elucidate it as best we can so that the differences between the systems will be made clear as well.

CHAPTER 1

HUMAN RELATION
WITH THE COSMOS IN MAYAN
AND CHINESE MEDICINE

THE HUMAN AND THE COSMOS IN MAYAN CULTURE

MAYAN CULTURE maintains a holistic view of the world, in which every aspect of existence bears relation to every other. Strong relations exist between the human being and all of nature and the cosmos: the gods, the celestial bodies, the animals, plants, and other human beings. No individual is isolated from the world; everything one does affects other people, animals, and objects, as well as spirits or supernatural beings. Conversely, every action of the universe, or of other people, affects the individual. The universe is a great unity which embraces nature and society; in the immediate view we, as human beings, have no metaphysical priority over all the rest. Natural phenomena and the things of the cosmos that make up the Mayan universe—the planets, mountains, rivers, fields, and so on—are personified and deified. These phenomena have power and will. The human animal exists in an intimate interdependence with them, and so natural and social phenomena are tightly bound, inextricably linked.

THE HUMAN AND THE COSMOS IN CHINESE CULTURE

In the Chinese view we see a similar holistic concept in which the human being forms a part of the cosmos and exists in intimate relation with all of its elements. Traditional Chinese medicine considers the individual to be part and parcel of nature—to such an extent that the individual's way-of-being affects all of nature—and the forces of the natural world, conversely, affect the well-being of the individual.

1

Mayan Mythology

Before the current state of decadence, the ancient Maya recognized that the universe was ruled by a supreme god who retired to the depths of the heavens, leaving in his place an anonymous substitute, *Ahau, el señor,* to watch over and govern the heavens and the earth. Below him, nine gods watched over the affairs of the earth. On the earth was planted the tree of the beginning, the great world-tree, the *ceiba,* which reached to the top of the heavens. The *ceiba* unites the earth with the heavens; it brings food for people to eat and bridges the heavens' different levels, reaching to the most high. Four guardians, the *bacabob,* were posted in the four corners of the universe, upholding heaven. Heaven itself was made up of various planes or levels placed one atop the other. The earth was a square with its corners pointing to the four cardinal directions, each corner relating to a color. The center formed a fifth point and a fifth color, through which passed the axis of the universe, the umbilicus of the world. In the *Popul Vuh,*[11] a Quiche Maya text from the seventeenth century, it is told that the universe was created from corn—the same corn from which humans were made. After the creation, the levels of heaven were elevated to their present position, where they were held in place by the *ceiba.* Four more *ceiba* grew to uphold each of the edges of the heavens standing over the earth.

Chinese Mythology

The mythology of ancient China that has come down to us[12] speaks to us of a four-cornered universe, with the corners oriented to the cardinal directions, each one corresponding to a color. In the center, in a fifth point corresponding to a fifth color, reigned *Huang Di,* the supreme god. His celestial palace was in the heights of a mountain with nine peaks. His administrator watched over the borders of the nine celestial countries. He had four heads with which to see in the four directions, and he ruled simultaneously the heavens and the land of the dead. In his gardens grew immense trees, among them the tree of immortality. Once, one of the gods led a human uprising against *Huang Di.* The next day *Huang Di* retired from celestial affairs, choosing a substitute who from that day forth ruled in his place over the heavens and the country of the dead. Command over the four cardinal points was shared among four gods who bestowed upon humanity all of the elements of civilization.

Chinese cosmology gives us a vision of the tree of immortality standing at the axis of the world—uniting the earth with the heavens—and atop the heights an enormous rice plant, symbol of nourishment. Heaven itself was divided into nine provinces whose frontiers were jealously guarded by the servant of *Huang Di*. "The nine heavens" also denoted the imperial court where the emperor, "the son of heaven," ruled as the representative of heavenly and earthly powers.

THE MAYAN COSMOS

The Mayan people speak of a world divided into three main regions: the heavens, the earth, and the underworld.

There is disagreement regarding the number of heavens. Sometimes there are understood to be seven, and other times nine or thirteen celestial planes. Montoliu Villar[13] suggests that the most accepted version is that there are thirteen gods: the *oxlahun ti ku*, the representatives of the heavens and the *bolon ti ku*, the representatives of the subterranean worlds. Eric S. Thompson,[14] on the other hand, proposes that the ancient Maya saw the universe as a kind of mountain or stepped pyramid composed of six ascending and six descending steps and an upper level. The sum of the levels is thirteen, comprised of seven above ground and six below. Paul Arnold[15] maintains that there were originally nine gods venerated by the Maya—the *bolon ti ku*, who formed a council to rule over human affairs—but that they were displaced by the thirteen Toltec gods who came later with the Aztec domination.

The Maya call each of the heavens *taz* (cloak or mantel), from which we might deduce that what is imagined are various capes or mantels superimposed one upon the other. Presently it is believed in some communities that the highest heaven is inhabited by Jesus Christ. The celestial plane is hot, but it is in charge of cold phenomena as well. It governs the day and is ruled by the sun. The subterranean region ruled by the *bolon ti ku* is known by the Maya as *metnal* or *xibalbá*, and recognized by Christians as Hell. In the underworld night and darkness rule. It is a world of water. The nine gods take turns ruling, one night at a time. The underworld is the kingdom of the *aluxob*—dwarf-like beings or spirits equivalent to the *chanekes* and *achenes* of other Mesoamerican cultures. It is said that the interior of the earth is hot, along with its rulers and those who dwell there, but that the surface is cold. There are various animals that belong to the underworld: the *moan*, a mythic bird which helps the soul on its journey

Human Relation
with the Cosmos

of rebirth, and which is similar in appearance to a pterodactyl; the *xoch*, or owl, emissary of illness and death; the *tzotz*, or bat, bringer of bad omens and death; the *xnuk*, a small owl, auger of illness; the *sak'i'*, a beneficial white seabird; and various snakes, among others.

Human beings exist in a state of balance in the center of the world, on the surface of the earth, between the heavens and the underworld. The human body is hot, though in the night it can become imbalanced and grow cold.

THE CHINESE COSMOS

The cosmology of ancient China has the cosmos divided into Heaven, Earth, and the Country of the Dead. The celestial palace of the supreme God was in the heights of a mountain with nine peaks. His secretary, or servant, watched over the borders of the nine celestial lands, each with its own guardian.

The number nine, aside from being the assignation of the heavenly provinces, was given a primordial religious significance among the ancient dynasties. Nine sacrificial vessels were passed as talismans from one dynasty to the next, and the number nine was recognized as a signifier of *yang* qualities.

THE MAYAN GODS

Each plane of Heaven and Earth has its god in charge of looking over one part of the universe. The majority of the gods have dual characteristics; if they can bring health and fertility they are equally capable of provoking disease, failure of the harvest, and other evils. Of the thirteen celestial deities, our friends among the Maya called to mind several, though not all: *Junab kuj*, the Creator; *Aj K'iin*, the sun; *Aj Uj*, the moon; *Jool Poop*, Head Governor, He of the Sleeping Mat; *Aj Ixche*, Goddess of Fertility and Medicine; *Aj Ek'*, Lord of the Stars; *Aj Iik'*, Lord of the Winds; *Aj Luum*, Lord of the Earth; *Aj Káax*, Lord of the Mountains and Forests; *Aj Chak*, Lord of the Rain; *Aj Ja'*, Lord of Water; and *Aj Itz'am Na'*, Lord of the Arts and of Writing. The deity of corn is a beneficent god known as *Yumi Kaax*, Lord of the *Milpa*.

In the *metnal*, or underworld, there are nine gods. The principal god is *Aj Puuch*, God of Death. He is followed in importance by *Aj Kimil*, God of

Burials, *Aj Jich K'aal,* God of Suicide and the Hanged, and *Aj Muk'nal,* Lord of the Tombs, among others. Each one of the four cardinal directions has its own god as well. These are the four *Balamob* who protect the earth; thus one does not take anything away from the mountains or the earth without first seeking their permission. The *Balamob* are: *Aj Kalan Chako'ob, Aj Kalan Lu'uinob, Aj Kalan Balam,* and *Aj Kalan K'aak'.*

Of the celestial deities, *Itzamna* and *Ixchel* are responsible for questions of health and illness. *Itzamna* represents the principal deity. Besides his function as Creator, he is the Master of Rain, representing fertility, the sun, health, and disease. In the form of a reptile he represents the rains in the four corners of the world. He may be invoked in some rituals by his animal names *Kinich Ahau Itzamná* or *Itzamná face of the sun. Ixchel* is the goddess of the moon, the waters, births, weaving, and medicine.

Bacab is an important god who divided himself into four parts so that he could watch over each of the four directions. The four *bacabes* or *bacabob* seem to have a close relation with the gods of wind, rain, and lightning. The *Ritual of the Bacabes,*[16] written in the state of Campeche, contains psalms and orations dedicated to these gods to combat illness.

The most popular gods are the *chakob,* or rain gods. There is one *chak* for each cosmic direction. An ancient myth holds that frogs, which sing before the rain, are sons of the *chak* whose province is in the east—the direction of the color red, the place of the rain gods' paradise.

The gods or guardian spirits of the woods, towns, and *milpas* are called in Yucatec Maya *Balamob,* meaning "jaguars" in the common language, but taking on special significance with regard to these guardians. These deities watch over the moral and social behavior of men and women, and when it is necessary they punish them with illness and accidents.

The *aluxob* guard the woods, jungles, springs, and stone mounds known by earlier Maya as *cuyo*s. According to some Mayan people, the *aluxob* are the leftover men of clay from the third creation[17] and they remain on earth as helpers of the underworld gods. They are cold beings who live in the realm of night; by day they are like clay figures without life. As cold beings they are in charge of illnesses which produce fever. At night they guard sacred places and give warnings by throwing stones and making strange noises. Hunters offer them cigars and incense to keep them at bay. The *aluxob* are commonly seen and commonly heard by people who live near them; when people speak of the *aluxob* they speak with a certainty that signals absolute faith in their presence. Some describe them as trouble-makers who, from time to time, enter houses and bother the inhabitants, like gnomes or gremlins; they are occasionally known to steal children.

Human Relation
with the Cosmos

The guardians of the day are the snakes, especially the *itz'a k'an,* the rattlesnake, and the black-tailed *eek unej.* They are emissaries of the Lords of the Earth who guard the hills, springs, and streams by day.

THE CHINESE GODS

Four gods ruled the four cardinal directions and the four seasons. In the east reigned a god who was the god of spring, who had given the human race fire and a net to catch fish. He had the head of a man and the body of a serpent. In the west reigned a god who looked like a bird. He was responsible for the sunset, making sure it set every night with regularity. His helper, his son, was the god of metal. The south was under the dominion of a god with the head of an ox. His charge was the summer and the summer sun, and he had by his side the god of fire. He was the god of medicine and he taught the human race how to cultivate the five grains. The ruler of the north was a god with a human face and the snout and hooves of a pig. With the help of the gods of the water, the winds, and the sea he watched over the winter months. It was this god who was chosen by *Huang Di* as his successor after the uprising of mortal humans.

In the mythology of ancient China the forces of nature and the stars were deified. All things depended on the gods: all life and all reproduction—human, animal or vegetable—the arrival of the rains to bring a good harvest, peace between city-states, the discord that brings war among peoples, the blessings of health, and the curse of disease.

A strong pragmatic tendency which largely did away with the gods germinated in the *Zhou* dynasty (1066 BC–221 BC), saw its consolidation during the *Qin* and *Han* (221 BC–220 AD) dynasties, and endures to the present day. This current found its roots in Taoism: studying the relations between nature, the cosmos, and the human spirit, and finding it essential to explain phenomena and live without metaphysical concepts in a simple, rational manner. Due to this pragmatic rationalism, the arrival of Buddhism in China encountered strong opposition that lasted more than three centuries and necessitated vast cultural transformation before the new religion could be established.

THE FOUR DIRECTIONS OF THE MAYAN UNIVERSE

The vast space of the Mayan universe is divided into five sacred regions. This division begins in the terrestrial plane and continues into the heavens. Each region is represented by specific attributes and a color: red, black, white, yellow and green.

Red is the color of the eastern horizon *(laak'in)*. In it gather the *chakob,* the rain gods, and the god of agriculture *Bolon Tz'a-kab,* who brings prosperity. In the east it is hot, and in the orations this direction is always referred to as *no'lajin,* the Great East. In the east are born the sun, the moon, the stars, the clouds, and the rain. The winds *(iik'o'ob)* and the rains *(chakob)* are, for the most part, beneficial and welcome. Winds from the east are hot, and when they collide with air from the south the rain comes. Altars are oriented towards the east. The animal that lives in the east is the *koj,* or mountain lion.

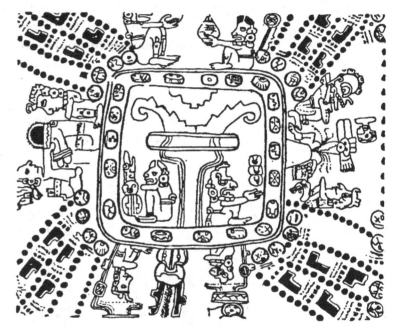

Drawing from the Dresden Codex representing the four directions of the cosmos.

The color white descends from the north *(xaman).* The north is cold, and is the birthplace of harmful winds. The wind from the north *(xaman iik)* blows from October to December—*los nortes*—and sometimes, together with the *chikin iik,* the west wind, brings judgment and bodes ill. It is because of this that animals must be vaccinated in the autumn.

The black direction, direction of death, is the west *(chik'in),* fountain of ill winds, birthplace of disgrace, region of the dead, horizon where the sun sets. The western animal is the serpent. The wind that blows from the west *(chik'in iik)* is the most dangerous, blowing from the end of December through January, bringing asthma and other illnesses. The west wind is born low, from the earth, and blows out to sea. This wind acts to detoxify the earth, and it is for this reason that it is so harmful.

The south *(nojol)* is hot and corresponds to the color yellow. The infrequent rain and winds from the south are beneficial for the planting and cultivation of crops. The arrival of the south wind *(nojol iik)* is seen as an opportunity to burn land for the planting of the *milpa.* The animal that dwells in the south is the green bird *x'kok'.*

Human Relation
with the Cosmos

For the Maya the center of the world is green like the *ceiba,* tree of the beginning which unites the earth with the heavens. There is some disagreement as to whether center is gauged according to the cardinal points (east, west, north and south) or to the solstice points (the points where the sun tops the horizon on the solstices and equinoxes).

The Mayan universe consists of an inferior and superior part, four edges, and a center. The four surrounding directions, or cardinal points—*laak'in, chik'in, nojol* and *xaman* —are also referred to as "the four winds." This cosmic geometry is applied to the establishment of communities, the construction of living areas, the *milpa,* the altar and the human body. The word *kantis,* signaling the four directions or four corners of the universe, is a widely used word in the vocabulary, suggesting the importance, to the present day, of this geometric concept of cosmic and social space.

THE FOUR CARDINAL POINTS IN CHINESE CULTURE

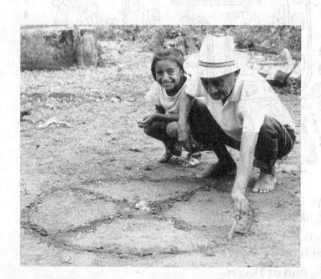

Each cardinal direction corresponds to a color, an animal, and a host of other characteristics. The north is the direction of the color black, the turtle, and death. From the north come harmful winds. The west belongs to the tiger and the color white; the south is the province of the color red and the phoenix; the east is blue and home to the dragon which brings a beneficial rain; the center corresponds to the color yellow and to the emperor, umbilicus of the human world.

The Chinese attribute energetic properties to the four cardinal points. Early in the morning the sun rises in the east, bearing energy in the form of *chi,* together with the energy known as *shaoyang,* the energy of birth, the germination of the day. At midday the sun hangs in the south. The energy of the southern sun is known as *laoyang* and controls the process or development of the day. In the afternoon the sun turns to the west where the energy is known as *shaoyin,* an astringent power, closing the day. At night the sun rests in the north, where energy is guarded and tended; this process of preserving and conserving power is known as *laoyin.*

The Chinese recognize that the energy in the human body flows just as it does in the rest of the natural world, lending great importance to the four directions and the hours of the day in the process of curing and tending to disease.

The Mayan calendar consists of various cycles, among them a cycle of three hundred sixty five days, known as the *haab*—eighteen months of twenty days and one additional month of five ill-starred days. The names of the months are: *pop, uo, zip, zotz, tzec, xul, yaxkin, mol, chen, yax, zac, ceh, mac, kankin, muan, pax, kayab, cumbu* and *uayeb*. The names of the days are: *ik, akbal, kan, chicchán, cimí, manik, lamat, muluk, oc, chuen, eb, ben, ix, men, cib, cabán, edznab, cauac, ahau,* and *imix*.[18]

Another cycle, that which governs the ceremonial calendar, is the *Tzolkin*. The *Tzolkin* is composed of a succession of 260 days in which the twenty day names are combined with a series of thirteen numbers; for example one *ik*, two *akbal*, three *kan*, up to the number thirteen accompanied by a day name—*ix*, in the case of the list above—at which point the count begins again at one. A complete date in the Mayan calendar comprises the combination of the days and months of both cycles—for example two *ik*, zero *pop*, as the Mayan numerical system begins with zero. Each day of the month is oriented according to the four directions and is influenced by an animal, a plant, and a deity. *Kan, chicchán, manik* and *lamat* belong to the east; *muluc, oc, chuen, eb* and *ben* to the north; *ix, men, cib, caban* and *edznab* to the west; and *cauac, ahau, imix, ik* and *akbal* to the south.

Years *(haab)* are also oriented according to the cosmic directions and are influenced in turn by certain deities. The year *muluk* (water), for example, is presided over by the red *bacab* of the east. This year, when it comes around, falls also under the influence of *Kinich Ahau*, Our Lord Whose Face is the Sun, and these years witness an excess of sun showers, sparse plant growth, and an increase in cases of evil eye *(mal de ojo)*. The year *ix* (white) is governed by the white *bacab* of the north and brings a good harvest of cotton, a poor harvest of maize, and many deaths. The year *kauak* (lightning or storm) is ruled by the black *bacab* of the west, influenced by *Uakmitun Ahau*, Lord of Death, and is a year of plagues, drought, and death. The year *kan*, presided over by the yellow *bacab* of the south and influenced by *Bolon Tz'akab*, Lord of the Nine Resurrections, is considered a good year, although moral errors committed during this year may result in the unleashing of great harm upon the people.

The days Tuesday and Friday of each week are considered special days during which one is more vulnerable to illness—but which, at the same time, are propitious days to cure certain ills and counteract witchcraft.

Previously, when a Mayan child was born, his parents would consult a priest or daykeeper to learn the child's destiny. The priest was keeper of a

Human Relation
with the Cosmos

sacred almanac in which he would find the date and all of the pertinent information: its corresponding gods, plants, animals, objects, and the celestial direction. If the reading showed a bad or difficult destiny, the priest advised and performed rituals to ensure that the evils to come were lessened. Similarly, when someone fell ill, it was necessary, in order to establish the roots of the illness, to know the date of birth and consult the sacred almanac. This information was essential to the diagnosis and prognosis of the disease, and facilitated treatment.

THE CHINESE CALENDAR

In correspondence with *The Yellow Emperor's Classic of Medicine* (The *Neijing Suwen*), the ancient Chinese recognized vital relations between the *chi* and blood energy of the human body and the flow of energy in the natural world. In ancient China the year and the day were each divided into twelve periods. There are twelve months in a year and twelve divisions in a day. Similarly, as the twelve months comprise four distinct seasons, so the twelve hours of the day are divided into four "seasons." The four seasons pass, completing the year. In summer the days are long; in winter the days are short. Spring and fall are transitional seasons.

Of the twelve sections of the day *(zi, chou, yin, mao, chen, si, wu, wei, shen, you, xu, hai)* each temporal unit comprises two hours. The first period, *zi*, runs from eleven PM to one o'clock AM. During these two hours, *yin* energy is exhausted and *yang* grows; during the period *wu*, in the middle of the daylight hours, *yang*, conversely, exhausts itself and turns to *yin*. During the first half of the day, from the darkness of the morning hours to the bright light of noon, atmospheric temperature rises and natural light grows. *Yang* increases and *yin* decreases.

In ancient China the day was divided further into twenty-four equal divisions along the lines of the twenty-four solar periods in the year. The first, seventh, thirteenth, and nineteenth indicate the beginnings of spring, summer, autumn, and winter, respectively. The fourth, tenth, sixteenth, and twenty-second solar periods are times when seasonal changes are at their height. Humanity moves to these cyclical rhythms. The *Neijing* says, "The cycles of heaven and earth reflect in the constant changes in nature," and again, "Because of the natural movement of heaven and earth and the sun and moon, we experience a change of long months and short months and go through three hundred and sixty-five days, which form one year in the Chinese calendar. The energy flow within the human body through the channels corresponds to this."[19]

THE MAYAN DUALITY: HEAT AND COLD

The Mayan cosmovision has the world divided in two—heaven and earth—in which various other relations of contraries are at play. The superior half is high, hot, positive and active, while the inferior is below the earth, cold, negative, and passive. This duality finds its most common and useful expression in the notions of hot and cold. Practically everything in the Mayan world is classified according to its thermal nature. Plants are catalogued as *tzig u cuch* (cold) and *choko cuch* or *kinal cuch* (hot). In general, cold plants hold a lot of water, are green, and grow alongside rivers, lakes, and streams. Some Mayan *campesinos* say that cold plants symbolize rain because they grow near water, and are therefore plants of the *chakob*, the rain gods. The spirits of mountains, springs and rivers—the *aluxob*—are considered cold, and thus are often seen as bringers of illness.

The human being, as well, is composed of elements hot and cold, harmonized in a state of equilibrium. This equilibrium can be lost due to external or internal forces, and can be regained as well by actions, meditations, or external factors affecting the body.

The air can be cold or hot. Liquids are generally taken lukewarm so as not to cause any imbalance. Food, as well, is understood to be hot or cold (generally cold). Offerings that are used in traditional ritual are also recognized as hot or cold, and are used according to the nature of the ritual.

THE CHINESE DUALITY: YIN AND YANG

The basic duality of the Chinese world view, in accord with that of the Mayan view, is the notion of *yin* and *yang,* the principle of opposites intertwined which permeate every aspect of the Chinese medical and metaphysical system. The concept finds its roots in a meticulous vision of the dualities of natural phenomena such as day-night, heat-cold, heaven-earth, and wet-dry. The theory of *yin* and *yang* holds that all phenomena in the universe are formed by the union of opposing elements, which find

Human Relation
with the Cosmos

themselves at once in a state of contradiction and interdependence; their interaction is the basis of the change and development of all things.

For the ancient Chinese, water and fire symbolized the basic properties of *yin* and *yang*. The fundamental characteristics of *yin* are those of water-cold, darkness, and the tendency to sink—while *yang*, like fire, tends to be hot, bright, rising, and expansive. From these characteristics others are inferred: looking at *yin*, we see interiors and a tendency towards the insides of things, inferiority, passivity, inhibition, slowness, substance, and femininity. Similarly, tendencies towards movement, superiority, exteriority, vitality, excitation, speed, transience, and masculinity belong to *yang*. *Yin* and *yang* depend upon each other; neither exists in isolation. Without day there is no night, without excitation no inhibition. The two forces exist eternally in contradiction, interdependence, and constant transformation.

These forces exist in all of the cosmos, in all of nature, and in the human body. When *yin* and *yang* are in a state of equilibrium, the body is in a state of health; when this balance is lost, disease sets in and illness takes over. This imbalance can be brought about by internal or external factors. Treatment and prevention in Chinese medicine work towards regaining lost equilibrium and conserving the harmony between *yin* and *yang* as it finds itself expressed in various forms.

MAIZE IN MAYAN CULTURE

Like all of the people of Mesoamerica, the Mayan people have at the center of their world, of their vision of the world in its terrestrial and cosmic aspects, the cultivation of maize. The Maya transform the nutrients of mountain and valley, lowland swamp and highland precipice, into maize—and so give back their own blood and heat to the corn, which in turn becomes the blood and heat of their bodies. After several years of production the soil of the *milpa* (the traditonal agricultural method in which corn, beans and squash are grown in an integrated system) must be left to rest so that the jungle may grow back. In the *milpa* grow plants which are used as medicine, including the *maíz, calabaza* and *frijol* (corn, beans and squash) that are the three sacred sisters; the *milpa* is the sacred space where the Mayan *campesino* exists in unity with the natural world. As long as the cultivation of maize persists, social and cultural relations are maintained and the survival of ethnic identity and traditional practices, including traditional medicine, are strengthened.[20]

Mayan culture has always relied upon the development of a maize-based agriculture and to this day maize remains the economic and social base of the culture. Questions of human health and ecology revolve entirely around the cultivation of maize. To the present day the *j'meen*—the Maya shaman or priest whose role has persisted over the course of 500 years of Spanish Catholic domination, and who is currently best known as *curandero*—has as his chief occupation the practice of agricultural rituals to ensure good harvest and good relation with the *dueños* and spirits of the earth in general and the *milpa* in particular. He is responsible, in short, for the health of the land, and of the community of people who depend on the land for their survival.

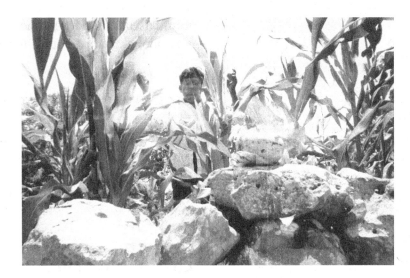

The paradigm of the processes of creation in Mayan theology has its roots in the annual cycle of death and resurrection of maize.[21] In the process of generation of maize, creation necessarily implies the sacrifice by burial of the living seed. In each cycle the plant itself dies and vanishes completely; the seed, which is buried in the earth, travels to the underworld, and then returns to be born again from the body of the earth.

> *Each year the seed of maize is introduced into a hole or fissure which breaks the earth's surface, and after eight days in the underworld, the fruit resurges from the depths, opening the earth a second time to allow the plant to surge into the light. The burial of the seed in the earth and its amazing rebirth in the form of the life-giving plant is a cycle which implies the rigors of sacrifice. In order that there be maize to eat in the autumn, each spring a part of the previous harvest—the seed—must be sacrificed to the earth, where it undergoes a process of decomposition and transformation that converts the buried seed into the vital plant, the fruit which forms the fundament of Mayan life.*

This cycle of maize implies notions of sacrifice, death, and resurrection which resonate throughout the cosmic and social understandings of the Mayan people.

> *The hungry earth gives and takes of vegetation as of all life; men who have died are reborn in their sons, as the stars return to light the night sky after their daily journey in the underworld, but in their transit they leave something of their brilliance, of their cosmic vitality, in the belly of the earth. Death, the periodic sacrifice of everything that lives, regularly consumes the living into the entrails of the living planet, and the*

Human Relation
with the Cosmos

buried seed gestates there to be reborn into life in the continuous and unalterable cycle.[22]

As a fundamental part of the culture in the classic epoch of Mayan civilization, maize also greatly influenced notions of what constituted beauty. The shape of the ear of corn—its long body and thin, diminishing form—found itself reproduced in household objects and human statues, and was a symbol of beauty, youth, regeneration, and vitality.

RICE IN CHINESE CULTURE

Rice, the basis of the Chinese diet, is considered sacred, and holds a place in Chinese culture very similar to the place held by corn in the culture of the Mayan people. This basic grain is surrounded by a series of myths and rituals, and is the center of many cultural practices too extensive to detail here.

COSMIC INFLUENCE IN MAYAN CULTURE

The vision of the Mayan people is one in which the human being exists as an intimate part of the workings of all of nature—to the extent that the health and well-being of the individual is effected equally by daily contact with other people and objects, weather, and work, as by the gods and supernatural forces, the planets, plants, animals, and all of the movements of the cosmos. These relations give rise to a series of behaviors, attitudes, norms, and rituals that ensure the harmony of the individual with every aspect of the universe, from the most mundane to the most remote.

There exists a series of behaviors and infractions which can draw the wrath or ill-will of the *"dueños de los lugares peligrosos"*—the spirits of dangerous places—like the *bacabob, balamob, aluxob,* and *yumob,* who live in the *milpa,* in the mountains, in springs and watering holes, in the rains, in the ancestral ruins, and in all wild places. If one neglects to pray and ask permission to pass through, to cut back the forest for planting, if certain rules of the wild plants and animals are not respected, the spirits of these places and of these beings may be angered and may cause disease or suffering in the transgressor. Above all they may affect or damage the *ool* of the transgressor or his family members, bringing about the loss of crops or the coming of plagues and calamities.

Among the Mayan people of the Yucatán Peninsula there still exists a strong, conscious relation with the plants and animals. It is believed that the higher animals—snakes being the "lowest" of the superior beasts—are reincarnations of people. This, of course, implies a radically different relationship with the animals than that in industrial Western culture, manifesting as a personification of the animals. In places where these traditions are still strong, for example, the hunter asks permission of his prey before the hunt, respecting traditional precepts that ensure harmony and future abundance. In this sense the myth of *Kukulcán*—the deity responsible for the agricultural cycle, who was known as *Quetzalcoatl* among the Toltecs and other northern peoples—is familiar to those Maya who retain a strong sense of tradition.

Similarly, one prays to plants before cutting them to ensure that they retain their nutritional or medicinal value. Before treating a person with medicinal plants, the *curandero* asks for the favor of the gods—now of God the Father and Jesus Christ—to ensure that the remedy is effective.

A clear example of the influence of the planets is the effect of the moon on the gender of newborn infants. If conception occurs beneath a new or waxing moon, a girl is expected; if it occurs beneath a full or waning moon, the promise is of a boy. The moon has an especially strong influence over individuals with a weak *ool*. The planting of the *milpa* is timed to coincide with the new moon. It is also generally understood that if wood for building is cut during the waxing crescent, the wood will be stronger and more resistant to rot.

The sun, as the father and creator of the winds, is responsible for the weather patterns that affect the earth. The influence of the stars and their positions in the sky is very important to the agricultural cycle. For example, when the Pleiades is at its zenith it signals that it is time to harvest *camote* (sweet potato).

Objects in the natural world take on a mythic significance that is played out in ritual. Some brief examples include tying a newborn boy's umbilical cord high in a tree to ensure the boy's strong will and bravery, and burying a newborn girl's umbilical cord beside the family hearth to ensure that she be industrious. In a similar magical vein, a woman never leaves a scrap of burnt food stuck to the pot, because she will run the risk that, on giving birth, the placenta will not come free from the womb. If one points at an unripe fruit hanging from a tree, the fruit will fall; if a woman urinates near melons growing in the *milpa,* the melons will split. If a lightning bug enters the house, someone in the family will fall ill with a fever; if a dragonfly enters the house, visitors are to be expected.

Human Relation
with the Cosmos

Between individuals there exists, as well, a series of "magical" relations and customs that imply the interconnectedness of the individual with her family and society in general. Many small actions or behaviors exist to ensure the well-being of the society. Some examples: the family's first annual harvest from the *milpa* is shared equally with the closest neighbors. If a man is sweating upon finishing work in the field, he should cool down in the shade before going home so as not to bring illness to his wife and children. If a person with a condition of excess heat (menstruation, pregnancy, hunger, drunkenness) comes in contact with a malnourished child who has a weak *ool,* and if the former looks upon the child with affection, this can bring about *"mal de ojo,"* the evil eye, in the child. However, if the person hugs the child and touches him affectionately, the danger of evil eye passes. All of this implies a series of rules and rites that ensure the well-being of the society and all beings. It is a conception of the human being and the world that strongly emphasizes the importance of social harmony in the harmony of all things.

One of the most popular myths in the central Yucatán is that of *kuki kan,* "the bird of death." Since time immemorial a giant bird with the body of a serpent has appeared in the east batting its wings and making a tremendous noise. Those who look upon *kuki kan* grow ill and die of a pain in the stomach. But, a long time ago, the gods enchanted and captured *kuki kan,* and he now lives in captivity where he can do no harm. He can still be heard, however, squawking and howling fiercely in the distance, threatening to break free when rain clouds gather and thunder rolls in the hot months of the year, from June to September. As with many traditional beliefs this one has taken on a Judeo-Christian feature over the past centuries—it is said that Saint George, the dragon slayer, is the keeper of *kuki kan.*

COSMIC INFLUENCE
IN CHINESE CULTURE

Taoism, one of the fundamental currents of Chinese thought, and the current upon which the history of medical knowledge is based, is a philosophy of the whole in which every terrestrial action affects the energy of the entire cosmos to a greater or lesser degree. As in Mayan thought, the actions of the individual have a great effect on social and universal balance.

Throughout much of China the life of the people is strongly influenced by the adversity of drastic climate changes. In winter the cold is intense:

it snows, the rivers freeze, food becomes scarce, and activities like food storage, collection of firewood, and preparation of warm clothes become crucial. The winter's dryness warps and cracks the wood of houses. The north winds blow down from Siberia, driving a cold air which cuts right through the bones. In the northern regions where the cold is most intense, a heat treatment—moxibustion—was developed to combat diseases of a cold nature. In the summer the humid heat is equally unbearable and the torrential rains come, bringing a damp that never quits.

Ancient Chinese doctors, peasants, and sages realized that these changes in climate not only affect the body from the outside in, but from the inside out as well. Each element affects the body in a different way. The wind, whose characteristic is constant movement, produces traveling ailments like headaches—as wind blows over a mountain top—and pains which move over and through the body. Cold, which tends to freeze and sink, manifests in illnesses which settle in one part of the body, or pains which remain in one spot—a stuck energy. Damp conditions are characterized by rigidity, lack of mobility in the limbs and joints, and sensations of heaviness in the body—as dampness, like water itself, tends to sink.

Traditional Chinese doctors, the ancient sages, for their strict observance of natural phenomena, believed that respecting the natural world rather than combating it, adapting to its changes rather than forcing it to adapt to the human will, was the only way to attain harmony in the human body and the human spirit. Notions of medicine involved a profound understanding of natural phenomena; the way to prevent and cure illnesses was to mimic the processes of nature herself, and to restore balance in the least disruptive manner possible. Traditional Chinese medicine maintains a very different understanding of the human body than that of Western medicine and bears a different understanding of health and illness, treatment, prevention, and cure. Rather than treating symptoms as part of an overall strategy to cure a specifically defined disease, Chinese medicine treats a series of imbalances that may exist throughout the body, or within and between the various organs and organ-networks. In the Chinese system we do not see diseases with common names and discrete, recognizable symptoms such as "rheumatism," "cirrhosis," or "insomnia;" rather we see syndromes of organ imbalances such as "deficient heart fire," "excess liver *yang*," or "stomach heat rising," which manifest in various symptoms that might range from poor appetite and loose bowels to excessive anger, agitation, spotty skin coloring, and headaches.

CHINESE FIVE-ELEMENT THEORY

According to Chinese five-element theory the physical world is made of wood, fire, earth, metal, and water. Water and fire make our food; wood and metal are our houses and our cities; from the earth all things are born. The theory of the five elements has been referred to since antiquity, and it constitutes the basis of Chinese materialist philosophy. The interaction of these five basic elements brings about all of the complexity of the world; the infinite subtle combinations of these substances form the fundament of all knowledge and all matter. The five elements are not merely physical elements; they exist as well on a metaphysical plane, describing the properties of all things in the realms of heaven and earth.

Corresponding with the five elements, which are born of the movements of *yin* and *yang,* are other classifications such as colors—"the five elements of the visual field"—the five flavors, the five sounds, the five virtues, the five seasons, and the five cardinal directions (taking into account the earth itself, the center).

> *Water descends and is salty*
> *Fire ascends and is bitter*
> *Wood is straight or crooked and is sour*
> *Metal transforms and is pungent*
> *Earth bears fruit and is sweet*

FIVE ELEMENT CLASSIFICATION

Element	Wood	Fire	Earth	Metal	Water
Flavor	sour	bitter	sweet	pungent/spicy	salty
Color	green	red	yellow	white	black
Change	birth	growth	mutation	receptivity	retention
Climate	wind	heat	humidity	dryness	cold
Direction	east	south	center	west	north
Season	spring	summer	late summer	autumn	winter
Organ	liver	heart	spleen	lung	kidney
Tissue	gall bladder	sm. intestine	stomach	lg. intestine	bladder
Sense Organ	eyes	tongue	mouth	nose	ears
Connective Tissue	tendons	blood vessels	muscles	skin	bones
Emotion	anger	joy	sympathy	melancholy	fear
Sound	shouting	laughter	singing	weeping	moaning
Motion	grasping		hiccup	cough	shaking

The five elements are referred to when explaining human physiology, pathology, and the relations between humans and their environment. Each of the elements possesses a chain of characteristics:

Wood — Planning, communication, cleansing of toxins
Fire — Heat, spirit, ascension
Earth — Growth and nutrition
Metal — Purity and transformation
Water — Dampness and downward movement

The organs are classified as the vital centers of energy in the body, and are viewed in relation to their (internal) functions and their (external) actions. For example: as the wood element pertains to the springtime, in the spring the liver is vigorous—either in health or in disease; the characteristic of wood is communication; the wood element sweeps up from the earth and grows towards the heavens; in the spring the wind is strong and *yang* is ascendant; plants see their burst of growth, they reinvigorate themselves, bear new greenery, and begin the process of making fruit; this young fruit is sour, and so we see the connection of wood with the spring, the wind, the color green and the sour flavor, the process of birth, and the relation of all things that are reflected therein.

The liver has the function of harmonizing the body's elements, of ordering communication, and of cleansing toxins. The liver is responsible for making sure that the blood remains clean and free of obstacles so that it will circulate freely and bring harmony and energy to all parts of the body. Liver energy tends to rise—it is a *yin* organ—and it is closely related with the gall bladder. Liver energy can be seen in the eyes, and the liver is the governor of the tendons. In its pathology, the liver is very susceptible to wind—it produces nervous energy, convulsions, and tics.

The elements of each section in the previous diagram are related in a way similar to those below. The five elements of each vertical section present

Element	Characteristic	Organ	Function
Wood	Communication, birth, the movement of blood and fluids.	Liver	Harmonizes, drains excess. Governs the ascent and distribution of energy.
Fire	Heat, ascension.	Heart	Heats *yang*.
Earth	Growth and alimentation of all things.	Spleen	Moves and transforms the essence of grains and fluids. The fountain of transformation of *chi* and blood.
Metal	Clarification, elimination.	Lung	Controls respiration and descending energies.
Water	Keeps the body moist, governs descending energies.	Kidney	Governs the metabolism of fluids in the body. Brings fluids down and eliminates them.

Human Relation
with the Cosmos

among themselves a relation of generation and control. The characteristics of the five elements demonstrate the functional physiology of the five organs.

Among the five elements we see various types of relation, the most prevalent being the cycles of creation and control. The inter-generation or breeding of the five elements signifies that each element is born out of the previous—a "mother-son" relationship.

The Creation Cycle
Wood burns to create Fire
Fire consumes wood creating ashes or Earth
Earth compacts itself giving birth to Metal
Metal in the mountains generates and enriches Water
Water engenders trees which are Wood

Creation and Control Cycles

The Control Cycle
Metal dominates Wood; Wood is cut by Metal
Water dominates Fire; Fire is extinguished by Water
Wood dominates Earth; Earth is penetrated by Wood
Fire dominates Metal; Metal is melted by Fire
Earth dominates Water; Water is contained by Earth

Five Element Theory.

These relations of inter-generation and dominance maintain equilibrium. If excess or deficiency occurs, the cycle is disturbed. Excess in domination means that the mother is overbearing with her son, while the opposite would have the son dominating the mother. The cycles of Creation and Control are inseparable. If there is no birth, there is no production and growth of things; if there is no order there will be no equilibrium in the change and development of all things. Only in breeding is there order, and only in order are all things born.

CHAPTER 2

THE HUMAN BODY

THE HUMAN BODY IN TRADITIONAL MAYAN MEDICINE

THE ANCIENT MAYA conceived of the body in the same terms in which they conceived of the universe. The body, like the cosmos, has a superior and an inferior part, and four sacred directions radiating out from the center. To the present day the Mayan conception of the body is as an entity integral to the cosmos as a whole, and as such the body is an instrument under the influence—for good or ill—of all of the forces of the universe: the gods, the planets, weather and atmospheric phenomena, the seasons, and the world of animals, plants, and humans. The behavior of the individual bears on the energies at work in all of the universe. This being the case, the individual is only healthy when she or he lives in harmony with the gods, the natural world, and the community—complying with moral, social, and environmental precepts. Traditionally, the Mayan healer interviewed his patient about his personal life by conducting a sort of confessional in which the patient discussed his behavior, his actions, and their roots in terms of the social and moral precepts of the community. This tradition still exists, though in a subtle form.

THE HUMAN BODY IN TRADITIONAL CHINESE MEDICINE

In *The Yellow Emperor's Classic of Medicine (Neijing Suwen)*, there is a basic understanding that humans could not exist apart from the natural world. This understanding is repeated throughout the book: "From ancient times it has been recognized that there is an intimate relationship between the activity and life of human beings and their natural environment."[23] "All things in nature derive their form from the *chi* of heaven and earth. Because the *chi* of heaven and earth transforms and changes and is so variable, the forms of nature and living things are also variable."[24]

The body is viewed as a replica of the universe, as its double in miniature. In the *Huai nan zi* (a Taoist encyclopedia from the second century, AD) it is noted: *"his rounded head is the celestial arch, his square feet are made in the image of the earth; his hair is the stars, his eyes, the sun and moon; his eyebrows are the Great Bear Ursa Major; his nose is a mountain; his four extremities are the seasons of the year; his five vital organs, the five elements."*

One of the central principles of Chinese medicine is the conceptualization of the body as a single totality. There is a holistic, dialectic vision of the human body. It is said that each part of the body is in union and in counterpoint with every other in the conception of the whole. Likewise, the individual and her natural environment form an integrated whole; the change of any of the parts affects the whole. And so the ancients said *"As above, so below; as within, so without."*

The activity of the internal organs is reflected not only on the body's surface, but also in every other organ. Change in any of the organs manifests in external body parts such as the tongue, the ears, the hands, the soles of the feet, the nose, or the forehead. These external signs are used as diagnostic aids to treat corresponding internal syndromes. The diagnostic method is generally based on a holistic vision of all of the meridian channels, the organs, and the movements of internal *chi*. Such a holistic diagnosis leads to the development of a complex and balanced treatment and cure.

In ancient Chinese medicine, the intention was to achieve a perfect balance of physical and spiritual energies, the terrestrial and the celestial; this was the epitome of the state of health. The two—terrestrial and celestial—were not dichotomized, as in occidental medicine; the body was not given sinful, hateful properties, as in Judeo-Christian culture and its roots in the Greco-Roman world. Traditional Chinese medicine maintains that if the body is ill, the soul is affected, and if the soul is ill, the body will likely become diseased.

Ancient Chinese medicine began with treatments related to religious practice. The curative practice of *Chi kung* had its origins in Buddhist and Taoist practice. Other Eastern healing arts, as well, developed in conjunction with religion; East Indian Ayurveda developed alongside Buddhism and Hinduism; Japanese Traditional medicine *(Kanpo)* has its roots in Shinto and Japanese Buddhism. A basis of all of these traditions is the understanding of the body's divinity, and the notion that purification of the body is purification of the soul.

TIME AND THE BODY: MAYA

Each of the gods of each of the 20-day months of the Maya influences a specific part of the human body—exemplifying, again, the relation between the gods of the world without and the nature of the world within. These divine beings shed their influence over the temporal world from the distant directions, from the corners of the heavens and earth where they live. The implication is that, in each given month, a particular organ will be especially sensitive, or susceptible to the influence of the gods and the natural world, and thus will be that much more likely to become weakened or ill. This is found in the Codex Pérez (also known as the Paris Codex) and the Codex Vaticanus.

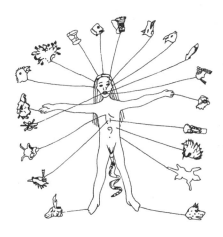

The Codex Vaticanus contains the image of a man surrounded by the symbols of each of the gods, each god representing a month of the year, and each one attached to a particular part of the body. The Codex Pérez, a colonial manuscript containing prehispanic elements in Mayan language, contains information relating particular illnesses with particular days, months, and years. It speaks of the relation of each month of the Gregorian calendar with certain illnesses and certain parts of the body. The following list is taken from the Codex Pérez:

January—Tumor in the side
February—Headache, neuralgia, swollen feet
March—Sore throat, neuralgia
April—Sore throat
May—Pain in the arms
June—Bloody vomit
July—Pain in the liver and stomach
August—Bladder infection, urine in the blood
September—Asthma
October—Swollen genitalia
November—Pain in the thigh
December—Rheumatism, knee pain

Obviously, in order to fit the Mayan scheme into the Gregorian calendar, some extrapolation would have been necessary.

The same text contains descriptions of the relations between the parts of the body, certain illnesses, and the hours of the day. Some hours are more likely than others to see the appearance of chills, colds, sinusitis,

The Human Body

chills, and swelling in the throat or the genital region, or pain in the knees or heels, for example.

TIME AND THE BODY: CHINA

Energy in Chinese medicine flows through the body just as it flows through the universe, and great emphasis is placed on the cardinal directions and the hours of the day in effecting cures. Changes in the seasons such as germination (spring), growth (summer), harvest (autumn), and dormancy (winter) also have their equivalents and effects in the human body. The various bodily organs, the blood, and *chi* in the twelve meridians that circulate through the body change according to the season of the year and the twenty-four energetic periods into which the year is divided.

In Chinese medicine the liver and gall bladder have the characteristics of wood and in the spring they dominate the energy in the five organs and the six viscera. The heart and small intestine are fire and summer is the season in which they dominate the bodily energy. The spleen and stomach represent the earth and are most influential during late summer, or Indian summer. The lungs and large intestine belong to the metal element, and their season is autumn. The kidney and bladder are water and their time is the winter.

The day is divided into four seasons: the morning is spring, midday is summer, the evening is autumn, and the middle of the night is the winter. During the dawn and the morning hours the body's *yang* energy rises; at midday it prospers; in the afternoon and evening *yang* is descending; at night the *yang* energy is at its lowest while *yin* energy comes to dominate.

The ancient Chinese determined when and in which meridian the *chi* and blood ascend and descend according to the hours of the day. For example, the stomach meridian is in its state of highest energy between seven and nine o'clock in the morning. *Chi* and blood in any given organ network achieve their maximum energy at the peak hour of that organ, and this energy begins to descend immediately after the passing of the hour.

The processes of a disease move according to the movement of *chi* and blood in the corresponding organ network; by this logic a patient may demonstrate changes such as high spirits in the morning, calm during the day, increasing aggravation of symptoms in the evening, and difficulties at night. Consequently, the treatment should follow celestial and terrestrial laws and should be enacted according to its proper moment in the day. The healing power of acupuncture becomes particularly evident when

PERIOD	DATE	POPULAR NAME	SEASON
One	December 22	*Tung chih*	Winter solstice
Two	January 6	*Hsiao han*	Little cold
Three	January 21	*Ta han*	Great cold
Four	February 4	*Li chuen*	Birth of spring
Five	February 20	*Yu shui*	Rains
Six	March 5	*Ching che*	Insects awake
Seven	March 20	*Chu uen fen*	Spring equinox
Eight	April 5	*Chi ing ming*	Pure light
Nine	April 20	*Ku yu*	Cereal rains
Ten	May 6	*Li hsia*	Birth of summer
Eleven	May 21	*Hsiao man*	Small maturation
Twelve	June 6	*Mangchong*	Ribbed grain
Thirteen	June 21	*Hsia chih*	Summer solstice
Fourteen	July 7	*Hsiao shu*	Little heat
Fifteen	July 23	*Da shu*	Great heat
Sixteen	August 8	*Li ch'in*	Birth of autumn
Seventeen	August 23	*Ch'u shu*	Dog days
Eighteen	September 7	*Pai lu*	White dew
Nineteen	September 23	*Ch'iu fen*	Autumn equinox
Twenty	October 8	*Han lu*	Cold dew
Twenty-One	October 23	*Shuang chiang*	Fall of the frost
Twenty-Two	November 7	*Li tung*	Birth of winter
Twenty-Three	November 22	*Hsiao hsue*	Small snow
Twenty-Four	December 7	*Ta hsue*	Great snow

it is effected during the optimum hours of the day. It is conjectured that this has to do with the influence of variations in atmospheric temperature and natural light as well as with the functioning status of the internal organs and the distribution of *chi* and blood through the body.

Quan bing[25] maintains that the state of illness varies between night and day in the majority of patients. For example, asthmatics frequently suffer attacks before sunrise, and people with tuberculosis often develop fever in the afternoon. It has been observed, as well, that most deaths occur between eleven o'clock at night and one in the morning, while the fewest occur between five and ten o'clock in the morning.

To make a good diagnosis, besides observing the four forms of examining the patient, traditional Chinese doctors must take into account factors like the weather, the season, the phase of the moon, and if the seasonal energy is superficial or profound. Given that physiological functions and pathological changes are tightly bound with the season, the weather and the time of day, traditional Chinese doctors, taking these points into account, prescribe treatments according to chronobiological rhythms in order to improve therapeutic results. Diseases of the small intestine and bladder *(taiyang)* meridians should be treated between nine in the morning and three o'clock in the afternoon; diseases of the stomach and large intestine meridians *(yangming)* can be treated between three o'clock in the afternoon and nine o'clock at night; diseases of the gall bladder and triple heater meridians *(shaoyang)* should be treated between three and nine o'clock in the morning; those of the spleen and lung meridians *(taiyin)* between nine o'clock at night and three in the morning; the kidney and heart meridians *(shaoyin)* should be treated between eleven at night and five in the morning; and the meridians of the liver and pericardium *(jueyin)* are treated between one and seven in the morning.

THE BODY, HOT AND COLD: MAYA

Like the universe itself, the human body is composed of the two principles hot and cold, which exist in a state of balance with each other. This equilibrium can be lost due to both internal and external factors. Similarly, the balance can be restored by these factors, and by actions taken by the patient.

The cause of illness most frequently cited in the indigenous communities is the imbalance of heat and cold in the body. With respect to this equilibrium, a series of rules and preventive habits—very different from occidental sanitary norms—are prescribed. These standards revolve around nutrition—or more specifically *alimentation,* that is, a general set of rules regarding food intake—methods of prevention in dealing with weather conditions and transitions of the body between conditions of heat and cold, patterns of work and rest, and the relation with other people according to their state of heat or cold.

The air can be cold or hot, though generally it is responsible for cold conditions. It is the custom to drink water lukewarm so as not to bring on chills. Food, as well, can be either hot or cold, though most foods are considered cold—one generally should not combine hot and cold foods, as the combination can result in *chot' nak*—twisted intestines, or cramps.

Conditions like pregnancy, drunkenness, and exhaustion are considered hot, and precautions must be taken to avoid foods and medicines of a cold nature, which may result in illness. An excess of heat is considered contagious, and precautions are taken to avoid the spread of the condition. Mayan culture places strong emphasis on conditions in which the body is imbalanced towards the hot extreme, for which one is more likely to be attacked by diseases of a cold nature. Because of this, many precautions are taken to avoid hot conditions, or to protect oneself when signs of heat are observed. Due to the dialogic conception underlying the actual practice of medicine in the Maya world, remedies and medicines are indicated more by their nature as hot or cold than by their chemical properties.

Another duality that plays an important role in the Mayan conception is the opposition of "dirty" and "clean" *(limpieza* and *suciedad)*. These conditions apply to the internal organs, which can tend to become "dirty" due the nature of their function and thus provoke illness. In cases of dirtiness of the organs, one might use medicinal infusions with a cleaning action to reestablish cleanliness in the body.

Another prevalent duality that exists is that between strength and weakness. Sicknesses have been known to be caused by people with a strong gaze but a weak *ool*. Similarly, a person may exhibit signs of weakness in a given organ, which might then be treated by a medicine with a very gentle action.

THE BODY, HOT AND COLD, YIN AND YANG: CHINA

Although the structures of the body and the conception of health and disease are extremely complex in Chinese traditional medicine, every condition can be resolved into its fundamental condition of *yin* or *yang.* The *Neijing Suwen* says, "Heaven and earth, the *chi* and the blood all reflect the interplay of *yin* and *yang.* Water has the property of coldness, fire the property of heat. The interdependence of *yin* and *yang* is reflected in all things in the universe and cannot be separated."[26]

Yang carries always within it an element of *yin,* and *yin,* likewise, bears a grain of *yang.* The two are interdependent, the two are one. The movement and interchange between the two energies constitutes the whole of the organic human body. "The key to mastering health is to regulate the *yin* and *yang* of the body. If the *yin* and *yang* balance is disrupted, it is like going through a year with spring but no winter, or winter but no summer.

When the *yang* is excessive and cannot contain itself, the *yin* will become consumed. Only when the *yin* remains calm and harmonious will the *yang chi* be contained and not be overly expansive, the spirit normal, and the mind clear."[27] When *yin* and *yang* fall out of balance, the individual falls into a state of disease, and may even meet her illness-unto-death.

Cold is the principal energy of the winter, as heat is of the summer. Cold is *yin,* heat *yang.* If the ambient temperature suddenly drops, the body is challenged in maintaining its homeostasis, and illness may occur. Being dampened by rain or sweating in the wind are examples of common situations which bring about imbalance and illness.

Diseases of heat and of cold are divided into two types: external heat or cold, and internal heat or cold. Similarly, external heat or cold have two forms of bringing about illness: one superficial, attacking the surface of the body, and one profound, directly affecting the organs and tissues. If there is an intense condition of *yin*-cold, it can damage the body's *yang* energy; if *yang*-heat is excessive, it can harm the *yin.* Internal heat or cold are pathological reflections of the insufficiency of *yin* or *yang* energy. Although damage by internal or external heat or cold have their differences, both symptomatically and fundamentally, they have mutual relations and influences. A deficiency of *yang* can provoke internal cold, making the body more susceptible to external cold. A deficiency of *yin* can provoke an excess of internal heat, causing vulnerability to external heat. Similarly, if the body is attacked by an external cold which is not repelled after some time, the body's *yang* energy may be damaged, leading to a pathology of internal cold. Likewise, external heat for an extended period may affect the body's deep reserves of *yin,* bringing about signs of excessive internal heat.

TUCH AND TIPTÉ AMONG THE MAYA

The *tuch* (umbilicus, or navel) is considered to be a strongly erogenous zone, similar to the breasts in occidental culture. The umbilical region radiates an energy—*u muuk' nak*—which beats with life and is fundamental to the health of the body. The energy, *u muuk' nak,* is located in an organ known as the *tipté* in the local language but commonly referred to as *cirro,* a word from colonial-era Spanish. This energy gives a woman the capacity to procreate, and in general is essential to the strength or weakness of a person. It is believed that the navel is the center and the beginning of life in the body, and there are various illnesses that attack this part of the body: "collapse of the *cirro,*" "*cirro* untied," *chich naak* (melancholy, or depression), problems which have to do with wind, and states of weakness and female infertility. Diseases related to the *tipté* are predominantly treated with massage and herbal therapies, although many cases call for the traditional therapy of the shaman's prayer. Starting from the navel, health or disease radiate towards the four cardinal directions.

THE DAN TIAN OF THE CHINESE

The Chinese recognize an area located just below the navel as being "the gate of life." This spot is known as the *dan tian,* though it is perhaps better recognized in the West by its Japanese name, *hara.* In the *dan tian* is stored the primordial *chi*—the fundamental material of life and the motor force which maintains the proper functioning of the organs and connective tissue. If the energy in the *dan tian* is vigorous, the organs function properly and the individual is healthy; if, on the contrary, the primordial *chi* is deficient, long-tern illness may result.

THE JOINTS: MAYA

The joints or "keys"(*llaves* in Spanish) called *uwuatzi* in Yucatec Maya, are considered to be vulnerable areas where the body folds over on itself: elbow, knee, wrist, ankle, etcetera, are points where illness may easily pass into the body. They are similarly related to the four cardinal directions.

THE RIGHT SIDE OF THE BODY: MAYA

Among the Maya of Yucatán the right side of the body is associated with health and success and the left side of the body carries the stigma of illness and failure. For this reason it is recommended, for example, to sleep lying on the right side, and to begin any given work with the right hand. These customs have been observed in Chiapas, as well, among the Tzotzil Maya of Zinacantan.

PARTS OF THE BODY: CHINA

For the Chinese, the body is recognized as a whole wherein the right side is *yin* and the left side *yang*. The back of the body is *yang* and the front is *yin*, the upper half is *yang*, the lower half, *yin*; the exterior of the extremities is *yang*, the interior, *yin*. The viscera are *yang*, the organs are *yin*. The body's surface and the four limbs are *yang*, while the internal workings are *yin*.

VITAL PRINCIPLES: MAYA

A question which is essential to the understanding of traditional medicines in general and, in our case, to Mayan medicine in particular (and which is often devalued or disregarded altogether), is the question of the soul and the world of the supernatural.

With the conquest, the spiritual world of Spanish Catholicism came to dominate the Mayan world, and traditional notions of the human vital principle or animating force became eclipsed by the "Christian soul." In spite of this, what is known as "the Christian soul" retained, for the indigenous people, meanings other than that which the church assigned. Indigenous notions of the soul involve concepts that differ greatly from the Judeo-Christian concept with regards to the body, the body's vital energy, and the physical world.

In contemporary Mayan culture on the Yucatán Peninsula we have identified two animating forces: the *pixán* and the *ool*. Spanish colonial culture tended to ignore the distinctions between the Christian soul and the indigenous soul, and much moreso the differences between these two indigenous concepts. That is to say that the Mayan concept of a dual animating force never entered the Spanish colonial mentality, which gave space in the body to only one soul. Curiously—though not surprisingly—the misunderstanding and accompanying misrepresentation of the Mayan conception of a dual animating force has impregnated medical anthropology up to the present day. When mention is made in the literature to spiritual or supernatural illnesses, these are generally credited to problems rooted in the *ool*.

The problem resides largely in translation. When we asked the Mayans to explain to us, in Spanish, what are the *pixán* and the *ool,* they responded simply that they are the soul ("the *pixán* is the soul and the *ool. . . .* is also the soul"). But when the question and answer are posed in their language, the results are very different. The explanation is complex and elaborate, and many concepts simply don't translate into Castillian Spanish. Cultural differences prevent the easy translation into an occidental language of concepts which are bound to the complex cultural fabric of the Maya. Simplified by the limitations which bind their translation into Spanish [and, further, into English], we will look at these two different vital forces.

One of these vital forces, the *pixán* (which seems to find its equivalent in the Nahuatl *teyolía),* exists from before birth; during pregnancy it is introduced into the body, giving it life. At death the *pixán* abandons the body and goes to the land of the dead where it can be reincarnated in another person. The most common definition of the *pixán* in Maya is *"leti le ku jok'ol ken kimi ken"*—"that which leaves me when I die." In the case of accidental death the *pixán* remains suspended in a state of torment until a *j'meen* helps to bear the spirit to its resting place. Otherwise, the spirit would become a ghost, trapped in the air.

In the cycles of reincarnation there is one stage in which the *pixán* returns as an animal. If one has led a bad life, she will return as a bad animal, for example a serpent; if she was good, her reincarnation will be a good animal. After this stage, she will return again as a human. Again, in the case of accidental death (and presumably treatment by a *j'meen)* the *pixán,* for not having completed its destiny, will return rapidly in the form of another human being.

The *pixán* makes its home in the entire body, but is concentrated in the head. It is the substrate of life. Of *pixán* and *ool,* it is the *pixán* which most closely resembles the Christian soul.

The other vital force is the *ool* (which finds its equivalent in the Nahuatl *tonalli).* A reasonable translation might be "the wind of life" or "the air of life." The *ool* is gathered into the body by way of the breath. It enters the lungs, passes to the heart where it finds its home, and from there its vital energy is distributed, in the blood, through the whole of the body. *Le oolo' in kuxtal* is spirit—the vital impulse—which governs the state of health, the body's strength, and emotional balance. The opposite of *le oolo' in kuxtal* is weakness, sadness of spirit, melancholy. The *ool* is concentrated in the heart, but affects the head as well in its job of maintaining the will.

The *ool* is a warm or hot energy, and is susceptible to countless illnesses such as fear *(susto)* and the evil eye *(ojo).* The latter is produced in people (generally children) with a weak *ool,* by people with a strong *ool.* The *ool* is affected, as well, by the "winds" that inhabit sacred places such as the hills, the ancient stone burial mounds *(los cuyos),* and the *milpa,* which all have their attendants. These winds principally affect hunters and others who pass through these places without observing sacred precepts (for example failing to give thanks for the harvest in the *milpa*). The *ool* of one person, as a hot energy, can cause disease in other people. It can also leave the body in dreams. When the body dies, the *ool* dissipates into the atmosphere like a hot wind.

Christianity introduced by the Spanish conquest deformed these basic indigenous concepts by confusing the *ool* with the soul—giving it spiritual and supernatural connotations which it simply does not have. The Maya say "these forces don't simply leave the body—you have to throw them out" *("lie mukoo maseu joko ju junoo, yana joska u muuk"),* meaning that one must work consciously to maintain the health of the *ool*—that to abandon its care is to allow the *ool* to abandon the body.

VITAL PRINCIPLES: CHINA

Chinese culture recognizes three basic vital principles: energy *(chi)*, essence *(jing)*, and spirit *(shen)*—besides the five superior spiritual energies which include the last two: *shen, jing, xin, hun* and *po.* These concepts are essentially untranslatable, having no equivalent in occidental terms. Unlike the Mayan vital forces, the *pixán* and the *ool,* the Chinese concepts have had the good fortune of remaining untranslated by the Christian mind, and thus we receive them more-or-less intact.

Ancient Chinese healers concluded that a sort of vital fluid or vital breath known as *chi* circulates within the body. In China, *chi* is associated with air and is the motivating force of the body, entering by way of the breath and the food. The translation often appears as "vital energy" or "vital force," though the best interpretation may be simply "energy." *Chi* is the primordial energy of the universe. *Chi* is unique, but depending on its function or constitution it can take various names. If we take the Western definition of energy as that which is capable of working or developing, that which *moves,* then we can consider the Chinese concept of *chi* more or less equivalent, and go with the simple term, *energy.* Along with the flux of *yin* and *yang, chi* is always in motion, containing diverse elements and characteristics (among these the qualities of cold and heat).

In Chinese traditional medicine, energy—as opposed to matter—is recognized as the basis of all things natural. Everything that *is* is produced by the flux of energy in the universe. The body is energy incarnate; vital activity is the manifestation of body-as-energy. Over time, the Chinese deepened the concept of *chi* and defined the different forms it manifests. The translation as "energy" came but a few hundred years ago, while the concept of *chi* has thousands of years of growth in the medium of Chinese medical and spiritual thought.

In China it is considered that only when the body is filled with the *chi* of heaven—from the breath—and the *chi* of earth—from the food—can it develop its functions in a healthy, balanced way. While the prenatal *chi* is fundamental—the basic motor force—it is the postnatal *chi* upon which the sustenance of life depends. The life of a human being and all of her activities are motivated by prenatal *chi* and supplemented by postnatal *chi*. The two are interdependent and interacting, forming the *"true chi."*

Essence, or *jing,* is the material substrate of energy, and is what, in the body, converts into energy. *Jing* is the basic substance, the primeval force that gives birth to all life. It is the essential energy—the part that constitutes the organs, the structure, the living material that corresponds to the union of sperm and egg—the union of man and woman—that forms a new being with new *jing*. The fountain of essence and the formation of energy in the body can be prenatal or postnatal. *Jing* dwells in the kidney, source of the deep energy associated with the element water and with the deep well of the body's *yin*.

Spirit, *shen,* is exercised by vital activity, and lives principally in the heart. It is the active expression of life. *Shen* is born of the living union of the essences of man and woman. *Shen* finds its most extraordinary expression in fantasies, waking dreams, forces of creativity, and the imagination. It is associated with fire and the heart, the storehouse of *yang,* the body's male principle.

Apart from the three basic principles, Chinese traditional medicine classifies five superior spiritual activities. *Shen* and *jing* aside, we have *xin, hun* and *po.*

Xin is defined as the heart, the axle upon which all activity revolves. *Xin* is the emperor of the body, dominating the emotions, and the function of generating ideas, reflection, will, wisdom, memory, and intelligence.

Hun is perpetual companion to the spirit. It comes and goes with *shen*. *Hun* resides in the liver, being most active in the spring, *yang* inside of *yang*. It is the guardian of the spirit, the warrior soul. *Hun* is the traveling restless wanderer, the force that refuses to surrender. In other cultures we might see *hun* as the force behind reincarnation, that-which-refuses-to-die. The pathology known as *gang bu cang hun* (the liver expels *hun* from its house) finds its manifestation in sleeptalking, somnambulism, and hyperactive dreaming.

Po is that which enters and leaves together with the *jing* essence. It is stored inside the lung, *yin* inside of *yin*. *Po* corresponds to the living mate-

The Human Body

rial, the balance that keeps the body alive. It is the white soul, the soul that lives in the bones and goes to the grave with them. *Po* regulates the conditioned reflexes as well as instinctive reflexes (breathing and swallowing, for example).

POINTS AND WIND CHANNELS IN MAYAN MEDICINE

The various traditional Mayan therapies recognize the existence of a series of points on the body through which a doctor or *curandero* can manipulate the "wind" through bleedings and the application of needles. We have identified approximately fifty points, which will be discussed in the next chapter. Some *curanderos* refer to canals, or channels, along which the wind circulates through the back, arms and legs. When there is pain in a joint or articulation, the doctor mighty apply a needle to a point in the articulation that follows in that particular channel.

POINTS AND MERIDIANS IN TRADITIONAL CHINESE MEDICINE

The channels, or meridians, are passages which connect the energetic points, by way of which energy circulates throughout the body. These meridians form a network connecting the superior part of the body with the inferior, the right side with the left, internal with external—bringing each part of the body into balance with every other part. By way of this network, for example, a headache can be treated by inserting a needle into a point on the foot.

In very general terms, the system of meridians is defined as the pathways through which travel the blood and *chi*. This series of canals connects a multitude of points on both the exterior and interior of the body. Along these pathways are found the different points of major energy concentration (mistakenly known as acupuncture points). This energy, as previously stated, is built by way of the breath and the food; if the energy in a given meridian increases or decreases dramatically this causes illness, and the treatment consists of regulating the energy back to its normal state, by way of acupuncture, moxibustion, massage, herbal therapy, diet, and exercises such as *chi kung*.

An estimated 365 points cover twelve principal and two extraordinary meridians; but, including collateral and extra meridians as well as points that lie off of the specific meridians, some two thousand points can be counted. The principal twelve meridians are: lung, large intestine, stomach, spleen-pancreas, heart, small intestine, liver, gall bladder, triple heater, pericardium, kidney, and bladder. Besides these we have the central channel, the most important of the extraordinary meridians, comprised of the governing and conception vessels. These meridians, all interconnected, form a unified field across which the body's energy moves continually. In this way the organs are interconnected: lung with large intestine, large intestine with stomach, and so on. These meridians are neither blood vessels nor nerves, but an entirely different sort of entity distinct from any anatomical system.

Eight other important meridians include the extraordinary vessels and the collateral vessels. By "collateral vessels" (luo) we refer to a specific network consisting of branches of the meridians. The meridians and collaterals cross the entire body, making an organic union of the diverse parts. The eight extraordinary vessels are not directly connected to the organ networks and are not restricted by the sequence of the twelve principal channels. They take diverse routes and flow in an irregular pattern; hence the term "extraordinary vessels." They are, in Chinese, *dumai, ren, chong, dai, yinquiao, yangqiao, yinwei* and *yangwei*.

When the flow of *chi* and blood in the twelve channels is excessive, the extra energy flows over into the extraordinary channels to be stored there. When the *chi* in the twelve channels is insufficient, the extra *chi* from the extraordinary vessels flows back into the principal channels. The twelve channels are like rivers, the eight are like lakes. The function of the eight extra channels is to maintain and regulate the twelve. The eight extraordinary vessels have their own routes and the internal *chi* stored there influences the internal organs and the exterior of the body in its own fashion.

THE TONGUE IN CHINESE MEDICINE

A close connection exists between the tongue and the internal organs. The heart meridian connects with the root of the tongue, as do the meridians of the spleen and the kidney. The five organs and six viscera connect directly or indirectly with the tongue. The energy or essence of the organs and viscera rise to feed the tongue. Because of this, pathological changes in the various organs produce changes which manifest on the tongue.

The tongue has principal relations with the stomach, spleen, and heart. The heart governs the blood vessels and the tongue is abundantly irrigated by the heart; the heart governs the spirit, which has to do with the mobility of the tongue and the faculty of speech, for which it is said that the tongue reflects primarily the functional condition of the heart. Among organs and viscera, the heart is the emperor.

In the tongue we find that the sense of taste, with its influence over the desire to eat, has a relation with the acceptance or rejection of various foods, their digestion and transport, functions realized by the stomach and spleen. The stomach and spleen are the base of postnatal energies, the fountain of transformation of blood and energy; therefore the condition of these organs and the strength or weakness of the blood and *chi* of the whole body are reflected in the tongue.

It is said that the front of the tongue reflects the condition of the upper burner (heart and lungs), that the center of the tongue corresponds to the middle burner (spleen and stomach), and the root of the tongue is related to the lower burner (liver and kidney). The sides of the tongue reflect the condition of the liver and gall-bladder, and the root of the tongue reflects the kidney.

FIVE ELEMENT THEORY
AND THE HUMAN BODY
IN CHINESE CULTURE

As we mentioned earlier, Chinese culture recognizes that all of nature is composed of the five elements, and the human body is no exception. The five elements must not be considered as materials, but rather as forces or tendencies. Each element presents certain properties. So we see that the body houses five organs and six viscera, each relating to a particular element. The liver and gall bladder are wood, the heart and small intestine are fire, the spleen-pancreas and stomach are earth, the lungs and large intestine are metal, and the kidney and bladder are water.

The generative relation, or Creation Cycle, between the five elements shows us that the liver is mother to the heart and son of the kidney; the heart is mother of the spleen and son of the liver; the spleen is mother to the lung and son to the heart, etcetera. The relation of dominance, or Control Cycle, tells us that the liver dominates the spleen, the heart dominates the lungs, the spleen dominates the kidney, the lung dominates the liver, the kidney dominates the heart.

This theory represents and has represented, for Chinese medical practice, the fundamentals of acupuncture. The five element relational theory aids in diagnostics and prognosis, showing the course of an illness among the organs, and guiding the observant doctor to the methodology by which he or she will apply the needles.

THE ORGANS, EMOTIONS, AND VITAL PRINCIPLES IN TRADITIONAL CHINESE MEDICINE

In Chinese traditional medicine, inside of the body are found the five organs and six viscera, like special tissue. The five organs are the heart, lung, spleen, liver, and kidney. Their general function is to store energy; they are the places where all of the nutrifying substances necessary to the performance of vital activity—such as blood, energy, essence, spirit, and the various fluids—are stored. All of the organs exhibit a relation with the heart-mind. Their most important function is the storage of *jing* essence.

The viscera are: bladder, stomach, small and large intestines, gall bladder, and triple burner. Their general function is that of receiving and transferring the contents of the other viscera along their pathway. They govern the alimentary canal and the acceptance of food—its transmission, transformation, and excretion.

The five organs store essence and energy but cannot transport and transfer fluids and substances; the six viscera can transfer their contents but cannot store them.

The extraordinary organs are: the brain, the medulla oblongata, the bones, and the uterus. These special tissue seem like organs, but are not. They seem like viscera but are not. Their function is to store *yin* and essence. In this function they are similar to the five organs, but they maintain a unique relationship with the organs.

Each of the five organs has control or action over a particular emotion and a particular spiritual activity. The heart is related to sadness, joy, and tears. In this it is in charge of housing the spirit, or *shen,* and the capacity to dream, to fantasize. The heart is also in charge of mental activities, including consciousness and thought, as well as governing the blood vessels and relations with the sweat, the tongue, the skin, and its parent viscera, the small intestine.

Altering the heart's function causes mental disorders. In the case of a *yang* deficiency in the heart, symptoms might include heart palpitations, fear, and memory loss, corresponding to a malfunction in the cerebral cortex. In the case of a *yin* deficiency in the heart, one becomes subject to night sweats and insomnia, symptoms of a problem in the nervous system.

The liver governs the blood and houses the soul *(hun)*. It regulates the flow of blood through all of the tissues and organs, adjusting the flow according to the requirements of the body's activities. It also controls the dispersion and distribution of *chi*, controls the movements of the joints and tendons; it is related to the function of sight, the reproductive organs, and its partner viscera, the gall bladder. Emotionally, it is responsible for judgment, anger, rage, and the ability to make decisions. When the liver's function is impaired there is difficulty in the management of emotions in general, and in particular there are problems with depression and irritability.

The spleen stores ideas and is responsible for the transportation and digestion of food. The spleen administers the properties and essence of our food to the entire body, and transports and transforms fluids to maintain normal metabolism. This job is brought to bear with the combined force of the lung, the kidney, the triple burner, the heart, and the bladder. The spleen regulates the circulation of blood and its absorption by the muscles. Along with the stomach it is in charge of digestion and absorption. In terms of spiritual influence, the spleen lends us the capacity for abstract thought. As the governor of nutrition in the body, the spleen generates ideas so there is no lack of spiritual sustenance. When spleen energy is deficient, there will be indigestion, abdominal distention, and diarrhea—as well as edema and all sorts of water retention. When there is a problem in the spleen, one tends to worry and become preoccupied with a single idea, unable to let it go.

The lungs control the *chi* and house *po,* the white soul, or internal vigor. The lungs have to do with the clarification and descent of spiritual energy from the heavens, they are associated with surface protection by way of the skin and the pores. The lungs open to the air by way of the nose, and their partner viscera is the large intestine. The lungs are related to melancholy and grief—the inability to leave the past behind, to let go of sadnesses, to move on.

The kidney stores the will *(zhi)* and governs deep essence. The essences of all of the organs, as well as of the kidney, are controlled here. The kidney is the base of the reproductive system. Its role is to develop all of the functions for maintaining the individual and the species, which explains its relation with the will. The kidney is related to the brain and the nervous system, the production of hormones, the growth of bones, the metabolism of water, and the absorption of air from the lungs. The kidney controls the vital gate, the entrance into life. The kidney's function includes as well that of the adrenal glands. The kidney's partner is the bladder, whose function involves urination and opens to the outside by way of the anus and urethra. When the kidney is stagnant or weak, the will is affected, and one is susceptible to fear, panic and terror, losing the will to live in the face of frightening obstacles.

The triple burner is formed of three parts: the upper, middle, and lower burners. The upper burner functions like a fountain, the heart and lungs dispersing their energies. The middle burner is where the spleen and stomach digest the food and absorb the earthly *chi*. The lower burner is the drainage, where the kidney and bladder excrete the remains. The triple burner is closely related to the pericardium, whose function is to protect the heart.

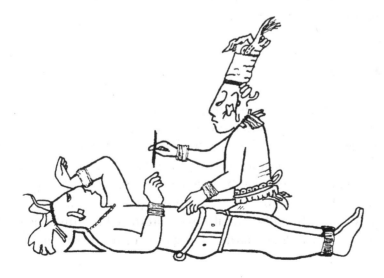

The Human Body

CHAPTER 3

CAUSALITY AND ILLNESS

CAUSALITY IN MAYAN TRADITIONAL MEDICINE

THE CONTEMPORARY MAYAN cosmovision offers a rich system of explanations about phenomena of health and disease, whose complexity is compounded by syncretism with other cultural systems. Due to the course of historical interactions with conquest-era Spanish medicine and current Western concepts, the interweaving of cultures gives rise to a medical system which presents the characteristics of each of its tributaries. Due to the complexities of historical process, the notion of "traditional medicine" is more complicated than it might at first appear. Nevertheless, we will attempt here to make a basic classification of the causal factors of disease based on concepts referred to by the *curanderos*. It must be noted that our Western sensibilities are the medium through which these concepts have been selected and classified—adding another layer to the weave of syncretism that both enriches and obscures the traditional concepts.

ORGANIC CAUSES

By "organic causes" we mean those factors which are related to an imbalance in physical or terrestrial phenomena, such as the flux of heat and cold, movements of air, changes in diet and dietary habits, as well as other mechanisms such as posture, extreme or brusque movements, wounds, excess work, lack of rest, and bad hygiene. These factors produce imbalances in the body which affect the physiology and cause changes both internally and externally. The illnesses produced by this type of phenomena are considered "natural," organic, or mundane *(luum kabil)*.

SUPERNATURAL CAUSES
(IIK NAAL—"ILLNESS FROM
THE WORLD OF THE WINDS")

Supernatural or spiritual causes are those which are related to influences or "winds" produced by people, animals, plants, or objects, or directly by supernatural beings (gods, saints, spirits, *aluxob*) by way of the winds which affect the body and break its equilibrium.

In our work with the *curanderos* we infer that what we here differentiate as "organic" and "spiritual" causes of disease are actually quite intimately related; it is not easy to separate them in practice. Whether "organic" or "spiritual" causes are discovered to be at the root of the disease depends on the particular case, as the symptoms may be the same. On many occasions a particular illness may have both types of causes. There does not exist, either, a clear demarcation between internal and external causes, although in any particular case the *curandero* will know very well, and will proceed with the treatment accordingly.

Similarly, both organic and supernatural illnesses may be caused by interactions with one's family, community, with nature or the gods, or by sentiments or thoughts which arise within oneself. Actions that show a lack of respect for familial, common, or divine elements—breaking with family ties, social codes, natural or cosmic law—can generate harmful energies in the protagonist, causing an imbalance that leads to illness. Lack of respect for a family member is a factor which may lead to "natural" illness—because it is a terrestrial or mundane relation—but at the same time the gods demand that family ties be respected, and thus supernatural factors may come into play as well. Illness is thus defined as an imbalance between the individual and his social or natural surroundings.

This understanding of illness comes from an intimate relation with the natural world and the social community, a firm understanding of natural and social law, and an intricate understanding of the workings of the human body. As in Western medicine where we believe in microbes and their influence on health because they have a basis in experience and experiment, the Mayan people base their beliefs on empirical evidence and the experience of generations of *curanderos.*

To facilitate the organization of intricate and detailed information we present the diverse explications of causality in the appendix on traditional Mayan disease classification. The descriptions found there are translations from the Mayan dialect spoken in Campeche, and should be consulted for a more specific understanding of the origins of disease in the Mayan system.

HEAT AND COLD IMBALANCE

With respect to the entirety of causes, one relation is outstanding and seems to be integral to the entire body of Mayan medical thought: the concept of hot and cold. It seems that a great part of the causes of illness—dietary disorders, emotional imbalance, excess of work, weakness, etcetera—can be seen as representing qualities either hot or cold. Conditions, objects, food—all are classified as hot or cold and under certain conditions arise as the potential cause of illness. Both natural and supernatural winds are also considered to fit within this concept.

The term "warm," as we translate it, is used by the Maya to refer to a physical state, produced by heat, in which the organism is in imbalance and is susceptible to illness. When the body is hot—from having awakened rapidly without proper stretching to circulate the blood, from being exposed to the sun, from working in the city or in the *milpa,* from having received a massage, eaten warming foods or taking "hot" medicines, or from having warm conditions like pregnancy or menstruation—one is most susceptible to illness due to winds and cold foods. During these times, great attention is given to avoiding foods which are considered very cold, like limes and oranges. There are other cold fruits and vegetables but none so extreme as these, to which health restrictions only apply in cases of pregnancy or puerpery (considered delicate warm conditions). This goes directly against the occidental medical understanding that one should consume foods rich in vitamins during these periods.

External cold is considered to cause stagnant blood—a condition of physically darkened blood which produces internal wind. Hot and cold phenomena affect the entire body, but most notably the blood and certain organs such as the brain, the stomach, the *tipté,* and the joints. Some examples of this group of causes:

Diarrhea *(wach kajan)* and dysentery *(kiik naak)* can be caused by:

- Drinking ice water or eating cold food while the stomach is in a warm state. This produces air in the stomach.
- A baby suckling the breast of its mother in the hot air. This air passes into the baby's belly.
- Drinking water from a warm pot.

- Eating foods of a hot nature, especially if they are cooked and tender.
- Eating hot foods with cold liquids. Care is given to guard against children doing this before they know better.

Chill in the stomach *(xaka ta'a)* can be caused by eating warm citrus fruit. Stomach ache *(chiibal naak)* is often the result of mixing hot foods with cold conditions, or vice versa. Painful urination *(yaya wix)* can be provoked by mixing too many condiments in one meal, causing the food to become hot. Intestinal fever *(tu chokui tu choche)* is a condition of thirst brought on by heat in the belly. Sourness in the stomach *(tu kee)* is caused by chilling the food by mixing it with cold water. Different types of headaches *(kinan pool, chiba pool, kinan pach ka* and *jolon al)* can be caused by:

- The heat of the sun, especially when one suffers from weak blood.
- When one is working in the *milpa* or in the sun and a mist or light rain falls. This doesn't happen in the case of a thunder shower because the rain brings the entire body to an even temperature.
- When one is hot and a cool wind crosses one's head. This wind enters the head, causing the blood to stagnate and become dark.
- When one leaves the house warm.
- When one bathes but does not wet the hair (this heats up the head).
- When a woman has just given birth and she is hit by a cold wind. The first two days after giving birth, a woman is hot and weak for the loss of blood. For these reasons she is especially susceptible to harm by the cold air.

Dry cough *(se'en)* and rheumatism *(reuma ik')* can be caused by:

- Being hot after receiving a massage and being hit by a wind.
- Bathing in warm water and stepping out into the air. When the air cools the body, the blood stagnates and doesn't circulate well.
- Eating oranges while hot.
- When one walks barefoot on cool, humid earth, or in mud.
- Returning hot from work and washing the hands.

Night sweat *(k'il kab)* can be caused by:

- Rocking a baby when it is recently bathed.
- The mother sleeping with her baby—the excess heat causing the baby discomfort.
- Changing clothes in the open air.

Irregular menstruation *(mesankil)* can be caused by:

- Bathing in cold water just prior to a period.
- When a woman is menstruating and drinks cold water, eats lemon, or washes her hair. The maturation of the ovules does not happen normally because of chill or weakness.

DIGESTIVE AND NUTRITIONAL DISORDERS

The *curanderos* and the Mayan people in general place great importance on eating habits. Some problematic eating habits might include: eating too little or too much, eating at odd hours or in a rush, eating an inappropriate kind of food (heavy, sweet, greasy, or spicy), consuming refrigerated foods, working immediately after a meal, or overly indulging in alcohol.

Diarrhea *(wach kajan)* can be provoked by:

- Eating to excess.
- Eating at an odd hour, especially after having strong hunger.
- When the mother eats heavy foods and breastfeeds her baby.

Changes in the *tipté* can be due to:

- Eating a large meal after the hour for eating has passed. If one eats at an inappropriate time the weakened *tipté* contracts and tightens.
- Excess hunger.
- Hard work or effort immediately after eating.

Eating heavy foods that the stomach rejects can cause indigestion *(chi'bal naak')*. Dysentery *(kiik naak)* can be caused by excess grease, excess spice, or by abuse of alcohol. Diabetes can be provoked by eating an excess of sweet foods. Eating meat that has been refrigerated can cause tightness in the stomach. Painful urination *(yaya wix)* can be caused by the accumulation of residues from the fluids that one drinks. Eating limes in the days immediately following menstruation can cause irregular menstruation *(mesankil)*. Bladder infection *(k'an chi kin)* can be caused by not purging for an excess period—causing an accumulation of residues and bile in the stomach and bladder.

Posture and Movement

Brusque movements, falls, and contusions can cause diarrhea, dysentery, and irregularities of the *tipté*. It is said that with brusque movement and bruises the *tipté* or *cirro* may loosen and the intestines may shift position.

Diarrhea *(wach kajan)* can be caused by remaining seated for a long time when one is not accustomed to it, or by lifting heavy objects. Collapse of the crown in children *(tzan nu yaal* or *caida de mollera)* is caused when a child is lifted too rapidly or is treated with brusque movements. Neck and shoulder pain *(kinan pach wa)* are caused by blows to the back or inflammation of the shoulder blade. Irregular menstruation *(mesankil)* is caused when a woman falls and twists her hip.

Excessive Work

Work is considered to cause heat, and to weaken and tire the body. A tired back from excess work can bring about dysentery *(kiik naak)*. Similarly, hard work can cause irregular menstruation *(mesankil)* in women. People who work a lot also tend to suffer from neck pain *(kinan pach ka')*.

Contamination

It is a common understanding among *curanderos* and the people that many maladies arise from dirtiness, or contamination. The concept of contamination, however, generally doesn't refer to germ theory or microbiology. The *curanderos* never use the word "microbe" as part of the explanation of this phenomenon. Over the course of many community meetings, when we asked the causes of diarrheas and other illnesses which in our understanding are germ-related, microbes were never mentioned. A few of the *curanderos* were familiar with the term, but only used it when questioned explicitly about microbes. We noted that it was generally used out of context (for example, referring to an animal, plant, object, substance, or food, we were told that "it has a lot of microbes" if it had poisonous or harmful properties). On the other hand, the concept of contamination was used in many cases that are strictly related to Western notions of germ theory (for example, weak stomach and sour taste in the mouth [*tu kee*]). Following are some examples:

Diarrhea *(wach kajan),* nocturnal defecation *(xaca taá),* and dysentery *(kiik naak)* can be caused by:

- Eating rotten, dirty, or uncooked food or drinking contaminated water.
- Drinking raw milk.
- Not washing food and dishes before eating.
- Children eating dirt, garbage, or other things that aren't food.
- Drinking standing rain water.
- Eating food infected by flies, dust, or parasites.

Weak stomach and sour taste in the mouth *(tu kee)* can be due to:

- A dog or other animal licking the silverware and dishes.
- Using dirty plates and dishes.

LACK OF PREVENTIVE CARE

Other illnesses are strictly related to the failure to take preventive measures of varied sorts and degrees. If one fails to urinate when the bladder is full, it can result in excess bile *(k'an chik'in).* If one does not keep generally sanitary habits, at least once a year he may experience painful urination and bladder infection *(yaya wix).* Failure to take adequate care during pregnancy and failure to breastfeed a baby immediately after birth can result in a lack of mother's milk *(sa'p u k'aab u yim).*

WEAKNESS

Among the Mayan people there exists no concept of malnutrition. We have observed that it is a very difficult concept to get across in educational campaigns on nutrition. However, the term "weakness" is commonly used and understood, and is generally related to a lack of healthy food.

Another important concept in the area of nutrition is anemia, known as "hollow blood," and recognized to produce weakness. When one is weak, there is a greater chance of contracting an organic illness, such as diabetes *(chujuk wix),* headache *(chiba pool* and *kinan pool),* menstrual irregularities *(mesankil),* and lack of mother's milk *(sa'p u k'aab u yim).* Weakness can also precipitate other illnesses, such as problems with the *cirro,* evil eye, bleeding from the umbilicus in newborns, desire, fear, and evil wind. With hunger the *cirro* becomes weak. But if one suddenly appeases one's hunger with a large meal eaten rapidly, the food is heavy on the body and can bring about a tightening of the *cirro*.

Evil eye in infants can be caused by weakness and malnutrition in the mother; the child in turn becomes weak. Put in contact with someone of strong disposition or with a strong gaze, an imbalance in the child's body temperature comes about. Since the child is in a fragile state, his blood is weak and cannot resist the change in temperature.

Bleeding from the umbilicus in infants *(jo'k'o k'iik tu tuch)* might come about when the path of a child whose blood is weak is crossed by a young woman menstruating, a pregnant woman, or a pregnant animal. This happens because the blood moving in the women or the animal is hot. This illness is only seen in children of weak disposition.

Skin lesions *(chupul yo'ola poch)* more commonly known as *dzibolal* (desire for food), appear when someone with a strong *ool* or a strong gaze desires a certain food, and this desire goes unsatisfied, and is met by someone with a weak *ool,* generally a younger relative or a child.

Fear comes about when a shock of some sort occurs to children with a weak *ool.* Those with a weak *ool* are nervous by nature, and thus are more susceptible to this kind of attack. When one is weak in general, one is more susceptible to attack by the winds.

EMOTIONAL STATE

In the causal conception of certain illnesses we find the notion that negative emotions can bring about imbalance in the body which in turn leads to illness. States like spite, anger, annoyance, and resentment can lead to illness as readily as changes in temperature or climate. Some examples follow:

- When a woman argues spitefully with her husband or with a neighbor, and then breastfeeds her baby, *wach kajan* (diarrhea) can develop in the infant.
- Worry and disgust can lead to *xaka ta'a* (dysentery).
- A specific fear or anger can cause *k'an chik'in* (overflow of bile), *chujuk wix* (diabetes), and *sa'p u k'aab u yim* (absence of mother's milk).

Kinan pool (a type of headache) can appear:

- In general illnesses like "bile," in which one's temperature rises due to anger.
- When a general weakness has set in due to feelings of disgust.

Causality and Illness

Kinan pach na (neck and shoulder pain) can be caused by nerves, anger, thinking too much, exhaustion, or overwork.

It is believed that strong emotional impressions can directly affect the *ool* and result in the medical condition known as fear. Fear is a disease of the *ool*, a state simultaneously described as *xma ool* (perturbed *ool*), which affects the will and the emotions in general. Fear tends to attack children with a weak *ool* and people of a generally nervous condition. Fear can be transmitted from mother to child during pregnancy and into the early years of infancy. Fear can come about from "natural" situations, in which one receives a shock or strong impression, as well as from circumstances involving supernatural beings. Examples of the natural causes of fear are:

- When a pregnant woman receives a serious fright. It is more grave in the early stages of pregnancy, because the illness develops with the fetus. When the child is born, it is born with fear. The name of this condition is *jak'iool*.
- If the mother is in a nervous or frightened state, this can be transferred to her infant or young child (known as *jak'ola'*).
- When the mother is struck by fear while lactating and the fear passes to the infant by way of the milk, this is known as *jasaool*.
- When a child or newborn directly receives a fright which develops into fear, this is known as *xpak'i'*.

Examples of supernatural situations include the following:

- Fear can be caused by the bird known as *coos* or "witch bird." This bird has nocturnal habits and attacks chickens. When killing them it tears out the throat first so they make no noise. The cry of the *coos* bird frightens children, especially newborns.
- When one comes across the *alkab k'ok ob iik'*, a snake or green iguana that speaks or laughs like a woman.
- Any appearance of *aluxob, bacabob*, etcetera.

INVOLUNTARY HUMAN ACTIONS

Under some conditions one may involuntarily cause an imbalance in another person which may result in illness. This understanding, basic to Mayan culture, reads in its depths as an indication that the human social subject is not and cannot be isolated; each individual bears an influence on the entirety of society. This view necessitates a series of social rules to avoid the potentially negative affects of certain human interactions and to heighten positive social interdependence.

When a person with a strong gaze looks with tenderness on a small child "with a desire to hug the child," but doesn't touch the child, this can bring about a temperature imbalance which affects the infant, causing *ee'k ich tabi* or *tu menta ojo*—evil eye. In this pathology, a sympathetic relation is established but unsatisfied—a relation of attraction, desire, or tenderness between the adult and the child; when the child is drawn into this relation with the adult, he loses heat and becomes ill. The condition is more common when the child is weak or malnourished, and if the other person is a woman who is pregnant or menstruating, if the person is hungry, drunk, or has a blemish in the eye. These states are characterized by excessive heat and some sort of change in the gaze. People with a strong gaze can cause *mal de ojo* not only in other people, but in animals and small birds as well.

A similar process is seen in cases of *jo'k'o k'iik tu tuch* (bleeding from the umbilicus in newborns)—in which a pregnant or menstruating woman or a pregnant animal passes near a newborn child and body heat transfers from the passerby to the child, affecting the child's blood. The same illness can befall a woman who has just had intercourse, has not bathed, and comes close to the baby. It is said that the effect is caused by the heat of the semen ("the dirtiness") that the woman carries inside her. In this way the man affects the child by way of the woman.

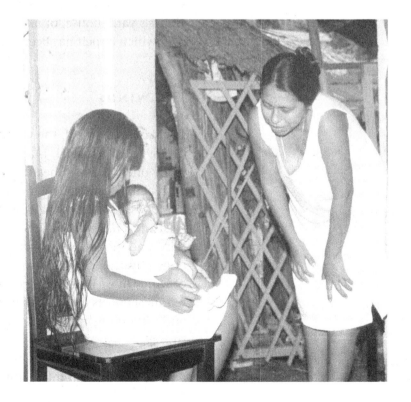

When a person with a strong *ool* or a strong gaze craves a particular food and this craving goes unsatisfied, this longing can be passed to a younger relative or a child, causing *chupul yo'ola poch* or *dzibolal* (desire for food). "Desire for food" is different from simple hunger, and manifests as lesions on the skin. It is said that these lesions take the appearance of the food that was craved.

ANIMALS, PLANTS, AND OBJECTS

It is believed that animals—birds, horses, dogs—can also cause *ojo,* evil eye, if they have a strong gaze or when they are in a state of excess. The evil eye caused by an animal is known as *ojoy balche'.*

There are occasions when plants may be affected by the weak or tired state of a passerby, and this state may then be passed from the plant to another person. There is also risk of this when a plant is accidentally splashed with alcohol used in a medical ritual, and later someone comes in contact with the plant.

VOLUNTARY HUMAN ACTIONS

One may cause illness with malicious intent when one feels envy, hate, or desire for vengeance towards another person and employs a witch or *"brujo" (way chivo)* who can cast spells *(meyak'as)* which cause illness. They commit the deeds at night, usually on a Tuesday or Friday, managing to sneak some substance into the victim's food, or throw something into the victim's yard, house, or *milpa.* A common totem is dirt from a cemetery over which a spell has been recited.

THE WINDS

The damaging wind, the wind that causes illness, a wind at once physical and metaphysical, is a concept in Mayan medicine which explains many phenomena in health, illness, death, and life. Everything is imbued with characteristics of wind: the air, the will, the entirety of life. Different foods and drinks can provoke wind or be part of its transmission. The west wind *(lakin iik),* the north wind *(saman iik),* "the wind that brings rain" and the "evil wind from the grave" can have for us explanations at once physical, chemical, and microbiological, but there are other types of wind whose meanings are more difficult to explain. These phenomena manifest effects over the entire human body, but especially in the blood and certain organs like the brain, the stomach, the *tipté,* the joints, and the *ool.*

The wind is an entity which unites the natural world with the supernatural world. The wind might be a physical phenomenon, like the imbalance between heat and cold in the body, it might be caused by another person, animal, or plant, or it might be considered a living phenomena sent by supernatural forces—the "owners or spirits of the wind." Water, woods, earth, and the sun all have their living spirits, and the wind as well is inhabited or "owned" by its spirit. Thus the wind has a multiple character, at once a living being and the effect of living beings.

The concept of "evil wind" generally encapsulates winds of a supernatural character. The *curanderos* understand that the wind or air has negative properties coming from living beings (gods, saints, spirits, *aluxob*) which are the owners of the various natural phenomena (water sources, woods, rain, wind, sun).

There exist a great variety of explanations of the "evil wind": it can originate within the person, it can be caused by other people in a manner either voluntary or involuntary, by objects, plants, and animals, by actual winds (especially the west wind and the north wind), by the spirits of a place, by incompleted promises, and by different sorts of work.

Evil wind is related to the evil eye. Evil eye can be caused by a sort of gaze from another person, but it may also be produced by a supernatural being or by a wind. Winds and supernatural beings can also cause fear when they provoke a shock or strong reaction that affects a person's *ool*.

In general the evil winds are cold, but there exist hot winds as well. Like other hot and cold phenomena, these winds break the body's balance, causing illness when the person is thrown into a state of excess heat or excess cold.

Following is an enumeration and classification of causes of evil wind:

Winds of Internal Origin
An internal wind may be caused when, due to carelessness, one begins the day with activities using "the contrary side of the body" (the left side).

The Wind as a Physical Phenomenon
As mentioned previously, many illnesses, such as diarrhea, flu, rheumatism, and menstrual irregularities can be caused by stepping out into a cold wind. A mother returning from the mountains or the woods and breastfeeding her child before getting warm can cause the child to contract the species of diarrhea known as *wach kajan*. *Wach kajan* and *se'en* (a dry cough) are also caused by the wet wind and the wind that brings rain.

The Evil Wind Inside the Wind

We have heard talk of some winds which are worse than others, as if the evil wind were carried on the back of the worldly wind. Many illnesses, such as *wach kajan,* are more commonly caused by the evil wind from certain cardinal directions, like the *chikin iik'* or *k'an chik'in*; the west wind or "red cloud," and the *xaman iik'* or *xamankan,* or north wind. Some illnesses are born by whirlwinds or dust devils *(tu jentan ta iik'al mozón).* Whirlwinds are generally manifestations of malevolent supernatural energy. Each type of whirlwind has its name and its "owner." During late summer there are evil winds that commonly cause illness and death in both children and adults.

The Spirits and the Winds

Various spirits tend to generate harmful influences or forces that travel on the winds. It is said that the nature of spirits is wind: "If it travels in the air, it comes from heaven." Thus the winds and the air are pathways over which travel forces both beneficial and harmful.

Like all phenomena in nature, the winds have their particular spirits or owners—principal deities who keep servants and helpers. The gods, spirits, and caretakers can produce winds, which serve them. Some examples of winds which are the servants of spirits are the *k'akal iik* (wind of the burial mounds), *iik k'aja'* (the wet wind), the *rekai muyal* (evil of the red cloud), the *u yi k'a luum* (air off the earth), and the *xtuu'* (the evil solar wind).

Winds are produced by the sun. The sun, *kin,* is the father of all things. Every color that the sun produces creates an effect and an illness. The worst is the color purple, which is the color of the body's heat. The sun can also produce the evil eye *(ojoy kiin).*

When a promise made to some force or supernatural being is not kept, this being or force may send an evil wind as punishment. This is known as *xlu muk* or *xk'amuk ool.* Some examples of this are:

- When one offers food to the *pixánes*—spirits of the dead—but fails to complete the offering; also when one receives an inheritance but fails to offer prayers of thanks.
- When one offers ritual food *(sakab)* to the saints, *balamob,* or spirits of the forests and mountains but the *sakab* is not accepted.
- Failure to "cure" the earth of the *milpa* by ingratiating oneself to its owner or spirit. Much damage is caused by the present generation's loss of these ritual traditions.

- Failure to make offerings of an animal and its blood to the spirits of the place where a corral is built, in the ceremony known as *wahikol* or *lo'-corral*. If the proper sacrifice is not made, the spirits will exact a price, bringing death to the animals and sickness to the people.
- Breaking certain rules of the spirits of the forest or the hills *(kakab)* or of ancestral burial mounds, as well as passing a sacred spot or taking something from it without permission.
- Cairns, or mounds of stone, produce illness (most notably the *k'ojani kakab iik'*), because these cairns house the remains of the ancestors, as well as their utensils and medicinal herbs. These places are guarded by the *aluxob*. It is most common to be attacked by this illness when passing by such a place at noon, six o'clock in the evening, and five o'clock in the morning.

Evil Eye Produced by the Winds

Since the winds are possessed of life, they can provoke evil eye just as people can. Sometimes a wind will pass over a small child and will hug the child, unwilling to let it go unless the wind is paid and given food. There are certain hours when it is more common for these winds to pass and cause illness.

The most frequent types of evil eye caused by the wind are: *ojoy k'a'an* (eye of the clouded sky), *ojoy luum* (eye of the earthly wind), *ojoy yi ka ja'* (eye of the water), *ojoy kiin* (eye of the sun), *ojoy mama uuj* (eye of the moon), *ojoy alux* (eye of the *alux*), and *ojoy balam* (eye of the *balam*).

Evil Wind Resulting from the Work of a Curandero

When a *j'meen* performs a cure, the evil wind that is expelled from the patient can pass into some object and be the cause of illness in another. Sometimes the ritual is performed using a traditional sugar cane alcohol called *xjool ja'*, and what is left over is thrown out. On other occasions, the *curandero* uses an animal or object to perform the cure *(k'ej)*. Whatever is used—alcohol, plant, animal, or object—becomes the recipient of the evil wind. If the *curandero* leaves these objects at the site of the ritual, any passerby may be struck by the illness.

Evil Wind Caused by Animals

Various animals are considered to be carriers of the evil wind-for being related to the spirits of a place, for being emmisaries from the underworld, or for some dangerous or harmful characteristic they possess. Some of these animals are *xoch* (owls), *coos* (witch birds), *chak dzi dzib* (cardinals), and *chapat* and *chimes* (varieties of centipedes).

Causality and Illness

OTHER CAUSES

It is common for the *curanderos* to explain evil wind in terms of inheritence, allergies, contagion, bites, accidents, and other illnesses. *Chujuk wix* (diabetes) can be inherited. *Se'en* (dry cough) can be caused by an allergy to dust or can be passed from person to person in the air. An excess of children in the house makes it difficult to clean, causing a susceptibility to *wach kajan* (diarrhea) and *kiik naak* (dysentery), among other illnesses. *Chiba pool* (headache) can be caused by bathing when one has a cough or by letting a toothache go untreated. *Chu'u chum* (tumors in the skin) can be caused by insect bites, scratching, or being pinched when the body is ill. *K'il kab* (night sweat) in children is caused when the child sleeps with the mother who passes her bad mood and her sweat to the child, and when someone sweeps the floor beneath a hammock in which the child sleeps.

CAUSALITY IN CHINESE TRADITIONAL MEDICINE

Chinese traditional medicine devotes considerable attention to the development and evolution of illnesses. Illness is recognized as the result of the rupture of the body's physiological balance—the concept "cause of disease" refers to conditions that bring about this rupture. When an organism's functions or internal structures are damaged, disease sets in. Abnormal climatic conditions are reflected in the body, and internal and external changes disrupt normal somatic activity, causing the body's resistance to drop, making one more susceptible to illness.

For the Chinese the basis of the development of all things resides not in the exterior but in the interior. Internal causes are changes in the root, the base, the essence. External causes are related to changes in the environment, in the circumstances of a life, but they bring about internal effects.

Externally, many factors can affect the body and cause illness. All involve the interaction between the conditions that produce illness and the physical condition of the person involved (their strength or weakness to resist illness). These factors introduce a destructive pathology in the interior of the organism, interrupting the inner harmony. This manifests as an imbalance in the blood, the *chi,* the *yin/yang,* the viscera, and the organs.

Internal causes have to do with an obstruction of *chi* (the *chi* of the food or the *chi* of the breath), and with its internal pathways and natural balance—all of which are affected by exercise, thought, the seven emotions (see below), and excesses in work, rest, or sexual activity.

External causes refer to "the six atmospheric influences" and "the six pathogenic factors" such as external trauma, damage caused by insects or animals, parasites and pestilence.

Internal Causes
MALNUTRITION

For Chinese traditional medicine, nutrition is fundamental to health, and lack of proper nutrition is a common internal cause of disease. Digestion and assimilation of foods is the job of the stomach and spleen; thus any illness due to changes, deficiencies, or excesses in nutrition affects first these organs, producing excess phlegm, water retention, and changes in body heat ultimately affecting other organs in their cycle. After great illness the pathogens involved might not be eliminated until the stomach and spleen recover strength enough to restore the body to its healthy patterns of nutrition.

For Chinese medicine, nutritional imbalance as a cause of illness has three general causes:

- Eating without control.
- Dietary preferences.
- Ingestion of impure or rotten foods.

Eating Without Control
Insufficient food causes weakness in the sources of *chi* and blood, bringing about developmental problems in children and chronic weakness in adults.

Eating to excess causes faulty digestion and accumulation of internal gases, provoking nutritional irregularities in children. Overeating in adults affects the spleen and stomach, dampening the digestive fire and stagnating blood and *chi*.

Dietary Preferences
For lack of a particular element in the diet, a variety of deficiency-related diseases, such as hypothyroidism and night blindness can result. Consuming cold or raw foods in an inadequate or random manner can damage the *yang* energy of the spleen and stomach, manifesting as cold symptoms in this organ network. Excess of hot and spicy foods provokes heat in the stomach and damages the body's fluid production. Too much sugar or

Causality and Illness

grease damages the spleen and stomach by accumulating damp that manifests as phlegm and excess heat that manifests as fire and damages the organ network.

Each of the five flavors corresponds to one of the five organ networks: the sour flavor corresponds to the liver network, bitter to the heart, sweet to the spleen, spicy to the lung, and salty to the kidney. When one tends to overly indulge in one of the five flavors it causes the energy in the associated organs to increase.

Alcohol abuse causes damp heat and turbid phlegm, which in turn provokes a variety of illnesses.

Ingestion of Impure or Rotten Foods
Eating food that has passed its prime inhibits the function of the stomach and spleen. Excessive ferment (intoxication) damages the stomach and spleen; if it is extreme it can endanger one's life. Food infested with parasites causes a variety of types of parasitosis.

THE SEVEN EMOTIONS

Interacting with her environment the human being manifests diverse emotions. An intense or prolonged emotional change can exhaust a person's emotional reserves, provoking an internal illness. In Chinese medicine the Seven Emotions are: joy and contentment *(xi)*; anger, rage, indignation, and disgust *(nu)*; melancholy, sadness, worry, depression, anguish *(you)*; anxiety, pensiveness, and fixed thought patterns *(si);* heaviness, distress, contrariness *(pei);* terror and fright from a specific cause or event *(kong);* fear and general tension *(jing).*

Emotional changes are reflected in the internal organs. It is said in the *Neijing* that "the *chi* of the five organs forms the five spirits and gives rise to the emotions"[28] and that every emotional stimulus has a function within its related organ.

The blood and *chi* form the material base of the body's emotional and spiritual activities. The *chi* works to heat and promote the primary functions of organs and viscera, while the blood works to nutrify and bring fluid energy to the organ and viscera networks.

Each organ has its correspondent emotional activity: heart, joy; liver, anger; spleen, worry; lung, grief; kidney, fear. When pathologies occur in the organs, viscera, *chi* or blood, their functions may be stimulated or weakened. These changes are reflected in the person's emotional state, which wil be heightened or diminished accordingly. Thus, just as emotional imbalance affects the organs, disease in the organs causes emotional imbalance; spiritual manifestations, mental state, and emotional flux all are determinitive in the etiology of illness.

The Seven Emotions cause illness and internal damage in two ways:

- Direct damage to the five organs. Sharp or sustained emotional stress can influence the physiological function of the internal organs, producing pathological changes. Each emotion damages a different organ—anger inflames the liver, excessive joy can damage the heart, worry troubles the spleen, melancholy hurts the lungs, and fear dominates the kidneys.
- Different effects are manifested in the organs according to the direction in which the energy moves—that is, whether it is ascending or descending. Anger causes energy from the liver to rise (contrary to its natural inclination); joy causes a slowness in the energy; melancholy tends to diminish the energy; fright causes energy to descend; panic confuses the energy (it rises or descends without reason); worry tends to bring stagnation.

The heart houses the spirit, acting as emperor among the organs; emotional stimuli affect first the heart and then all the rest. The liver, in its

Organ	Emotion	Change	Symptoms	Correspondence
Liver	Anger	Rising	Dizziness, headache	With lung: pale face, depression, tightness in chest, difficult breathing
Heart	Joy	Slowing	Agitation, laughter and tears without control, palpitations	
Spleen	Worry, preoccupation	Stagnation	Bloated abdomen, lack of appetite	With heart: restlessness, memory loss. With lung: chest tightness, difficult breathing
Lung	Grief, sadness	Dispersion	Difficulty breathing, depression, fatigue	
Kidney	Fear, terror	Descending or disordered energy (rising or sinking without control)	Menstrual disorders, diarrhea, incontinence, bladder infection, fright, abnormal behavior	With heart: palpitations, speaking in tongues, restlessness

Causality and Illness

function of keeping the *chi* and blood flowing smoothly through the body, works to regulate the emotions.

The preceding table shows the relation of each organ to its emotional activity (be it normal or excessive), the changes produced by the movement of energy, some symptoms that serve as examples, and the emotional relation between the organs themselves.

SEXUAL ACTIVITY, WORK AND LEISURE

Excessive Sexual Activity

Excessive sexual activity signals a person's lack of control over his or her desires, and brings about a loss of energy that can lead to various pathologies. Overindulgence in sex, like excessive work, occupies an important place in Chinese theory. Many authorities in every age have remarked upon the effects of excessive sexual activity. The *Neijing Suwen* explains: "A drunk man arrives at his house and makes love with his wife, exhausting his essence with furious energy, and he loses his reserves of *chi* and doesn't satisfy himself, he has no time to maintain his spirit, only to satisfy his desire, and this produces undue happiness."[29]

The sexual function has a close relation with the life of the five organs, especially the kidneys. This relation extends to *chi,* essence and spirit. It is said that the kidneys govern the hidden essence, that which is guarded; they are the storehouse of essence and *chi.* Essence and *chi* must be guarded, or hidden, so as not to be spent wastefully. Prenatal *chi* and essence form the material base for the kidneys' vital activity. When a man and a woman unite their *chi* in sexual passion, one result is the process of reproduction. The strength or weakness of kidney *chi* and essence is directly related to the constitution of the entire body, its growth, development, aging, and death.

Excess in sexual activity produces internal damage and leads to disease. In surrendering to desire, one wastes essence, damages *chi,* and loses spirit. The most direct effect is the spending of the kidney's vital essence. The kidney's nature is *yi,* and abuse of the kidney causes a loss of *yin.* Due to the interdependence of *yin* and *yang,* an imbalance is created which manifests as an overabundance of *yang.* Overabundant *yang* tends to rise, resulting in the syndrome known as heat rising due to deficient kidney *yin.* After time, both *yin* and *yang* become exhausted and a condition of deficiency appears, manifesting as chronic weakness and progressive exhaustion. Problems such as impotence, spermatorrhea, premature ejaculation in men, and leucorrhea and menstrual irregularities in women often find their cause in excessive sexual activity. Other symptoms include weak knees and hips, dizziness, and tinitis (ringing in the ears).

Although the kidney is the primary organ affected, the heart-mind, as emperor among the organs, is also affected; the ancients taught a series of exercises related to the sexual life which served to conserve sexual energy and protect the heart-mind.

Excessive Work and Excessive Rest

Physical labor, a normal and vital part of human life, helps to circulate the blood and *chi* and strengthens the body. Resting from work is also essential to the recuperation of essence and *chi,* but an excess either of work or of rest can result in illness.

According to Chinese medicine, excess work causes a deficiency in the body's vital energy, resulting in tired limbs, shortness of breath, mental exhaustion, and low voice. Excessive worry, which often accompanies overworking, causes a steady loss of blood and nutrients—producing palpitations, memory loss, insomnia, and nightmares.

Excessive rest provokes a state in which the blood and *chi* fail to circulate properly, resulting in weak digestion and deficiencies of *chi* and blood. The body's general energy level drops, one eats poorly and lacks strength, the muscles become weak, and there may be palpitations, insomnia, and sensations of depression and confusion.

External Causes
THE SIX ATMOSPHERIC INFLUENCES

The natural life of the individual and the communtiy is tightly bound to climatic and seasonal changes. The *Neijing Suwen* says: "The most important element in clinical diagnosis is to know the relationships between heaven, earth, and humankind."[30] In another chapter we find that "The seasons change with the six atmospheric influences giving rise to the birth, growth, decline, and death of all things in nature. Dryness withers, summer heat increases the temperature, wind promotes movement, dampness moistens, cold freezes, and fire hardens the earth."[31]

Each of the four seasons has its characteristic climate: spring is temperate, summer hot, autumn cool, and winter cold. In the process of climatic change, *yin* and *yang* grow or fade day by day. This natural process

Causality and Illness

influences the life of all natural beings, and humans are no exception. The *Neijing Suwen* says: "*Yin* provides form. *Yang* enables growth. Warmth of the spring gives rise to birth, the fire of the summer fuels rapid growth and development, the coolness of autumn matures all and provides harvest, and the coldness of winter forces inctivity and storing. This is the rhythmic change of nature. If the four seaons become disrupted, the weather becomes unpredictable and the energies of the universe will lose their normalcy. This principle also apples to the body."[32]

The ancient Chinese sages observed the climatic changes and created a metaphor for the cycle of all things, synthesizing the characteristics of the six types of climate or energy: the movement or flow of air is called "wind," low temperature is referred to as "cold," high temperature is known as "heat" or "summer heat." When the degree of humidity in the air rises, this is known as "dampness," (with it's opposite being dryness); if heat or summer heat develop further, they become "fire." In antiquity, these six phenomena-wind, cold, summer heat, dampness, dryness and fire, whose changes occur cyclically under normal circumstances—are known as "the six climates" or "the six atmospheric influences." Under normal circumstances, the six atmospheric influences do not attack the body and cause illness.

When we speak of the six climates, we mean to indicate a phenomenon in which the climate changes occur brusquely or violently. When the body's resistance is down, one cannot respond to severe changes in the environment, and illness is the result. When the six climates constitute the causes of disease they are known as "the six pernicious influences" or "pernicious factor of the six abnormal climates." They are considered abnormal when climatic changes are severe, or when there is some interference in the normal process of seasonal change. This abnormality occurs in two ways:

- When climatic changes occur in a form that is different from the normal order. For example, a cold snap in the spring, or a hot and dry spell in autumn or winter. These abnormal changes make it difficult for the body to adapt.
- When the change of seasons happens very brusquely and the body has no time to adjust properly to the change. This causes the body's resistance to drop, often leading to illness.

Therefore, if one does not live in accordance with the seasons, illness results. If one doesn't recognize, in daily life, the need for exercise, proper nutrition, and other standards of personal care, the body's resistance is lowered, and though climatic changes might be normal, the body still fails to adapt. The body has a built-in capacity to deal with these changes. Since the difference between normal climate and perverse climate is often not extreme, the most important factor is the body's ability to react.

There are certain common characteristics to the six atmospheric influences and the ways they produce illness. Each atmospheric influence bears relation to an elemental pattern of disharmony; that is, each of the seasons relates to a predominant climatic element which produces illnesses particular to that season. Thus we see that, because wind dominates in the Chinese springtime, wind-related illnesses are most common in the spring. In summer ambient heat causes heat-related illness. In the humid dog-days of summer dampness predominates, while in the autumn, dryness is the common disease pattern, and in the winter patterns of cold are provoked by the external cold. Nevertheless, the climatic changes are rather complicated, and it is the relation of the seasonal elements to the body's specific constitution that causes illness.

Seasonal pathogenic factors can cause illness by themselves or in combination; for example diarrhea can be a cold-related illness, while flu might be provoked by a wind-cold pattern, etcetera. Under certain conditions one pattern transforms into another; for example an external cold pattern might turn into internal heat upon entering the body.

The six pathogenic factors enter the body from the outside, moving from the surface to the interior; they enter the body through the skin or by way of the mouth or nose; occasionally, however, the internal organs may be affected though no external symptoms appear.

The different climates tend to affect the specific organs to which they correspond: in spring the liver is most subject to disease, in summer the heart, in autumn the lungs, in the maximum *yin* of the year's end the spleen, and in winter the kidneys. From a clinical perspective, the pathogenic factors of the six atmospheric influences can be seen as related to the lives of bacteria, viruses and parasites which enter the body when external factors lower the body's resistance.

Besides these external pathogenic elements, there are elements of internal origin that take the form of cold, heat, wind, dampness, dryness, and fire, but differ from the external elements in that they do not produce external symptoms; they generally produce symptoms of deficiency, or of deficiency and excess combined; external climatic factors often present external symptoms with patterns of excess.

Causality and Illness

WIND: QUALITIES AND ETIOLOGIES

Quality	Form of Causing Illness	Clinical Manifestation
The wind is *yang*; it opens and disperses, tending to move upwards and outwards.	It affects the *yang* parts, attacking the upper body, the surface, and the lungs.	Headache, dizziness, facial paralysis, sweat and aversion to wind; nasal obstruction, itchy throat, cough.
Wind moves and changes rapidly, and undergoes variable transformations.	The site of illness is mobile, lacking a fixed center; symptoms appear and disappear; illness is sharp and leaves quickly.	Muscle and joint pain which readily changes place, measles, itching; symptoms come and go.
Wind's principal quality is movement.	Spinning sensations, abnormal body movement.	Dizziness, tics, muscle spasm, numbness, stiff neck.
It combines easily with other pathogenic factors.	It is the precursor and chief of many types of illness, mixing easily with all of them.	Wind-cold, wind-damp, wind-heat, wind-dryness, etcetera.
The wind is related with the liver.	It produces excess in the liver.	Affecting the spleen and the earth element, diarrhea and abdominal distension occur.

Wind

Wind is the principal energy of the springtime, though it may cause illness in the other seasons as well. Among the climatic pathogens it is considered the most prevalent, mixing readily with the others. There are diseases caused by internal wind and by external wind. The external wind affects primarily the surface of the body, while the internal wind affects the essential functioning of the blood, the liver, and the *yin-yang* balance throughout the body.

Wind is considered to be *yang*. Its main characteristic is that of circulating and draining. It commonly attacks the *yang* parts of the body due to its tendency to rise upward and outward; wind therefore often manifests as illnesses of the upper body (head, thorax), the surface (skin, pores, muscles, and tendons), and the lungs.

Cold

Cold is the principal energy of winter, affecting the body's heat; thus many of the illnesses of winter are of a cold nature. Cold patterns also develop when one gets wet in the rain, sweats in the wind, or encounters similar situations.

Cold illnesses are divided into two types: external and internal. The first attacks the body in two ways—at the surface, or directly at the organs and viscera.

Internal cold is a pathological reflection of insufficient *yang*. Although internal and external cold often exhibit different symptomatic patterns, they are mutually influential. When a *yang* deficiency provokes internal cold, the body is more susceptible to external cold factors. Similarly, if external cold persists for a long time, it can weaken the *yang* and develop into internal cold. The physical manifestations of cold are *yin* in nature, metaphorically reflecting the signs of cold—stagnating, contracting, hardening, sinking.

COLD: QUALITIES AND ETIOLOGIES

Quality	Form of Causing Illness	Clinical Manifestation
Cold is a *yin* pathology.	Affects the surface *yang*; if cold affects the interior directly, the *yang* of the spleen or spleen-kidney are weakened, affecting the circulation of fluids and the digestion, absorption and distribution of foods.	Surface cold: fever and aversion to cold. Internal cold: abdominal pain and diarrhea. If cold affects the kidney and spleen there can be fear, cold extremities, and lumbar pain.
Cold characteristics include freezing, obstructing, and stagnating energy.	*Chi* and blood stagnate, there is no communication between organs, and pain occurs.	Surface cold: headaches and body pain. Cold in the meridians: pain in the bones, joints and muscles. Internal cold: abdominal pain, and digestive weakness.
The quality of cold is to contract, to close, and to limit.	The body's energy contracts and is extinguished, pores and vessels constrict causing muscle and tendon spasms.	Lack of sweat, headache, tight pulse, numbness, and muscle tension.
Cold is related to the kidneys.	Damp cold affects kidney and spleen. If there is deficient *yang* in the kidney, internal cold results.	Damp cold affects the kidney, resulting in edema, scanty urine, and lumbar pain.

Causality and Illness

SUMMER HEAT: QUALITIES AND ETIOLOGIES

Quality	Form of Causing Illness	Clinical Manifestation
Summer heat is *yang*.	Provokes an excess of *yang*.	Fever, sweat, thirst, strong pulse (*gong da*).
Summer heat works to elevate and disperse.	Damages fluids and *chi*, pores dilate and there is excessive sweat; when the body loses fluids it becomes weak; summer heat rises to affect spirit and consciousness.	Thirst, dry tongue and lips; shallow breath, weakness, loss of consciousness, confusion, irritability.
Summer heat often combines with dampness.	Combined with dampness the affects of summer heat become more generalized.	Fever, restlessness, thirst accompanied by weakness in the limbs, thoracic pain, vomiting, strong-smelling stools.

DRYNESS: QUALITIES AND ETIOLOGIES

Quality	Form of Causing Illness	Clinical Manifestation
Dryness is rough, grating.	Causes a loss of *yin* fluids.	Symptoms of a loss of fluids are: dry mouth, nose, lips and tongue; scanty urine, flaky skin, dry stools.
Dryness damages lung and kidney.	The lungs lose fluids and are not nourished. Their function of dispersing and descending is interrupted, resulting in deficient kidney *yin*.	Dry cough with little phlegm, difficult expectoration, phlegm with blood; panting and chest pain.

DAMPNESS: QUALITIES AND ETIOLOGIES

Quality	Form of Causing Illness	Clinical Manifestation
Dampness is heavy and turbid, descending, affecting *yin* organs.	Causes pain, heaviness, exhaustion. Tends to affect the lower body.	Surface manifestations: heavy head and limbs, exhaustion. Dampness in the meridians and joints causes joint pain and heaviness.
Dampness is heavy, stagnating and extending.	Illnesses are chronic and difficult to cure, moving to different parts of the body.	Internal dampness: pus, dark urine, leucorrhea, edema.
Dampness is *yin*, easily damaging *yang* organs.	When dampness obstructs the meridians, energy becomes blocked. *Yang* of the spleen is damaged and the function of transport and assimilation is hindered.	Excema, typhoid, chronic illnesses.
Dampness is related to the spleen.	Damages spleen *yang*.	

PATHOGENIC FIRE: QUALITIES AND ETIOLOGIES

Quality	Form of Causing Illness	Clinical Manifestation
Fire is *yang*; it rises and inflames.	Excitation and changes in the upper body.	Symptoms include high fever, aversion to heat, irritability and thirst, rapid pulse, red face and ears, ulcers in the mouth, inflamed gums.
Fire burning up *yin* fluids results in dry heat.	Damages *yin* fluids causing internal dryness.	Scanty, thick urine and feces, dry throat, heat in the mouth.
Fire produces wind, moves the blood, causes skin infections.	Overheats the liver meridian, burns *yin* fluids and burns off nutrition, produces wind, damages the blood, produces carbuncles and tumors.	If liver wind combines with heat: tics, tremors, stiff neck appear. When heat damages normal movement of the blood: bloody vomit, stools and urine, heavy menstruation, carbuncles, inflammation.
Fire belongs to the heart.	Affects the spirit and causes the blood to circulate more rapidly.	Restlessness and confusion, incoherent speech, palpitations, increased heart rate, rapid pulse.

Causality and Illness

CHAPTER 4

DIAGNOSTICS

DIAGNOSTICS IN MAYAN MEDICINE

TRADITIONAL PRACTITIONERS of Mayan medicine employ a wide variety of diagnostic methods drawn, over the long history of the medicine, from different cultural sources. Generally, each *curandero* specializes in one or several methods in her or his practice. For practical purposes, we have divided Mayan diagnostic methods into two large groups:

- Diagnosis by way of the patient's signs and symptoms.
- Diagnosis by divination.

SYMPTOMATIC DIAGNOSTICS

Herbalists, masseuses, and midwives generally base their diagnoses on the symptoms present in the patient and on general observations that occur in the course of examination. The process of observation and examination is carried on informally and lacks a defined structure. In this process, a *curandero* will note a series of signs and symptoms, many of which appear very similar to the markers of illness in occidental medicine—while others differ completely. These differences can be seen more clearly in the exposition of traditional illnesses in the appendix. Especially important are the events that lead up to the illness: cravings or desires, exposure to a particular wind, eating cold foods, and fits of anger are all possible examples.

Signs of Air or Wind

When the patient describes symptoms compatible with the characteristics of "air," like pains in the head and limbs, the *j'meen* or masseuse will proceed to perform a series of "listening palpations," palpating for sounds that will give a clue to the source and type of illness. If a "tympanic" sound occurs, the diagnosis is air and the *curandero* proceeds to exercise *tok* to release the stagnant blood. For Mayan healers, air or wind stagnates and "darkens" the blood.

The diagnosis of air stagnating the blood is confirmed by drawing a few drops of blood, listening to the sound as it leaves the body, and looking for dark coloring and viscous texture. When all of the air is drawn out, the blood returns to its normal color and texture; when the patient is palpated again the tympanic sound is gone. We have been witness to this procedure, and are convinced that, after curing, the sounds, color and texture do indeed change.

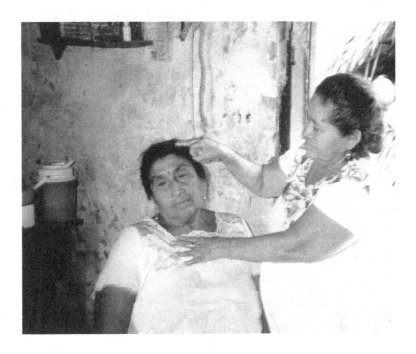

The Rhythm of the Tipté

Another process is used to establish changes in the *"cirro,"* or *tipté*. If, after a general examination and listening to the patient's body, the clinical manifestations of problems with the *tipté* become apparent, the *curandero* palpates the abdomen looking for a throbbing in the area of the abdominal aorta.

The doctor places one thumb above the umbilicus and with the other looks for a beating sensation by pressing lightly on the midline below the zyphoid process. He continues to palpate the two sides of the umbilicus, and above and below in the midline of the abdomen. The throbbing will normally be found just below the zyphoid process, independent of the patient's constitution. Any change—if the throbbing runs towards right or left, up or down—signifies that there is some anomaly. We are told that most commonly it will move up. In some cases, the rhythm—and therefore the *tipté*—may be properly located but be weak or "devoiced." When the sound is

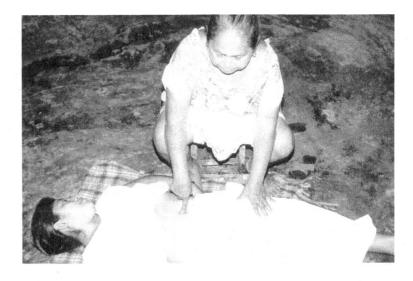

67

barely perceivable, it is said that the *cirro* is weak or tight; when it is said to be "devoiced," the *curandero* understands that the *cirro* is loose. With this understanding a diagnosis is established.

We have observed this process four times, palpating the aortic rhythm before and after the treatment. Each time the throbbing was encountered first to one side of the umbilicus and, after the treatment, in the midline directly above the navel.

Pulse Diagnosis

Pulse-takers will sometimes help the traditional doctor to reach a conclusive diagnosis. Most masseuses and *j'meenob* are familiar with at least

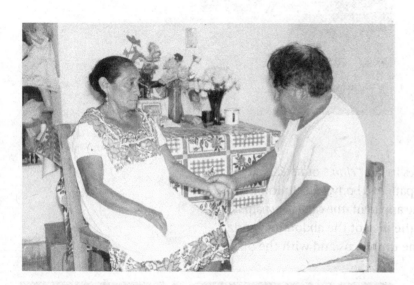

basic pulse diagnosis. It is common to be able to read a hot state, identified by a pronounced, rapid radial pulse "that feels as if it wants to leave the body." A *curandero* will generally confirm the diagnosis by reading the pulse in the temples.

Other *curanderos* recognize different diagnostic elements in the pulse. Some palpate the radial artery to detect a fever, and say that they feel "the silent beating of the heart" towards the middle of the wrist. One can determine the state of the lungs by reading the pulse "little by little," and a problem in the stomach when the pulse feels "as if it is returning into the body."

On other occasions it is difficult to distinguish between diagnostic observation and divination; the two seem to be often combined. Other *curanderos* have told us that the fingers feel "a voice that comes from the heart" to determine the ills of the patient. There comes a point where certain intuitive techniques cannot be distiguished as a single, specific tactile expression, and organic diagnosis becomes indistinguishable from divination. The *curanderos* we interviewed acknowledged that the art of reading pulses was, at one time, very advanced, but those who know it well are all very old or have passed on.

DIAGNOSIS BY DIVINATION

At times the *j'meen* makes a diagnosis using various divinatory techniques, often before the patient has explained his or her symptoms. Some *curanderos* refer to these processes—often related to supernatural illnesses—as "illumination." Techniques include reading shadows in a crystal sphere, reading kernels of corn, needles in water, eggs, animals' entrails, ashes, sparks of copal incense, and Spanish playing cards. Using these processes the *j'meenob* diagnose organic and spiritual diseases alike, identify the cause and gravity of the illness, and indicate other questions about the patient's life, love and fortune.

Diagnosis by Sastún

The *sastún*—a little glass ball—is one of the tools that distinguishes the *j'meen* from other traditional health workers. Some *sastúnes* or *sastúnob* appear to be spherical stone crystals or polished obsidian, while others might be simple glass balls or even the tops of perfume and medicine bottles.

To begin the diagnosis, the *sastún* is placed in a cup with three fingers of rum. Then it is held before the flame of a candle, preferably brought by the patient. The flame illuminates the *sastún,* which projects its shadow onto the clarity of the flame. The *curandero* holds the *sastún* in one hand before a candleflame, and makes an oration.

Observing the shadow in the *sastún,* the *j'meen* learns what sort of illness is at hand and what herbs to use. If a shadow in the form of a coffin appears it is said that the patient is going to die. A *curandero* will also consult the *sastún* to know if a patient is going to arrive at his house for treatment.

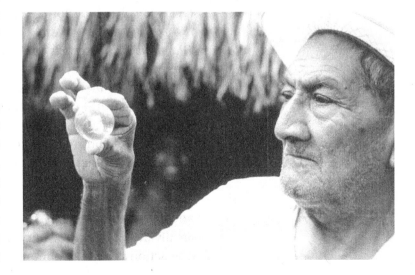

Diagnosis Using an Egg

This process is used specifically to confirm a diagnosis of evil wind. The *curandero* asks the subject to bring an egg to the session. The healer begins the ceremony, called *k'ej* or "change," by holding the egg and reciting the patient's name. The *j'meen* recites a series of psalms in which he names, in the Mayan language, each part of the body as he rubs it with the

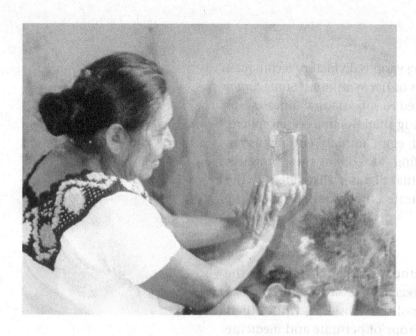

egg, making all his movements in the form of a cross.

After the "change," the egg is broken in a glass half-filled with water and the *j'meen* proceeds to read it. He can thus read the type of illness affecting the patient. Different forms commonly appear in the egg, including little black bodies and threads in the form of smoke, needles, a cross, a package, and other things, which the *curandero* interprets.

Some *j'meenob* prefer to break the egg into a clean jar, close it, and give it back to the patient. After nine days the patient returns to have the egg read. After the ritual it is important to burn or bury the egg and the jar.

Diagnosis by Reading the Entrails of an Animal

This technique is similar to that of the egg. If the patient is suspected to have a strong case of the evil wind, the *curandero* uses an animal (generally a chicken) to perform the *k'ej*. Some *curanderos* perform a formal ritual, at night, in which they sing eleven psalms while passing an animal and a plant—*tzipche,* or a rose—over the patient. At the end, after the animal dies "because it caught the evil wind," it is cut open to reveal the entrails. According to what is found there, the *curandero* makes his prognosis. Very few *j'meenob* still perform this ritual.

Diagnosis Using Kernels of Corn

There are various ways of diagnosing a patient using corn. In one of these methods the *curandero* strips forty grains off the corn—a symbol of life and rebirth—while invoking the gods and reciting the name of the patient. Various psalms are recited while the grains are shaken in the hand; the hand is moved brusquely to the left and a pile of corn is released. Another pile is made at the right, and this pile is read beginning with the number of kernels it contains. Other factors include the appearance of any horizontal or vertical lines in the pile, if the grains land in pairs or odd numbers, and if symbolic numbers, like three, seven, and nine appear. If the grains are divided into three distinct groups they are seen to represent the Trinity. The action is done two more times, and, taking into account the results of the three actions, the diagnosis is made.

Another technique is to throw a handful of grains into a drawing in the dirt of a circle divided into four parts by a cross, representing the earth and the four directions. Various psalms are uttered and the grains are read both according to their position with respect to the four directions, and the way they are grouped among themselves. This method of divination seems to be used only by the oldest of the *curanderos*.

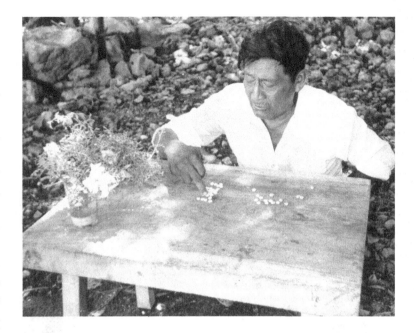

Another form, known as "oracle," consists of throwing nine grains of corn over a group of playing cards or a painting of animals. The results are read according to how the grains fall over the animals or the cards.

Diagnosis by Burning Copal

The gods are invoked by way of psalms, and the symbol of a cross is made over a censer filled with burning charcoal and bits of copal—a sweet-smelling, smoky resin. The copal is mixed with the charcoal to see how the sparks and smoke rise: if the smoke makes spirals, rises straight, or disperses horizontally. At the end the *curandero* looks at the pattern formed by the ashes; all of this is interpreted and becomes part of the diagnosis.

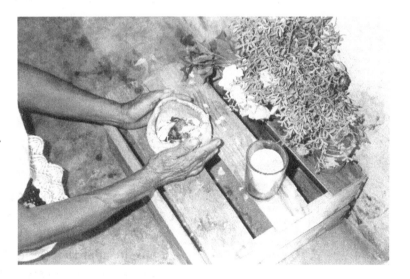

Diagnosis Using Needles in Water

After a series of orations invoking the gods to tell of the present, the future, and the past, a new embroidery needle is coated with fresh wax. The needle is called by the name of the patient. It is placed in a cup of water, where it generally will float, spinning horizontally. If the needle sinks it must be drawn out with a magnet without touching the water. If the needle sinks three times, the prognosis is very bad.

Diagnostics

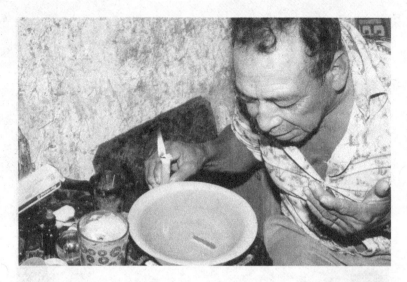

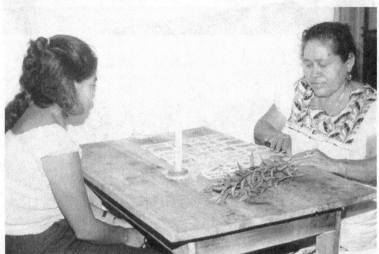

When one wants to know about the patient's relationships (generally with the opposite sex), another needle is placed in the water with the first. This needle is called by the name of the person in question. It is observed whether the needles repel or attract one another, if they cross or chase each other, and a diagnosis is made accordingly.

Diagnosis by Cards

Here we see one of the clearest cases of a ritual borrowed from another culture, in this case colonial Spanish culture. The *curandero* says the name of the patient while the patient cuts the deck. The *curandero* wishes the patient good luck and health; it is believed that the healer must think positively for this to succeed. The day and time of the patient's death can be read in the cards. Of all of the forms of divination described, this is the one most widely used in Campeche today.

DIAGNOSTICS IN CHINESE MEDICINE

As a holistic approach to healing, the Chinese system of diagnosis takes into account a wide range of information, from seasonal influences to the phase of the moon, from the time of day when the illness is worst to the patient's sleep and work patterns. The doctor looks for relations between the illness and the climate, the season, the social environment, and the patient's mental and spiritual condition. A Chinese traditional doctor will conduct an exploratory diagnostic session, but will not consider this diagnosis the final word on the patient's condition; rather, he will view the patient as a complex entity with a living history who is undergoing a specific imbalance related to her or his entire history.

In another way, as well, diagnostic etiology is not the final word for the Chinese doctor—different conditions may require attention at the same meridians and points, and, conversely, conditions which appear very similar may be treated by different methods and at different points. For example, a periarthritis of the shoulder and rheumatoid arthritis could require treatment at the same points, while two apparently identical cases of chronic bronchitis might need very different treatments.

The examination covers not only the current illness but the pathological tendencies of the patient—examining the patient's *yin* and *yang* characteristics, and regular patterns of excess and deficiency—using as signs all of the patient's physical characteristics as well as temperament, emotional state, and reactions to treatment. Other specifics of the diagnostic examination include attention to the sensitivity or pain in various meridians and points, abdominal palpation, and examination of the tongue and pulse. The objective is to establish a diagnosis of the general balance of energies in the body, first on a general level and then in each of the organs and meridians. It can even be said that the illness is not the primary indicator of an imbalance, and is not treated as the sole problem, because the illness will tend to change with the body's entire internal relations.

An example is to be found in an ancient text in a citation of a specific case: "The patient principally suffered from inadequate circulation of blood and *chi*. The relation between blood and *chi* was disordered, and neither could disperse properly; suddenly the problem came to the surface and the patient fainted. The ancestral or true *chi* could not contain the pathogen, thus the pathogen accumulated in the interior and could not be eliminated; in consequence the extraordinary vessel *yang quiao* became weakened and congested, resulting in a loss of consciousness."

TONGUE DIAGNOSIS

Examination of the tongue is one of the central methods of Chinese diagnosis. It is said that any change in the internal organs will be reflected in the tongue. Observing the tongue, the doctor will give attention to its color, form, and texture, and to the qualities of its coating, or fur. Changes in these qualities reflect the strength or weakness of the body's protective *chi,* whether the illness is internal or external, what its general characteristics are, and if the illness is tending to improve or worsen.

Diagnostics

A normal tongue will be pale red, moist, neither very thick nor very thin, appearing neither fragile nor old, and with adequate flexibility of movement. If the tongue is especially red and wet, the *chi* and blood are strong. A dry, pale tongue indicates weakness of *chi* and blood. The coating, or fur, which covers the tongue is produced by ascending stomach *chi*. When the tongue fur is slightly white and moist, it means that the stomach *chi* or digestive fire is strong; if the tongue is brightly colored with no coating, it signifies weak stomach *chi* or damaged stomach *yin*. A very dark red tongue indicates that a pattern of excess heat penetrates to the level of the blood, and thus the illness is situated very deep in the body. If the tongue fur is thin it generally means that the illness is acute and externally situated. When the coating is thick it means that the pernicious influence has penetrated to the interior. A yellow coating indicates heat, a white coating indicates cold, and a greasy coating indicates stagnant digestion. In an acute heat-related illness, the tongue fur can change from white to yellow or black. This is due to the pathogenic influence penetrating from the surface to the interior. Internal cold transforms into heat when external heat is very acute and damages the body's fluid balance. When the tongue fur changes from thick to thin, from dry to damp, the illness is disappearing, and the body is recovering its fluid balance.

The location of the tongue fur is also significant; if the fur is strongest near the tip of the tongue, an external illness is signaled. If the fur is thickest towards the root of the tongue, it suggests a tendency for the illness to direct itself inward; there may be stagnancy in the stomach or persistent phlegm. If the fur is strongest on the left side of the tongue, the organs are affected, and if it tends toward the right, the illness is at once internal and external. The two sides of the tongue indicate pathologies in the gall bladder and liver. If a thick coating is distributed over the entire tongue, there is persistent phlegm and accumulated dampness in the middle burner.

The doctor will also note the grade of dampness, stiffness, the shape of the tongue, the appearance of cracks, the size of the taste buds, impressions of the teeth in the sides of the tongue (scalloping), inflammation on the underside of the tongue, bleeding, abscesses or ulcers, if it appears excessively long or short, if it hangs to one side or exhibits signs of numbness, swelling, or paralysis.

In grave illnesses the tongue does not give adequate indications, but rather exhibits independent or contradictory signs; for this reason it is essential that the tongue examination be part, but not all, of the diagnosis.

PULSE DIAGNOSIS

The radial pulse also gives the traditional doctor important information about the patient's state of health. The pulse will indicate if an illness is internal (deep pulse) or external (shallow pulse); it helps to judge if the illness is deficiency-related (weak pulse) or excess-related (strong pulse); if there is heat (rapid pulse) or cold (slow pulse). The pulse can indicate the causal factors of an illness (for example, a rapid, slippery pulse speaks of an excess of hot phlegm as part of the base of illness), it can aid in observing the mechanics of an illness (for example, if on one side the pulse is stronger than the other—say the left side strong and the right side weak—then it could be the spleen affecting the liver); and can lead the doctor to a prognosis of the illness.

There are three places in the body to take a pulse: the head, which is the superior part corresponding to heaven; the wrists, in the center of the body corresponding to the human being; and the feet, the inferior part of the body which corresponds to the earth. In the head, the pulse can be taken in the temples or in the carotid artery in the neck; in the middle part of the body, the radial pulse is taken; and in the inferior region, the pulse is found in the dorsal part of the foot. Almost all of the locations for reading the pulse correspond to important points used in acupuncture treatment.

The most commonly used site of pulse-reading is the radial artery, the same used by occidental medicine, but three pulses are taken rather than just one. The doctor places three fingers—index, middle and ring finger—over the artery so that the middle finger is at the level of the radial protrusion. Each of the three sites on the artery has a different name—*cun, guan,* and *chi*—and each location manifests the state of a particular organ and viscera pair (different in the two wrists). The deep pulses—found when the doctor applies a bit of pressure in finding the pulse—indicate the functioning state of the six *yin* organs; the surface pulses—found when very little pressure is applied—indicate the condition of the six *yang* viscera, thus corresponding to the twelve organs and viscera.

Hand	*Cun*	*Guan*	*Chi*
Left	Heart/Small Intestine	Liver/Gall bladder	Kidney/Bladder
Right	Lung/Large Intestine	Spleen/Stomach	Pericardium/Triple Heater

The best time for reading the pulses is in the morning between five and seven o'clock, because the *yang* energy has just begun to circulate, there hasn't been excess movement, and the patient will not have eaten and will be very calm. If we want to gauge the state of the *yin*, the best time is between seven and nine o'clock in the evening. In either case, the patient should be relaxed, and should be situated so that her heart and the doctor's heart come to the same height.

A normal pulse will have sufficient force and be rhythmic without being tense. This normal pulse can exhibit changes due to various factors, like the climate and change of seasons. In spring the energy tends to be external, and the superficial pulses will be stronger. In winter, the energy retreats to the inside, and the deep pulses will be stronger.

Geography, as well, can affect the pulse. It is said that in the south people have a stronger superficial pulse, and in the north the deep pulse is stronger. Other variations are caused by differences in age, sex, stature, type and grade of activity, and physical states like pregnancy or menstruation.

Chinese medical history has various treatises about the pulses. The *Shang Han Lun* (Han Zhang Zhonjing, c. 220) speaks of 26 different types of pulses, while the *Mai Jing* (Jin Wang Shuhe, c. 300) speaks of 24. The *Bian Zhen Lun* speaks of 38 different pulses.

There are a series of basic pulses which can be characterized according to their nature as *yin* or *yang*, as follows:

Yin	Deep	Slow	Deficient	Short	Very weak	Smooth	Weak
Yang	Shallow	Rapid	Solid	Long	Full	Tense	Strong

CHAPTER 5

THERAPEUTICS

MAYAN THERAPIES

CONTEMPORARY MAYAN medicine demonstrates a host of diverse medical therapies. These depend on the character and specialization of the *curandero* (whether he or she is an herbalist, a bone setter, a *j'meen,* etcetera), the type of illness (organic or spiritual), and whether the *curandero* chooses to maintain a "pure" treatment or to mix the treatment with other types of therapy (pharmaceutical medicines or practices from other specialists or other cultures). In dealing with a specific illness it is rare that only one sort of treatment will be applied; rather, it is common to apply multiple therapies. The doctor might apply *tok,* sing various incantations, and prescribe herbs all in the same session.

For practical purposes, we have separated the therapeutic elements into the following practices:

- Herbology
- Application of massages known as *"talladas"* (rubbings) or *jet*
- Two variants of puncturing the body in specific points: *jup* and *tok*
- Application of cupping glasses (together with *jup* and *tok*)
- Application of poultices and plasters
- Incantations and cleansings *(limpias)*, in their diverse forms: *lu'usa' k'ee-baan* and *k'ej*

To facilitate an understanding and analysis of the various practices, we will compare each, in turn, with traditional Chinese practices.

CHINESE THERAPIES

Chinese medicine consists of a field of knowledge and practice collected and unified over thousands of years of study and experimentation by ancient and modern masters. As an art, it expresses itself as a collection of practices which share a common philosophy, but which are specialized in and of themselves. On some occasions the various therapies may be practiced separately, but it is much more common that the different treatments are practiced together to resolve a single case; they may even be practiced in conjunction with occidental treatments, as is the case with Mayan medicine.

In the West it is common to hear the word "acupuncture" erroneously used as a synonym for Chinese medicine in general. This reduces Chinese medicine to a single therapeutic modality, and leaves aside several other important therapies, which, though they have the same philosophical and systematic base as acupuncture, are quite different and are often practiced independently. Our usage of the word acupuncture, in both the Chinese and Mayan contexts, refers to its literal unravelling: "to pierce with an acute object."

Briefly, the chief therapies used in Chinese medicine are:

- Herbology
- Massage
- Acupuncture in its varying forms
- Application of cups (usually together with massage or acupuncture)
- Moxibustion and the use of plasters and poultices
- *Chi kung*

MAYAN HERBOLOGY

A vast number of medicinal plants are used by the Mayan *curanderos* of the Yucatán peninsula. We have counted as many as two hundred and fifty distinct species that are used medicinally to the present day. The actual number may be far greater. The plants used by the Maya are generally classified into two groups: *tzig u kuch* (cold plants) and *kinal kuch* or *choko kuch* (hot plants).

Plants classified as cold are, generally speaking, aqueous varieties; they grow in or near water, and are also referred to as being "cool" or "fresh." Their affect on the body is to inhibit illness by increasing the cold element in the body's harmonic balance. In Western terms they might be considered antipyretic (fever-reducing), antitussive (cough-relieving), and anti-inflammatory (reducing inflammations). Many of these plants have a sour flavor.

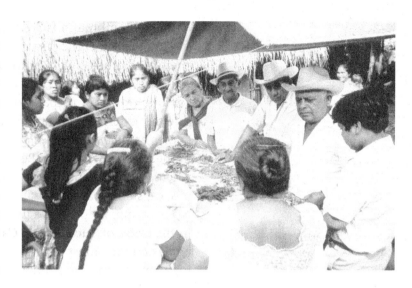

Plants considered *choko kuch,* or hot, are frequently dry, heavy, or have general heating and drying effect on the body. In general they stimulate organ function. As heating agents and stimulants, they can be used for "cold" in the womb, tightness in the *cirro,* general physical weakness, indigestion, and to fortify the various organs against infection.

On some occasions herbs are used not to counteract a cold or heat imbalance, but to stimulate it. For example infectious illnesses which cause a sudden rise in body temperature may be treated with a hot plant, like *ku'utz,* the leaf of wild tobacco *(Nicotiana tabacum,* L.) and *xmakulan,* to bring the fever still higher and cause it to break.

Along with the plants prescribed, the doctor may prescribe a diet which will work in conjunction with the herbs to bring about a synergy and to prevent an imbalance in the body. If the *curandero* prescribes hot plants, it will be important not to eat cold foods, and vice versa. Generally, to avoid stagnation and blockage of the stomach and intestines and to allow free passage of the medicinal substance to the blood, a medicinal diet will exclude fats and oils.

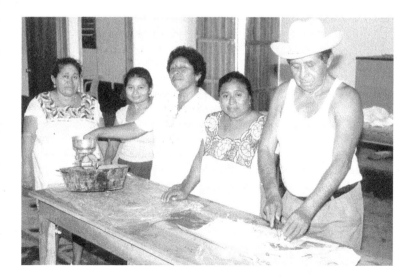

Plants classified among "plants for wind," like *tzipche' (Bunchosia swartziana,* Griseb), *chalché (Pluchea odorata,* L.) and *sinanche' (Zanthoxylum cuneata,* L.) are used against illnesses diagnosed as wind-related, although the clinical manifestation may be headache, stomach ache, or pain in the joints. With these plants, the Mayan masseuses make a pomade "against wind" that they apply to the head, the joints, or the belly. The same plants are used in ritual cleansings.

Herbal combinations are common, based on the doctor's experience and knowledge of the plants. It is understood that there are plants which "help each other," augmenting the affects of other plants in a synergistic way, and that there are other plants which are incompatible. The most common forms of preparation are infusions, alcohol-based salves, tinctures for external application, honey-based syrups—from the honey-bee known as *xunan kaab (melliponna beecheii)*—and balms traditionally based in the fat of cows or deer. Recently many of the *curanderos* in the villages where we worked have been trained in the making of extracts, tinctures, oils, capsules, soaps, and salves with a Vaseline base.

Following, we present a list of the medicinal plants used by *curanderos* in the states of Yucatán and Campeche, accompanied by their scientific name and their most common uses (for more detailed information regarding preparation, dose, and combinations, consult the appendix).

Mayan or Spanish Name	English Common Name	Scientific Name	Uses
Ajo	Garlic	*Allium sativum*	Rheumatism, bronchitis, asthma, burns
Ajonjoli	Sesame	*Sesamum orientale*	Absence of mother's milk
Altaniza		*Ambrosia artemisiaefolia*, L.	Irregular menstruation, skin abscess, vericose veins
Anís	Anis	*Pimpinella anisum*, L.	Diarrhea, *xaka ta'a*, dysentery, diabetes, *mesankil*, evil eye
Arnica		*Thitonia diversifolia*	Fever, bruises
Bakalché		*Bourreria pulchra*	Bronchitis, asthma
Beek'		*Eheretia tinifolia*, L.	Flu, cough, fever
Belsinik'che'		*Alvaradoa amorphoides*	Scabies

Mayan or Spanish Name	English Common Name	Scientific Name	Uses
Belladonna xiu		*Bryophyllum pinnatum*	Hemorrhoids, rheumatism
Boktún		*Anthurium*, spp.	Skin abscesses
Boldo	Boldo	*Peumus boldus*	Gall bladder diseases
Box ak' or *kantuul*		*Nissolia fruticosa*	Burns, pellagra
Boxchechem or *chechem*		*Metopium brownei*, Jacq.	Scarification
Bugambilia	Bougainvillea	*Bougainvillea spectabilis*	Cough, asthma, bronchitis
Cabello de elote	Cornsilk	*Zea mays*	Bladder infection, painful urination
Caimito	Star-apple	*Chrysophyllum cainito*, L.	Dysentery
Cilantro	Cilantro	*Coriandrum sativum*, L.	Gastritis
Coco	Coconut	*Cocos nucifera*, L.	Bladder infection, worms
Cola de Caballo	Horsetail	*Equisetum fluviatilis*, L.	Bladder infection
Cha'ak			Diarrhea
Chakchom, chan ch'om, or *piñuela*		*Bromelia karatas*, L.	Worms
Chak moltmuul		*Gomphrena dispersa*	Dysentery
Chak muk		*Rauvolfia hirsuta*	Menstrual irregularities
Chaktzitz or *uña de caballo*	Scarlet Sage	*Salvia coccinea*, L.	Nerves
Chakuoob or *pitaya*		*Cereus undatus*	Bladder infection

Therapeutics

81

Mayan or Spanish Name	English Common Name	Scientific Name	Uses
Chalché or *Santa Maria*		*Pluchea odorata,* L.	Irregular menstruation, vaginal discharge, infertility, bronchitis, asthma, evil eye, fear, evil wind
Chaya de monte		*Cidosculus aconitifolius*	Bladder infection
Chelen		*Agave silvestrus*	Menstrual irregularities
Chi abal, abal, or *ciruela*	Plum	*Spondias purpurea*	Bladder infection, gastritis, diarrhea
Chichibé		*Sida acuta*	Dysentery, vaginal discharge, nerves, evil eye
Chi, k'anibinche, or *nance*	Barbados cherry	*Malpighia glabra,* L.	Dysentery, evil eye, diarrhea
Chibo che			
Chi ke' or *árbol boca de venado*		*Chrysophyllum mexicanum*	Diarrhea, *xaka ta'a,* skin infections, pellagra
Chiople'		*Eupatorium hemipteropodum*	Irregular menstruation, vaginal discharge, asthma, rheumatism, nerves, evil wind
Chocuil xiu, pasmoxiu, or *claudiosa*		*Capraria biflora,* L.	Diarrhea, flu, cough, menstrual irregularities, vaginal discharge, rheumatism, dermatitis

Wind in the Blood

Mayan or Spanish Name	English Common Name	Scientific Name	Uses
Chokob kat		*Ipomea carnea*, J.	Rheumatism
Chooch		*Lucuma hipogluaca*	*Rheuma blanca* or white rheumatism
Chukum, chimay		*Pitecollobium albicans*	Diarrhea
Chulul		*Apoplanesia paniculata*	Dysentery
Chumo or *kanchunup*		*Clusia flava*	Cough
Ek', tinto ek', or *palo tinto*		*Haesatoxylon campechianus*, L.	Diarrhea, dysentery
Ek'k'ixil		*Bignonia unguis, Cati*, L.	Hemorrhage
Elel		*Oxalis latifolia*	Menstrual irregularities
Elemuy, sakelemuy or *yumel*		*Malmea depressa*	Bladder infection, high cholesterol
Frijolillo		*Lepidium intermedium*	Flu
Gobernadura		*Larrea divaratica*	Scabies
Guaco ek or *guaco kaax*		*Aristolochia pentandra*	Diarrhea, *xaca ta'a*, colic, diabetes, *mesankil*, fever, rheumatism
Guanábana	Guanabana, soursop	*Annona muricata*, L.	Diabetes
Ich juj, ojo de iguana		*Eugenia axillaris*	Diarrhea
Jabín	Jamaican Dogwood	*Piscidia piscipula*, L.	Dysentery, flu, cough, asthma, navel Hemhorrage in newborns

Therapeutics

83

Mayan or Spanish Name	English Common Name	Scientific Name	Uses
Jak'oolxiu or *dormilona*	Sensitive plant	*Mimosa pudica*, L.	Fear
Jalapa	Morning glory	*Convulvulus jalapa* or *Ipomoea purga*	Bladder problems
Jak'ool xiu or *jobonté*		*Euphorbia heterophylla*, L.	Skin abscesses
Jolol, cañotio or *roble yucateco*		*Bellotia campbelli*	Bladder infection, fever
Jumpetskín		*Tillandsia*, spp.	Skin abscesses, cough
Kabalyaxnik		*Ruellia nudiflora*	Evil eye
K'ak'ilxiu or *yerbabuena*	Peppermint	*Mentha piperita*, L.	Diarrhea, nausea, dermatitis in nursing mothers
K'alxixlooch, k'oochlé or *palo guarumbo*	Trumpet Tree	*Cecropia obtusifolia*, L. or *Cecropia peltata*	Diabetes, rheumatism, bladder infection, cough
Kanak		*Alchornea latifolia*	Nerves
Kanán		*Hamelia patens*	Scarring wounds
Kanantzín		*Lonchocarpus rugosus*	Premenstrual syndrome
Kanlol or *tronadora*		*Tecoma stans*, L.	Diabetes
Kantemok			Evil wind
Kep a'i or *pene de lagarto*			Menstrual irregularities
Ki or *henequen*	Henequen	*Agave* spp.	Burns
Kibix		*Dalbergia glabra*	Evil eye
Kokché	Croton	*Croton glabellus*, L.	Bronchitis, asthma

Mayan or Spanish Name	English Common Name	Scientific Name	Uses
K'ok'obche'	Jaborandi	*Pilocarpus racemosus*, Vahl.	Diarrhea, rheumatism
Kolokmaax		*Craxaeva tapia*, L.	Dysentery
Kopté or *ciricote*		*Cordia dodecandra*	Flu, cough, asthma
Kuché or *cedro*	Cedar	*Cedrella mexicana,* or *Cedrella odorata*	*Tu kee,* flu, cough, asthma, bladder infection, worms
Ku'che'		*Pseudobombax ellipticum*	*Xaka ta'a,* cough
Kukut or *cebolla*	Onion	*Allium ceppa*, L.	Vaginal discharge
K'uum or *calabaza*	Winter squash	*Cucurbita moschata*	Diabetes, burns, worms, nausea
K'uliche		*Astronium graveolens*	Scabies
Ku'utz, tobaco xiu or *tobaco cimarrón*	Tobacco	*Nicotiana tabacum,* L.	Rheumatism, fever, cough
Kuxub or *achiote*	Anatto	*Bixa orellan,* L.	Fever
Kuyche or *amapola blanca*		*Cedrella odorata,* L.	Cough, asthma
Laal or *hortiga*		*Tragia nepetaefolia*	Skin abscesses
Lima	Lemon	*Citrus limetta*	Diabetes
Limón	Lime	*Citrus aurantifolia*	Diarrhea, *xaka ta'a,* colic, *tu kee,* diabetes, flu, menstrual irregularities
Lo'l katzin			Evil wind
Lukum xiu or *apazote*	Epazote; wormseed	*Chenopodium ambrosioides,* L.	Diarrhea, *xaka ta'a,* dysentery, *tu kee,* worms, nerves
Luuch or *jícara*		*Crescentia cujete*	Fever, flu, evil eye, evil wind

Mayan or Spanish Name	English Common Name	Scientific Name	Uses
Llantén	Plantain	Plantago major, L.	Diarrhea, dysentery
Mak che		Ximenia americana, L.	Rheumatism
Makulis			Evil wind
Mejen x'tohkú	Datura, Jimson Weed	Datura stramonium, L.	Rheumatism
Mentha	Peppermint	Mentha piperita, L.	Colic, nerves
Misib kob		Turnera diffusa	Flu
Much kok, doradilla or flor de piedra		Orobanche, spp.	Bladder infection, flu, bronchitis, asthma
Mul och		Triumphetta semitriloba	Diarrhea
Mutz or dormilona			Nerves
Nabá or bálsamo xiu		Mycroxylon balsamum	Nausea
Nabanche', ojoi che', or zazafras		Bursera graveolens	Rheumatism, nerves, evil eye
Naranja agria	Sour orange	Citrus aurantium, L.	Xaka ta'a, colic, diabetes, mesankil, evil eye
Nemax		Heliotropum parviflorum, L.	Dysentery
Ojoi ak'			Evil eye
Ojoi kim			Evil eye
Ojoi xiu			Evil eye
On or aguacate	Avocado	Persea americana	Diabetes, flu, cough, rheumatism

Mayan or Spanish Name	English Common Name	Scientific Name	Uses
Oop or *anona*	Cherimoya, custard apple	*Annona cherimola*	Rheumatism, burns, dysentery
Orégano	Oregano	*Lippia berlandieri*	Menstrual irregularities
Orégano de monte, oregano grueso or *o'xiu*		*Lippia graveolens*	Diarrhea, flu, cough, asthma
Oruxús	Licorice	*Glycyrriza glabra,* L.	Flu, asthma
Ox or *ramón*		*Brisimum alicastrum* or *Trophis racemosa*	Diarrhea, flu, cough, asthma
Oxolak			Evil eye
Pa'aken or *nopal de monte*	Prickly Pear	*Opuntia cochenillifera,* L.	Diabetes
Pajalkam or *yerba mora*	Black Nightshade	*Solanum niggrum,* L.	Hemorrhoids
Pakal, china' or *naranja*		*Citrus sinensis*	Diarrhea, *tu kee,* flu, diabetes, *mesankil,* nerves, fear, dermatitis in lactating women
Payche'		*Petiveria alliacea*	Diarrhea, *tu kee,* flu, evil eye, *mesankil,* nerves
Preskúts			Flu
Peteltun, x'peteltunak' or *tz'utz'uk*		*Cissampelos pareira,* L.	Diarrhea, dysentery, *K'il kab,* evil eye
Pichí, guyaba	Guava	*Psidium guajava,* L.	Diarrhea, skin infections
Pitaya		*Cereus donkalarii*	Diabetes
Pixoy		*Guazuma ulmifolia,* L.	Dysentery

Therapeutics

8 7

Mayan or Spanish Name	English Common Name	Scientific Name	Uses
Pochot			Skin abscesses
Poleo	Pennyroyal	*Mentha pulegium*, L.	Diarrhea, nausea, cough
Pomolché		*Jathropa gaumeri*	Dysentery
Po pox		*Urera baccifera*, L.	Diarrhea, *xaka ta'a*, mesankil
Putxiu, putkan, lentejilla or *mastuerzo*		*Lepidium virginicum*, L.	Diarrhea, cough, bronchitis, asthma
Romero	Rosemary	*Rosmarinus officinalis*, L.	Diarrhea, diabetes, *mesankil*
Ruda	Rue	*Ruta graveolen*, L. and *Ruta chalepensis*	Nausea, fever, nerves, evil eye, fear, evil wind
Sábila	Aloe vera	*Aloe vulgaris*, L.	Diabetes, burns
Sak ak'			Flu
Sakatzín		*Mimosa hemiendyta*	Bronchitis, asthma
Sakbalbelkan or *pitaya*		*Hibantis yucatanensis*	Fever
Sak mul or *amor seco*		*Althernathera ramosissima*	Flu, cough, fever
Saksit		*Lasciasis divaricata*, L.	Skin abscesses, pellagra
Sak xiu		*Abutilan lignosum*	Diabetes
Sauco	Elder	*Sambucus mexicanus*	Rheumatism
Siit		*Lasciasis divaricata*, L.	Fever
Sinanche'		*Zanthoxylum cuneata*, L.	Diarrhea, dysentery, rheumatism

Mayan or Spanish Name	English Common Name	Scientific Name	Uses
Sinan ik			*K'il kab*
Tzipche'		*Bunchosia swartziana*	Rheumatism, nerves, evil eye, evil wind and wind-related illnesses
Sisal xiu		*Pilea microphylla*	Bronchitis, asthma
Son or guayacan		*Guaiacum sanctum*, L.	Diabetes, cough
Subín		*Acacia collinsii*	Bronchitis, asthma
Taa chak			Evil eye
Tankos che' or *tankasché*		*Zanthoxylum fagara*, L.	Diarrhea, nerves, diabetes, rheumatism
Ta'may		*Zeulania quidonia*	Menstrual irregularities
Té de China		*Micromeria browmei*	Diarrhea, cough
Té de limón	Lemon grass	*Cymbopogon nardus* or *Cymbopogon citratus*	Diarrhea, nausea, *xaka ta'a*
Tipt'e ak or *tipté ché*		*Jacquinia auriantiaca*	Cirro
Tomate verde	Tomatillo	*Physalis ixccarpa*	Diabetes
Toronjil		*Cedronella mexicana*	Diarrhea, nausea
Tu bux, engible, gengibre	Ginger	*Zingiber officinalis*	*Xaka ta'a*, colic
Tulub-balam		*Hippocratea celastroides*	Nerves

Mayan or Spanish Name	English Common Name	Scientific Name	Uses
Tusik xiu			Bronchitis, asthma
Tuxtache'			*K'il kab*
Tzinché or *tsuiché*		*Pithecollobiu-munguis cati*, L.	Dysentery
Tzitzil xiu		*Erigeron pusillus*	Fever
Tzitzín or *sisín*	Mugwort	*Artemisia vulgaris*, L.	Diarrhea, dysentery, *xaka ta'a*, worms, evil wind
Tzudspakal or *naranja*	Orange	*Citrus aurantium*, L.	Flu, nausea
Tzuluktok or *saktzulubtok*		*Baughinia divaricata*, L.	Bladder infection, flu, cough, asthma, fever
Tzunyá		*Pereskia*, spp.	Skin abscesses
Tzutup		*Calonyetion aculeatum*, L.	Bronchitis, asthma
Tzutzuk'			Evil eye
Utzupek'		*Tabernaemontana amygdalifolia*	Skin infections
Vasak xiu, chocuil xiu, xiusak or *malva*	Mallow	*Boerhavia erecta*, L.	Bronchitis, asthma
Vicaria	Periwinkle	*Vinca rosea* or *Catharanthus roseus*	Diabetes, vaginal discharge, dermatitis in lactating women
Xaché xtabay or *netolok'*		*Pitecoctenium echinatum*	Skin abscesses, pellagra
Xajauché or *xa'auche'*		*Tabebuia chrysantha*	Scabies
Xanabmukuy		*Euphorbia hirta*, L.	Skin infections

Mayan or Spanish Name	English Common Name	Scientific Name	Uses
Xbakenuo		*Peperomia pellucida*, L.	Fever
Xbeskan			*Kinan pool*
X'bobtun		*Anthurium*, spp.	Bladder infection
X'bolenti			Evil eye
Xbolontibil		*Cissus trifoliata*	*Kinan pool*
X'chay or *chaya*		*Cnidoscolus chayamansa*	Diabetes, bladder infection
X'chinto		*Krugiodendrum ferreum*	Bladder infection
X'etel			Absence of mother's milk
Xhalalnal		*Calosia virgata*	Diarrhea
Xik'inchaac		*Nymphaea ampla*	Bladder infection
Xik'inpek or *xikin*		*Calea zacatecich*	Diarrhea, skin infection
X'kabachi or *x kabá chichibé*		*Buchnera pusilla*	*Xaka ta'a*, diabetes
X-kakaltún or *kakaltún*, or *albahaca de monte*	Basil	*Ocimum micránthum*, L.	Diarrhea, dysentery, *k'il kab*, flu, skin infections, nerves, evil eye, evil wind
X-kambaljan, kambaljau, Xk'ambalkán or *contrayerba*		*Dorstenia contrayerva*, L.	Diarrhea, premenstrual cramps, skin abscesses, fever
Xkan lol		*Tecoma molis*	Flu
X'kat		*Parmentiera edulis*	Bladder infection
X-k'o'och, kooch or *higuerilla*	Castor	*Ricinus communis*, L.	*Tu kee*, fever

Mayan or Spanish Name	English Common Name	Scientific Name	Uses
X'koché, tayché or bokanché		Capparis indica	Bronchitis, asthma, fever
Xkukemba'		Phoradendron spp.	Skin abscesses
X'kulimsiis		Trichilia hirta, L.	Pellagra
X'mak'ulan or mak'ulan		Pipper auritum	Bronchitis, asthma, rheumatism, fever
Xmulix or mulix kaan		Tillandsia kaput-medusae	Postpartum headache, mesankil
X'nemis or Cola de Tejon		Cercus gaumeri	Rheumatism
Xoltexnuk		Lippia umbellata or Hyptis pectinata	Diarrhea, rheumatism
Xolte x'nuk		Lippia yucatanna	Bronchitis, asthma
X'paxak'il		Simarouba glauca	Dysentery
X'pechwukil or X'pechukil		Porophyllum punctatum	Diabetes, bladder infection
X'pichche' pach, pach chi, pach abal or pach pichi'		Psidium yucatanense	Diarrhea, diabetes, evil wind
X'pixton		Phyllantus glaucescens	Bladder infection
X'pujuk, maseual pujuk, or x'p'ot	French marigold	Tagetes patula, L.	Skin lesions or abscesses
Xpuk'im, xpukin or tzulubmay		Colubrina greggii or Calicarpa aciminata	Diarrhea, dysentery, diabetes
Xput balam		Solanum hispidum	Anginas, dermatitis
Xsakchaká or Chalchaká	Chibou	Bursera simaruba, L.	Diabetes, fever

Mayan or Spanish Name	English Common Name	Scientific Name	Uses
X'tabentun		Pittiera grandiflora or Turbina corymbosa, L.	Diabetes, bladder infection
X'tanlum		Ageratum gaumeri	Evil eye
Xtok'abal		Eupatorium odoratum, L.	Diarrhea
X'tokaban or xikinburro		Calea urticifolia	Diarrhea, diabetes, asthma, bladder infection
X'tujuyche'		Plumeria pudica	Flu
X'tujuy xiu		Lippia dulcis	Bronchitis, asthma
X'tukanil, pochpochk'ak or tuubto	Passionflower	Passiflora foethida, L.	Skin abscesses
X-tun che'		Chiococca alba, L.	Diarrhea, dysentery
Xukul		Portulaca oleracea, L.	Intestinal worms
Ya or Zapote	Sapodilla	Manilkara zapota, L.	Diarrhea, xaka ta'a, dysentery, bladder infection, high cholesterol, hypertension
Yaax che or ceibo	Ceiba	Ceiba pentandra, L.	Evil eye, evil wind
Yaxjalalché		Pedillantus itzaeus	Nervous tension, evil eye
Yaax k'iix		Buetnaria aculeata	Skin infection
Yaax-kiix-kanal or toxob		Caesalpinia vesicaria, L.	Evil eye

Mayan or Spanish Name	English Common Name	Scientific Name	Uses
Yak'unaax, yak'unak' or *cundeamor*		*Momordica charantia*, L.	Worms, vaginal discharge hemorrhoids
Yebek			Menstrual irregularities
Zacate pata de gallo or *grama*	Bermuda grass	*Cynodon dactylon*	Bladder infection

Besides the medicinal herbs, Mayan medicine uses a variety of products of animal or mineral origin. It is curious to note that these remedies lack common names, as exist in the herbology, to designate their medicinal uses. Although they do not belong, strictly speaking, to the botanical pharmacopoeia, we present here a list of animal or mineral products used in Mayan traditional medicine.

Ch'oon	Buzzard feathers		Fear
Kankab	Red clay		Insect bites, hot conditions of the skin
K'ok ak'	Turtle's blood		Asthma, bronchitis
Koos	Witch bird feathers		Fear
Kuite or *Tecolote* feathers			Fear
Pizot or *tejon*	Cuatemundi		Impotence
Tza kan or *víbora de cascabel*	Rattlesnake		Air, anemia, cancer, rheumatism
Tzu' or *liebre*	Rabbit (fur)		*Ak'an* or stutter
Tz'ulum or *colibri*	Hummingbird		Fits, seizures
Wakax or *rés (testiculos)*	Bull's testicles		Menstrual irregularities
Xich or *lechuza (plumas)*	Screech owl feathers		Fear
X-tzulu' or *legartija*	A type of lizard		*Mal de pinto*
Xunan kaab or *abeja melipona (miel)*	Honey bee (honey)	*Mellipona beecheii*	Flu, cough, menstrual irregularities
Yikel subin, hormigas de subin	Ants collected from the Ant Acacia	*Acacia collinsii*	Flu, impotence, weakness

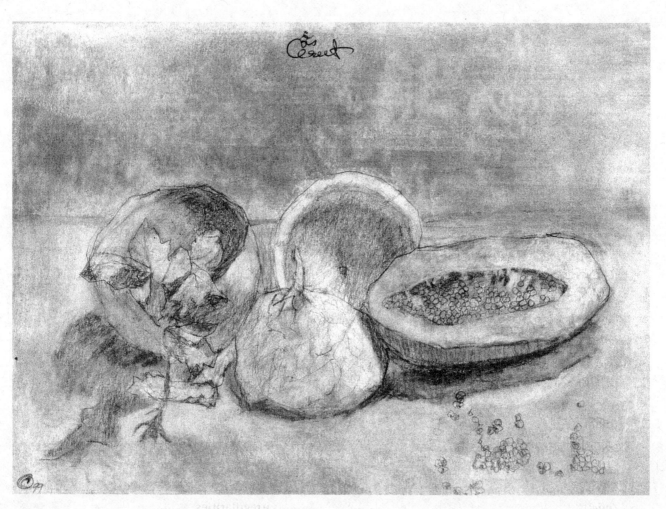

Acupuncture, heat treatment, and massage are forms of healing practiced on the exterior of the body that act towards the interior. If the illness is strongly rooted in the body, acupuncture or massage might not be sufficient therapies; in such a case, another form of cure might be effected using medicinal plants which produce changes from the inside of the body. The therapeutic function of herbs—besides drawing out the pathogen—is to eliminate the cause of the illness and restore the normal function of the organs and channels.

Since antiquity many books have appeared containing systematized information about medicines of diverse natures from the animal, vegetable, and mineral kingdoms. The compilation of these medical resources—the *materia medica*—is called *ben cao*. The *materia medica* of China is holistic and sophisticated, reaching far beyond simple herbology; the *ben cao* includes not only botanical medicines, but material from every realm of the natural world. During the period of the "fighting kings" or Warring States (403 BC–221 BC) and the *Qin* and *Han* dynasties (221 BC–220 AD), the *ben cao* was enriched and broadened by merchant exchange along the old Silk Road. This trade route introduced cardamon, grapes, walnuts, garlic, and many products of animal origin (like rhinoceros horn). During the *Tang* dynasty (618–907 AD) Chinese medicine welcomed the strong influence of Tibetan medicine. By the year 1082 the pharmacopoeia included more than 1558 medicinal products.

A concept fundamental to the *ben cao* is the hierarchy of remedies: the principal or emperor medicine, the assistant or minister, and the second assistant or subject. Combining herbs according to their nature and rank can produce mutual potentiality, mutual benefit, mutual exclusion, mutual fear, or mutual invalidation. This system works in conjunction with the four energies and the five flavors. In *The Agricultural King's Canon of Herbology,* medicines are classified according to their nature as superior, average, and inferior. Superior medicines are tonics which generally have low toxicity; some medicines considered average are toxic, some have tonic action, while others are sedative. Of the inferior medicines, most function to clear heat or cold or to break up stagnancy. Almost all of them have toxic long-term effects, and thus are used only short-term.

Tao Honjing (452–536 AD) reclassified the medicinal products into seven groups: stones (and jades), plants, trees, insects and animals, fruits, foods, and others. The nature of the medicines is divided into eight types: cold *(han),* slightly cold *(wei han),* very cold *(da han),* neutral *(ping),* warm *(wen),* slightly warm *(wei wen),* very warm *(da wen),* and very hot *(da re).*

The administration of herbs in Chinese traditional medicine is based in philosophical and energetic properties rather than in the pharmacological properties recognized by occidental science. Herbs are used either as an independent therapy or in conjunction with other modalities. Like other Chinese therapies, the application of medicinal herbs seeks to balance the energies in the body's different organs. Each plant has certain therapeutic characteristics, of which the ancients said "each herb has its own character, in accordance with the needs and the condition of the patient." The use of a given herb may be determined by its flavor, its thermal qualities, its actions (ascending/ descending, internal/external), its level of toxicity, or its relation to a determined organ network. According to the ancient writer Zhouli, illness is brought under control by considering the five flavors, the five grains, and the five medicines. It was said that every treatment should include five toxins to dominate the illness, five energies to nourish the body, five medicines to treat the illness, and five flavors to regulate the treatment.

A primary classification divides the plants among those with *yin* effects and those with *yang* effects. It is said that if a *yin* plant is administered in excess, it can have a *yang* effect (and vice versa). Generally a combination of plants will be prescribed—some to stimulate *yang* functions of weak organs, others to inhibit the *yang* of other organs (those which precipitate the imbalance), and others to strengthen the entire body. There are plants used to inhibit the *yang* of the liver or to stimulate the fire of the kidney, for example.

Each plant has a time and place when it should be gathered to insure maximum potency. An herbalist with a strong knowledge of the plants can combine them to complement their functions or heighten their properties. The systematization of this knowledge in its entirety is the origin of the theory of plant character. Plants of a cold or fresh nature have a *yin* character, those of a warm or hot nature are considered *yang,* and some are neutral and can tend to be either warm or cool, depending on the condition. The administration of plants of varying natures depends on the symptomatics of the illness. For example, if a patient demonstrates high fever, thirst, red ears and face, sore, inflamed throat—all of which are symptoms of a *yang* complex—plants of a cool thermal nature are prescribed to alleviate the symptoms and approach the roots of the illness.

In general, according to their function, plants of a cool thermal nature can be divided among plants which:

- clear heat and drain fire
- cool blood and relieve toxicity
- tonify *yin* and expel heat
- clear heat and dry dampness
- eliminate heat and favor diuresis
- cool and transform phlegm and heat
- nourish the heart and open the orifices
- cool the liver and extinguish wind

Hot and warm plants can be divided into those which:

- warm the interior and expel cold
- heat the liver and eliminate stagnancy
- tonify heat and build *yang*
- tonify *yang* and dispel dampness
- warm and connect the collateral channels
- help bring fire to the kidneys
- restore vitality

Among hot, cold, cool, and warm there are differences of degree; plants are used in accordance with the gravity of the illness. For example, if a plant with mild effects is prescribed for a serious illness, the disease will not be completely cured (or better put, will not receive complete treatment), and if a plant with a hot thermal nature is used where one of warm nature is needed, the *yin* of the patient may be damaged.

The theory of the five flavors was developed along with the understanding of the seasonal nature of foods. Plants are considered to have different flavors (sour, salty, bitter, sweet, and pungent); each flavor can be characterized as *yin* or *yang*. The pungent, sweet and salt flavors are *yang*; bitter and sour are *yin*. The five flavors are related to the five elements: bitter/wood, sour/fire, sweet/earth, pungent/metal, salty/water.

The *Neijing Suwen* gives each flavor a specific function:

- The pungent clears and expels, nourishing the tendons.
- The bitter contracts and nourishes *chi*.
- The sweet condenses.
- The sour elongates and nourishes the bones.
- The salty smoothes constriction and nourishes the vessels.

The pungent flavor functions to disperse, induce sweat, and circulate *chi* and blood. It is for these effects that hot plants like ginger or cayenne are used, for example, in flu with external symptoms and stagnation of *chi* and blood. Most of the herbs that promote sweat and circulation have a pungent flavor.

Sweet-natured plants nourish, balance, regulate, and disperse sharp pain. Plants with this nature are used when the protective *chi* is deficient, when there is internal pain, or when the body needs detoxification.

Bitterness contracts, shrinks, and fixes. In general it is used against cough, sweat, diarrhea, excess urination, and to stop excessive bleeding and leucorrhea; plants with these characteristics are used in cases of people with weak constitutions who demonstrate profuse sweat, chronic, tubercular cough, chronic diarrhea, spermatorrhea, and uterine hemorrhage.

The sour flavor clears heat, opens the orifices, and brings down energy that is rising against its nature. It is used against constipation, to eliminate heat, to diminish gasping in cases of asthma, to control nausea, to promote intestinal movement, and to dry damp conditions. It is used in cases of illness caused by heat or fire, asthma, edema, beriberi, difficulty in urination, overstrain, and diseases of dampness and *yin* deficiency.

The salty flavor diminishes constipation and smoothes obstacles. It is used for strain, tumors caused by blood stagnation, and muscle tension.

The five flavors align with the five elements and the five organs as well: bitter with the liver, sour with the heart, sweet with the spleen-pancreas, spicy with the lungs, salty with the kidney. Each plant, according to its flavor, tends to primarily effect one organ network; other effects of herbs in the internal workings of the body include ascending, descending, floating, and deepening.

These qualities are taken into account in dealing with illnesses in the upper body (cephalea) and the lower body (ascites), when there are manifestations of ascending energy (like vomiting, cough, or asthma), descending energy (as in diarrhea, uterine hemorrhage or anal protrusion), as well as in illnesses which tend to move outwards (like spontaneous sweating), or inwards (like constipation). In illnesses of the upper body or surface one uses plants which ascend or float rather than plants which descend or deepen. Flowers, leaves, bark, and shoots are the "light" parts of plants—corresponding with the actions of ascending or floating—while seeds, fruits, and minerals are heavy and serve to descend or deepen.

In Chinese herbology it is recognized that some plants have side effects—their toxic properties manifest alongside their beneficial properties. The stronger the effect of a plant, the more likely that it will produce collateral effects.

There are rules and contraindications regarding the combination of herbs. The forms of application include infusions, pills, powders, tinc-

tures, in baths and vapors, eye drops, nose drops, plasters, and supposi-
tories.

Following is a list of the animal and mineral products most commonly used in Chinese medicine:

Ephedra, cinnamon, perilla, ginger, elsholtzia, schizonepeta, *dong quai,* ligusticum, xanthium, magnolia, onion, cilantro, mint, raspberry leaf, chrysanthemum flowers, vitex fruit, pueraria, bupleurum, cimicifuga, horsetail, gypsum, *Anemarrhena trichosanthes,* jasmine, prunella, scutellaria, coptis, *Artemisia apiacea,* phellodentron, gentian, sophora, rhinocerous horn, rehmannia, scrophularia, peony, lithospermum, lonicera, forsythia, dandylion, ox gall, pulsatilla, bear gall, *Artemisa sinensis,* rhubarb, senna leaf, *Aloe vera,* cannabis seed, peach pit, euphorbia, croton, phitolacca, magnolia bark, alisma, coix, *Plantago mayor,* talc, aconite, fennel, black pepper, tangerine peel, orange, sprouted rice, radish seeds, cock's comb, squash seed, ligusticum *chuan xiang,* myrrh, sage, apricot pit, cardamon flower, Chinese rose petals, pinellia, datura, oyster shell, cassia, centipede, ginseng, astragalus, dioscorea, oroxylum, honey, deer antler, walnut hull, dog's testicles, donkey skin, turtle shell, nutmeg, opium poppy, melon pedicle, garlic, nux-vomica.

MAYAN MASSAGE: TALLADAS AND JET

The various forms of massage traditionally practiced in Mexican indigenous cultures are very little studied. Mayan massage is no exception. There is not a single, systematic form of Mayan massage, but rather a series of techniques directed towards specific problems. For reasons of clarity, we arrange them in the following manner:

- Massage to calm muscle spasms and tension, to relax the body and alleviate rheumatism. These forms are known as *talladas* or "rubbings."
- Massage intended to relocate tendons and bones.
- Massage in which specific points on the body are worked to produce generalized effects.
- Suctions, in the form of "cupping," applied against *tza nu yaal* (collapse of the crown).
- Massage for pregnant women to prepare them for birthing and to bring the child into position, and massage for women who have recently given birth (to bring them back to their previous state of health).

- Abdominal massage to accommodate the *cirro*—to tighten or loosen it according to the case, and to tune its rhythm or pulse.

Talladas *or Rubbings*

Rubbings are massages which are generally applied with the whole palm, placing the thumbs parallel and horizontal, spreading the hands across

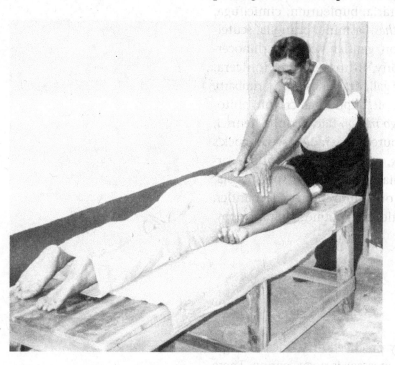

the body with firm pressure. This is used both to diagnose and to treat various muscular problems—especially localized aches and pains, as in *kinan pach ka'* (occipital headache) and backaches *(kam pach)*.

In performing the massage, various lines are followed along the different parts of the body. The most commonly used lines in the back run down the muscles on either side of the spine. Rubbings demand specific conditions. The patient cannot eat before the massage, and the work should not be performed where drafts or breezes are present. The preference among Mayan masseuses is to work with oil or balm of orange blossoms. Some traditional doctors make a balm of a plant known, on the Yucatán, as belladonna *(Bryophyllum pinnatum,* Kurz.), and another called *xkasi kuch,* neither of which is too warm. This is to avoid overheating the body and to prevent illness on contact with a cool-natured food or a cold wind.

For the Mayan masseuse there are two types of rheumatism. One is caused by night-time chill, and the other is characterized by joints aching in the daytime. Masseuses use plants, including: *tzipche' (Bunchosia swartziana,* Gr.), *sinanche' (Zanthoxylum cuneata,* L.), belladonna, garlic, *balsamito, guaco (Aristolochia pentandra), chamico,* 10and *guarumbo (Cecropia peltata).* For rheumatism due to cold, they use a balm of various plants cooked in a Vaseline base. For "hot" rheumatisms they use a tincture; the alcohol-based tincture is recognized as a "cool" remedy because there is no heat involved in the extraction process (because alcohol itself is a cold substance).

There are some masseuses who practice an "experimental" form of massage called *"jet." Jet* produces painful sensations at first, which, little by little, become more pleasurable and result in a deep sense of relaxation in the affected body part. A good deal of training and practice is required to develop the sensitivity to detect the required pressure, points of tension, knots, and inflammations.

Accommodations (Las Acomodadas)

Acomodadas (accomodations) are forms of massage which work dislocated tendons and bones back into place—accommodating them after stress, tension or accidents. These include *tronadas* or "snapping," chiropractic work, and traction to reduce luxations, heal fractures, and relieve stressed tendons. All of these forms of massage are performed by traditional bone setters. These doctors are often functionally illiterate and in almost all cases lack formal medical training; with this consideration in mind, the similarity of these practices with Western chiropractic and orthopedic work is astonishing.

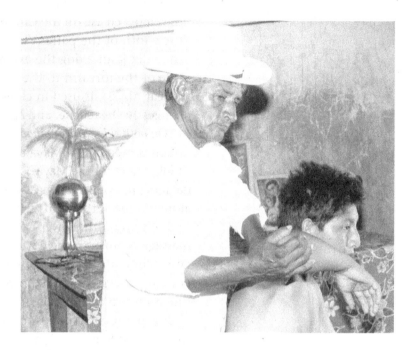

We had the opportunity, in 1992, to work with a bone setter who, performing a massage which had a very defined form and immediate effect, set the fractured shoulder of a woman in his village. She later consulted a medical orthopedist to check the results of the cure. After a series of x-rays and treatments costing thousands of dollars, the doctor told her that her shoulder was healing perfectly and that she should continue following the recommendations of the *curandero*.

Acupressure and Pinching of Points

There are various points on the body that are stimulated using pressure, moving the thumbs along the body, and pinching and pulling the skin to produce effects on the organs. The best known points are found:

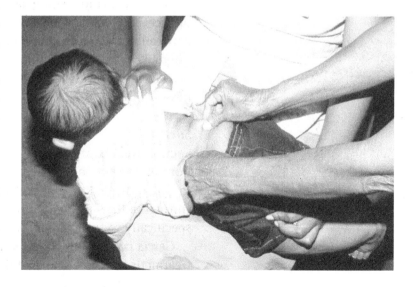

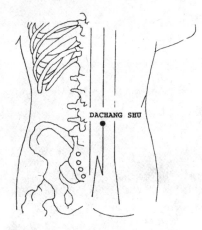

DACHANG SHU

On the medial aspect of the biceps. This point is used to "snap" inflammations and quickly reduce swelling. Pinching of this point is accompanied by rubbing the inner bicep and radial side of the forearm.

This point corresponds to the point *tian fu* (Celestial Storehouse or Lung 3 in Chinese medicine). It is found on the bicep, three *tsun* from the elbow crease (in the Chinese system one *tsun* or *cun* is equivalent to the width of the patient's thumb). The lung meridian runs from the shoulder joint along the external bicep and continues along the radial side of the forearm to the tip of the thumb. This final point, Lung 9 (Great Abyss), is used in cases of rhinitis, anginas, bronchitis, asthma, congestive headache, and epistaxis (nosebleed).

On both sides of the spinal column, below the fourth lumbar vertebrae. This point is used by the Maya to treat *manu jana* or "break" the indigestion. Indigestion, for the Maya, is a cold-natured illness, marked by lazy intestinal function. Generally in cases of indigestion the patient is given a rubbing along the back that ends with the treatment of pinching and pulling a fold of skin on the lower back in the area of the intestines. At times the massage is given in the entire lumbar region on both sides of the spine. Less frequently, though we have witnessed it on various occasions, the point is punctured with a thorn to treat indigestion. This form of acupuncture is known as *"jup."*

This point corresponds to the Chinese point *dachangshu* (Large Intestine *shu)* or Bladder 25, which is also the large intestine locus on the bladder meridian. Its function is to regulate the *chi* of the colon and stomach and to clear stagnation. It is used in the Chinese system for inflammation of the colon, strain, abdominal distention, rectal prolapse, incontinence, and lumbago. The local *(shu)* points directly stimulate connections between the nerves and the medulla oblongata, sending messages to the internal organs. The stimulation of these points helps balance energy in the meridian and is applied in chronic illnesses and in some acute illnesses.

Suction

Suction treatment is used by masseuses and midwives. Although variations exist from one *curandero* to another, in general suction treatment—in which the doctor applies his mouth to the crown of the patient's head through a fine-meshed fabric and draws two sucking breaths—is used specifically to treat *tzan nu yaal*, "collapse of the crown" (see appendix).

Garcia López[33] has done a study which proves the effectiveness of this treatment in various cases of diarrhea in children. He hypothesizes that the application of suction to the anterior fontanel stimulates points along the stomach meridian which, in Chinese traditional medicine, are used to treat nausea. In the Western tradition we associate depressions in the crown of the head with dehydration and the loss of electrolytes.

There is an ancient book in Chinese medicine called *Lu xin jing,* which means "Canon of the Crown of the Head."[34] The book elaborates a system of diagnosis by palpation of the fontanels in children and various treatments that are given in this region of the head.

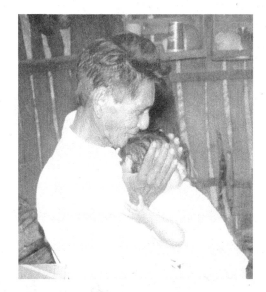

The Channeling of Winds: The Application of Cups

In some cases of back pain brought on by wind, the treatment is a massage by rubbing and the application of cups (similar to cupping in Chinese treatment). First, an herbal balm is applied to the back and the cup is moved over the parts affected. Before the treatment the cup, to clean it and empty it of vapor, is inverted over a lit candle placed atop a coin.

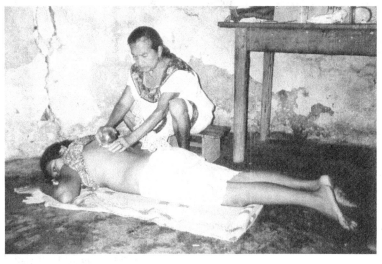

Preparation for Birthing; Recovery in New Mothers

Pregnant women are often aided by midwives who give massage and general check-ups and counsel after the first trimester. The traditional form of massage is given over the entire body. A specific technique intended to prepare the body, blood, and muscles is given once a month. Known as *jet,* it is considered the most important form of preventive medicine practiced during pregnancy. For many midwives it is the central facet of their practice.

Not all rubbings or massages are equal; each has its moment, and each moment in pregnancy has a specific technique attached to it. The work, however, always begins at the navel—the *tuch*—and at the four points or four sides surrounding the navel, and crosses the abdomen various times. Beginning after the third month, the massage and a salve of orange blossoms is applied to the back and the legs.

In the final trimester, some midwives practice a particular technique

105

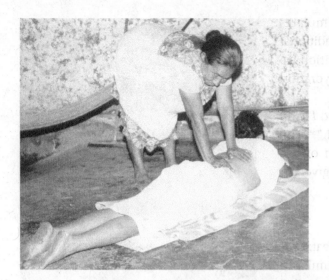

of massage to "accommodate" the fetus and facilitate smooth birth. Moments after birth, the midwife applies pressure upwards from the pubic bone to "raise" the womb. Nine days after labor the raising of the womb is repeated, followed by a massage to "tighten up" the body. The massage, applied first with the bare hands and then with a kerchief or cloth, is applied in the following order: head, neck, chest, waist, hips, buttocks, thighs, knees, ankles, and feet. The intention is to tighten up loose muscles and bones. Much attention is given to the hips, which are often wrapped with a sash to keep the pelvic arch from remaining "open."

After forty days a beating is performed on the back. The woman squats down with her arms crossed and with the midwife's knees pressing into her back. The midwife stretches the patient's arms, giving traction, while massaging the back with her knees.

In order to guarantee herself a role in the birth, a midwife is able to "bind" herself to the pregnant woman and the coming child. When a newly pregnant woman employs a particular midwife, the latter can give a massage accompanied by certain prayers which bind the child to the midwife—meaning that, at the hour of birth, no other midwife may attend, with the understanding that the invitation of another midwife may result in complications. If the mother decides beforehand that she doesn't want this arrangement, she can choose another midwife and break the bondage.

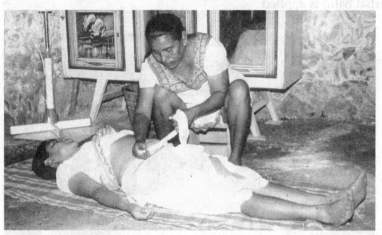

Postpartum massage.

The Accomodation of the Cirro

Another specialty of Mayan *sobadores* (masseuses), is returning the *cirro* or *tipté* to its normal state. The type of massage to be applied depends on whether the *cirro* is out of place, tight, or loose (see chapter 4).

If the *cirro* is out of place, it is accommodated by way of a massage which manipulates all of the organs in the abdomen. If it is loose, a massage is applied around the navel in a clockwise direction; if it is tight, the direction is counterclockwise. The massage is completed with a rubbing of the neck, shoulders, and back to open the flow of energy from the trunk to the head. Some herbalists prescribe a tea of *tipté ak (Jacquinia auriantiaca)* to be taken immediately after the massage.

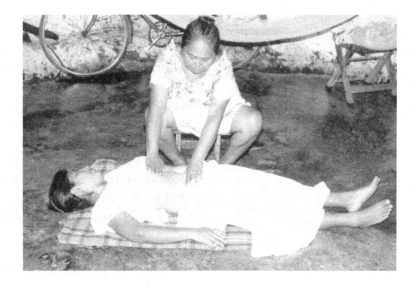

CHINESE MASSAGE (TUI NA)

For the Chinese doctor the body is supported by its muscles and bones. The brain, lungs, stomach, and heart take their place in an organic box of bone, cartilage, and connective tissue. The function of all of the organs is intimately related to the structure that supports them. Any dislocation or change in the position of bones and joints can affect the organs by way of the meridians. Similarly, internal illnesses can often be detected by surface palpation and manipulation of points on the exterior of the body. Irregularities such as the hardness or softness of particular pressure points can signal specific illnesses.

The skeleton functions to sustain and move the body and to protect the organs. Sometimes a brusque movement, a contusion, or rapid change of position can affect the muscles—affecting the nearby musculature and skeletal structure and causing repercussions in the rest of the skeleton, the blood vessels, and the organs (often bringing about the onset of disease).

In general, Chinese massage:

- Stimulates the circulation of blood in the capillaries, bringing blood to muscle tissue and joints.
- Facilitates the movement of lymph and the cleansing of lymph channels.
- Relaxes tense muscles, both internally and on the body's surface. Releasing muscle tension is known to release emotional stagnation as well.
- Gives increased flexibility to the tendons and joints.
- Allows the skeleton to find its natural posture.
- Improves and stimulates the function of internal organs by direct manipulation, improving digestion, assimilation, and elimination processes.
- Stimulates pressure points and meridians over the entire body, promoting the circulation of *chi* and the balancing of *yin* and *yang.*

107

- Augments the protective *chi,* thereby promoting resistance to illness.
- Serves as a surface analgesic to relieve pain from wounds and strains.

In the East, massage is used in virtually all forms of disease treatment. It serves as a form of physical exercise for those who cannot manage to get adequate aerobic activity, and is used in place of the more directed treatment of acupuncture in small children, elderly people and people of weak constitution for whom acupuncture is too strong. By simply using his hands to manipulate the patient's body, a doctor or therapist can aid the body in recovering from a great number of illnesses. It is commonly used in preventive health care and in general recovery from illness in China and Japan. There are forms of self-massage and exercise which allow individuals to treat themselves, thereby reducing dependence on doctors. Chinese health practitioners say that the more out of shape the body is, the sicker the person will be. Maintaining proper posture and form can improve health and prevent all manner of illness. It is up to each person to maintain her or his optimum state of health.

There exist a great variety of forms of massage in China and Japan— most of which share the same basic philosophy and understanding of the body. Eastern forms of massage include techniques of rubbing, beating, kneading, stretching, manipulation of articulations, and stimulation of points.

Depending on the method of pressure applied, the points and meridians can be sedated or tonified. To tonify a point and augment the *chi* moving through it, the point is massaged longitudinally along the meridian in the direction of the energy flow. The point is stimulated by rotating the pressure in a clockwise direction. The masseuse might, as well, use the flats of her fingers to manipulate the skin above, below and around the point, directing the pressure towards the center, working to concentrate the energy in the point.

To sedate or diminish the energy the massage is applied, again, along the line of the meridian, but this time contrary to the direction of *chi* flow; circular pressure is applied in a counter-clockwise direction. Finger pressure is applied around the point, pushing away from it as if to draw the energy out.

A form of cupping is applied to disperse heat and stagnation, particularly over the back and limbs. This technique dilates the blood vessels in the area affected, leaving the skin red and stimulated. The cups are made of bamboo or glass with a dull, rounded rim to prevent discomfort when they are removed. Before the cup is applied, the skin may be treated with a salve or oil; the inside of the cup is heated with a piece of burning cotton, and the cup is applied to the skin and moved rapidly across the body.

In China the study for a career in acupuncture lasts five years. It includes study of the theoretical base of medical practice as well as studies of herbology, massage, *chi kung* (an art of physical exercise discussed below), detailed studies of anatomy, and an understanding of particular patterns of disease.

MAYAN ACUPUNCTURE: TOK AND JUP

According to our investigations, Mayan medicine has the most developed autocthonous system of acupuncture in Mesoamerica, though it remains relatively unknown. Mayan acupuncture has two variants: *jup* and *tok.*

Though these practices are widespread among Mayan communities on the Yucatán peninsula, very little is known about them outside of these communities. The hermetic nature of this knowledge has to do in large part with the hesitance of the Mayan people to share their traditions with outsiders due to the persecution that began with the Spanish conquest and continued through the colonization. This persecution continues with the imposition of occidental traditions and practices on the Mayan people. Perhaps it is this hermeticism, this secrecy, that has allowed Mayan acupuncture—although rudimentary in comparison with Chinese practice—to remain alive as the most developed medical system in Mesoamerica.

In *The Ritual of the Bacabes,* written towards the end of the sixteenth century,[35] we find mentioned the use of *ix hun pudzub kik* (the needle which bleeds) and *ix hun pudzub olom* (the needle which frees the blood)—to treat various diseases. Currently, these acupuncture techniques are practiced with the spines and thorns of several varieties of plants (spines of henequen, *zubín,* and various bushes) and several animals (spines from the tail of the manta ray, *lebisa,* and *xtoon* [fish related to the manta ray], the fang of rattlesnake, tusk of peccary, the beak of the carpenter bird, and the quills of the porcupine).

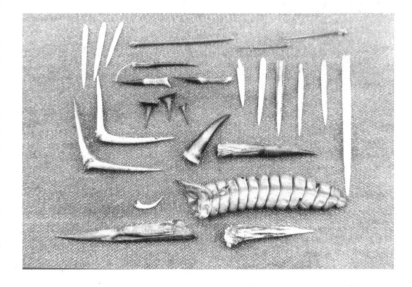

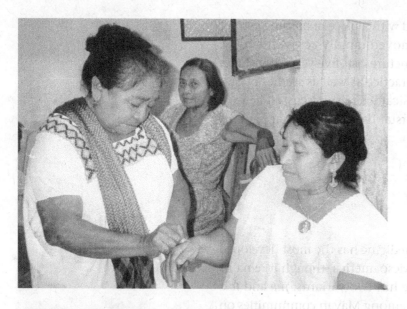

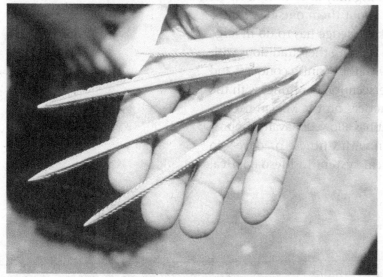

Many *curanderos* who perform *jup* and *tok* use the radial pulse to diagnose illnesses—demonstrating the unity of these practices in a single tradition. The practice known as *jup* involves the pricking of different points, without drawing blood, "to move the stagnant blood and air." Some points are specific for healing wounds or pains caused by air that has entered into the body. These are usually distal points—that is, the point that is punctured is not the location of the pain, but corresponds to it, though often the point being pricked will be in the general area of the wound or pain. In some communities acupuncture of this sort is not limited to clinical practice; mothers practice acupuncture on their children at home to cure such illnesses as indigestion and asthma.

There are two ways of practicing *jup*. One technique is to puncture the skin three times in the desired spot—lifting a fold of skin with the thumb and index finger and applying the spine with the other hand. The puncture is done with a rapid movement, punching and removing the spine three times, penetrating to a depth of almost a centimeter. This is usually done with the fang of a rattlesnake or the fine spines of some species of fish.

The other form of *jup* is effected with somewhat duller spines, like those of the *zubín* or the spur of wild turkey, with which the desired point is needled repeatedly without penetrating the skin, until the surface area is red and inflamed.

Tok, the other form of Mayan acupuncture, is expressly used to draw blood and is often combined with cupping to facilitate bleeding. The puncture is similar to *jup*, although in some cases penetration may be deeper and in others more superficial. *Tok* is used specifically in illnesses related to excess blood and internal winds. We have found that the points used in *tok,* and the use of the technique, correspond to the Chinese technique *ci xue liao fa,* a particular acupuncture method involved with bloodletting (which will be described further on).

The explanation given to us by Mayan *curanderos* is that *tok* is used to draw blood from the body when that blood is bad or stagnant, affected by the evil wind, and that the blood drawn in these cases is usually opaque and dark in color (it should be noted that they do not specifically interpret this as venous blood).

Tok is usually performed with the spines of fish (manta ray, *lebiza* and *xtoon,* to name a few) which because of their serrated edges produce a torn and open wound which facilitates the bleeding. In some points, the bleeding is accompanied by the application of a small cup, which is first heated over a small candle placed atop a coin and then applied to the region of the bleeding. This is believed to draw the blood more rapidly. Practitioners of *jup* and *tok* generally keep their needles or "spines" stuck into cloves of garlic; we imagine that this has an antiseptic action on the needles.

In our work with the *curanderos* we have identified over fifty points used in *tok,* rubbings, and the application of plasters. Of these fifty points, we will present a list of those used in acupuncture (with anatomical description) and look at the similarity of these points with those of the Chinese system.

Between the eyebrows

One of the most important points in traditional Mayan medicine is located in the midline of the face directly between the eyebrows. Some *curanderos* have no name for this point, others call it *tok lu ni'* (the *tok* of the nose) or *vena lu ni'* (the vein of the nose) or "it appeared." It is considered a crucial point because the blood of the head runs through it. Some say that when the hair begins to grow in infants a vein appears which runs to both temples—thus the name "it appeared."

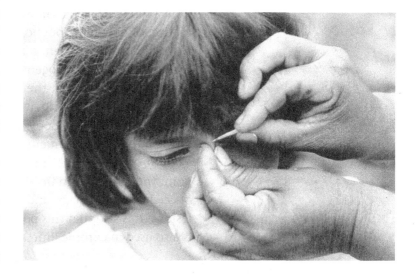

In the majority of Mayan communities in Campeche it is the custom to pierce this point in small children. A ceremony is performed each year on Holy Saturday in which the *j'meen* applies *tok* to this point in children who have not yet received the treatment. The idea is to draw a small quantity of blood which bears, from birth, an evil wind, and thus to prevent attacks and other illnesses in the future. It is a preventive measure that is only performed once in the life of the child.

If the wind stagnates in this point, it can stop the vein so that the individual cannot "breathe;" that is, no energy flows in this vein. This can cause symptoms of pain and, in some cases, a type of paralysis. Some *curanderos* also use this point to "open" the frontal *cephalus,* which radiates out from the nose, to stop attacks of the evil wind. A very fine needle, the spine of the *lebiza,* is used to puncture the little vein that runs above the nose. If an adult never received the piercing of this point as a child, he may suffer from headaches; a *j'meen* can perform *tok* to "open the breathing" of this point on any Friday.

In Chinese medicine the point located between the eyebrows, called *yintang* (Seal Hall), is considered very important. It is an extra point located on the Governing Vessel *(du)* which is used to eliminate wind-heat and to wake the spirit and the mind. The point is worked in cases of dizziness and chronic or acute convulsions. It is used also in cases of rhinitis, flu, insomnia, hypertension, frontal headache, illnesses of the nose and head, nervous vomiting and dizziness in childbirth.

Yintang unites the *ren* channel (conception vessel) with the *du* channel (governing vessel) and is considered to be the superior *dan tian,* or gate of life, an important point of confluence and storage of *chi.* Its function is to open and close the superior orifices, allowing the clear *yang* to freely ascend, governing the surface of the body and strengthening the extremities by fortifying the tendons. When the clear *yang* ascends it favors the inhalation of heavenly *chi* which leads to clarity of mind and aids the regulation of energy throughout the body. The *Neijing* tells us, "when the superior *dan tian* is open, it allows pathogens to be expelled," and "once the body is free of pathogens, it is best to close the superior *dan tian.*" The opening and closing of the three *dan tian* can be done by facing in the four directions, east, north, west, south, and again in the opposite sequence, to bring the *chi* in the body into harmony with the movement of energy in the natural environment.

In Hospital Annex #1 in Tianjen in the People's Republic of China, the point *yintang* is used in treating patients in the sub acute or chronic phases of cerebral hemorrhage, and in those who have recently suffered medullar lesions. It is said that this point wakes the brain and opens the orifices. It is also used in chronic illnesses—such as colitis or gastritis—in which the patient may unconsciously block her or his healing process. This point is used to remove the "object" that is blocking the treatment.

In the suprasternal notch

The majority of Mayan masseuses recognize a point at the top of the sternum, in the depression where the clavicles meet the breast bone. They perform *jup* on this point in cases of chronic asthma and for coughs and flu.

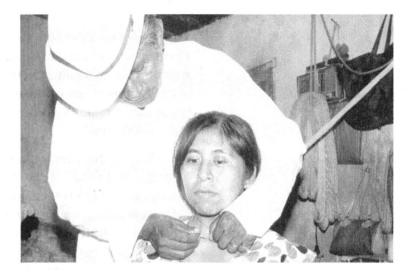

It is understood that asthma is caused by a wind, known as the asthma wind, and the suprasternal notch is opened so that the wind may be expelled from the body. It is punctured from above, below, the right, and the left, in accordance with the four cardinal directions. After the application of *jup* the throat is rubbed with deer fat and a few drops of the fat are taken internally by the patient.

Other *curanderos* also puncture the inferior part of the sternum, saying that illnesses are of the lungs and are caused by weakness. If the patient is very weak, however, this point is not punctured.

Another method for working this region in the treatment of asthma is to apply spines to the central forehead and both temples, or to puncture the region in the form of a cross—applying needles to the forehead, occipital region, shoulders, and the suprasternal notch.

Chinese traditional medicine recognizes this point as *tian tu* (Heaven's Prominence), or Conception Vessel 22, on the *ren* channel. Its function is to eliminate stagnation in the lungs, promote circulation and regulate *chi*. When this point is worked, adverse *chi* descends, dissipates phlegm, and clears the throat. The point is used in cases of asthma, cough, inflamed throat, laryngitis, spasms in the diaphragm, nausea, pharyngitis, tracheitis, bronchitis, asthmatic bronchitis, neurogenic vomiting, spasms of the esophagus, diseases of the vocal chords, and when there is a sensation of a foreign body in the throat. *Tian tu* is also a point of confluence with the extra channel, *yin wei*.

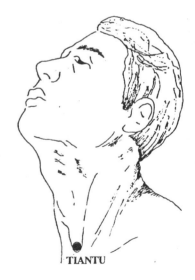

TIANTU

In the superior part of the sternum

The point located in the superior sternum which is used by some Mayan *curanderos* against asthma in combination with *tian tu* is called, in the Chinese system, *xuanji* (North Star). It corresponds to Conception Vessel 21 and is found immediately below *tian tu.* Its function is to regulate *chi*—causing rising energy to sink and detaining cough and asthma. It is indicated against cough, asthma, chest pain, and pharyngitis.

Five points found between the ribs to the sides of the sternum

These points are used by some *curanderos* to reinforce the treatment of asthma. They generally puncture all of the intercostal spaces on both sides of the sternum. Their Chinese equivalents are the points *yuxhong, shencan, lingxu, shenfeng,* and *bulan,* located alongside the sternum, two *tsun* outside of the *ren* channel.

- *Yuxhong* (Kidney 26—Amid Elegance) is found in the first intercostal space, on the side of the sternum. It works to regulate the *chi* of the lungs and to control cough and asthma. It is used in asthma, cough, hypochondria, tightness in the chest, and lack of appetite.
- *Shencang* (Kidney 25—Spirit's Storage) is located in the second intercostal space, two *tsun* from the *ren* channel. It is also used to regulate lung *chi* and respiratory function and to eliminate heat. It is indicated in cases of cough, asthma, chest pain, and nausea.
- *Lingxu* (Kidney 24—Spirit's Ruins) is located in the third intercostal space, alongside the sternum. It also functions to regulate the lungs and eliminate heat. It is indicated, similarly, in cases of asthma, cough, chest tightness, hypochondria, mastitis, and nausea without appetite.
- *Shenfeng* (Kidney 23—Spirit's Seal) is found in the fourth intercostal space, and its functions are identical to those of the above points. It also is used to control excess phlegm.
- *Bulang* (Kidney 22—Stepping Corridor), located in the fifth intercostal space, two *tsun* from the *ren* channel, also regulates lung *chi,* and is used to treat cough and asthma.

In the shoulder

A point below the clavicle towards the shoulder crease, which forms part of the above-mentioned cross, is also used to control cough and asthma.

This point is recognized in Chinese acupuncture as *shufu* (Kidney 27, or Hollow Residence). It regulates the *chi* throughout the body, eases breathing, calms nausea, and is used in cases of loss of appetite.

Behind the ear, below the mastoid process

Some Mayan *curanderos* recommend this point for hearing problems and for ringing and pain in the ears. It is said that by puncturing this point "the ear opens." It is punctured with the spine of a manta ray or the fang of a rattlesnake—after which deer fat is applied. The fat is heated, rubbed onto the area until it hardens, and covered to retain its heat.

It is understood that the point is located very close to a vein which runs directly to the heart, and care is taken to puncture only the skin, not the vein.

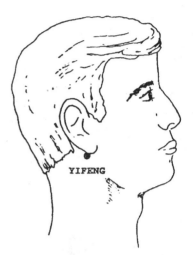

Chinese acupuncture locates the point *yifeng* (Shielding Wind), or Triple Heater 17, behind the earlobe in the depression that marks the mastoid process. *Yi* (from *yifeng*) means "medicine," and *feng* means "wind;" thus we see that this point is used to treat wind-related illnesses. Its function is to wake the ears and open the eyes; to eliminate heat and wind, to promote the circulation of *chi* throughout the meridians, to stimulate the sense organs, to heighten the sense of hearing, and to ease pain.

This point is indicated for tinitis, deafness, muteness, pain in the teeth or eyes, facial paralysis, inflammation of the mandible and the mastoid process, difficulty in swallowing or speaking, and neuralgia. In combination with the point *fengchi,* or Pool of Wind (Gall Bladder 20), this point is used in some cases of cerebral hemorrhage. Moxibustion is commonly used on this point for problems like buzzing and pain in the ears.

Between the upper lip and the nose

In Mayan medicine, in cases of flu with cough *(se'en)* the point just between the nose and upper lip is punctured. This point is also commonly used to treat headaches.

In Chinese medicine the point in the depression above the upper lip is known as *renzhong* or *shuigou* (Philtrum), or Governing Vessel 26. It is used to clear heat, open the orifices, and regulate *yang*. It is used for anosmia (loss of the sense of smell), inflammation of the face and lips, epilepsy, trismus (lockjaw), facial paralysis, jaundice, pain and rigidity in the spine, apoplexy, infantile convulsions, shock, diabetes, and mental disorders. It is useful in arousing people who have fainted, and it is the point of confluence with the large intestine and stomach meridians.

Beneath the lower lip, below and between the two incisors

In cases of toothache some *curanderos* puncture the point on the gums beneath the lower lip and (more-or-less) between the two lower incisors.

In Chinese medicine this point, inside the lower lip, is called *cheng jiang*

(Receiving Fluid), or Conception Vessel 24, and is used to disperse heat and wind and to calm the spirit. It is applied in the treatment of cavities and toothaches, gingivitis, excessive salivation, speaking difficulties, muteness, hemiplegia, trismus, torticolis, and mental disorders.

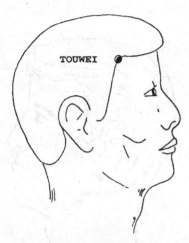

At the hairline on either side of the forehead

This point is often used by Mayan masseuses and *j'meenob* in cases of *chiba pool,* a type of headache in which the blood stagnates and becomes thick and dark due to the presence of a heating wind. *Chiba pool* is diagnosed by tapping the head with the knuckles and listening for a hollow, tympanic sound. The point is punctured with the spine of a manta ray.

In Chinese traditional medicine this point is known as *touwei* (Head Support), point 8 on the stomach meridian. It is found in the line where the first hairs grow on the temple, and its function is to eliminate wind, disperse heat, and clear the head and eyes. It is indicated in cases of congested head, facial paralysis, blurred vision, vertigo, excess weeping, and eye pain.

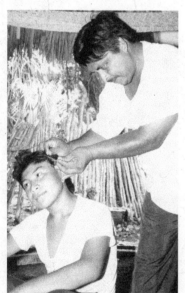

In the midline of the face, on the hairline of the forehead

This point is punctured in cases of headache and is generally used in conjunction with the preceding point.

In Chinese acupuncture the point located just behind the hairline in the midline of the face is called *shenting* (Spirit's Hall), Governing Vessel 24. It is punctured to clear the head and eyes and calm the heart-mind.

It is used in cases of headache with dizziness, inflammations in the eyes, weeping, insomnia, epilepsy, over-excitement, hysteria, rhinitis, sinus congestion, bloody nose, weak sense of smell, and asthma.

At the hairline in the temporal region of the head

This point is only used in conjunction with the two preceding points in cases of headache due to wind and stagnant blood *(chiba pool).* It is punctured with the spine of a manta ray.

The Chinese equivalent of this point is called *hanyan* (Jaw's Dislike), Gall Bladder 4, and is used in cases of migraine, painful or difficult vision, epilepsy, dizziness, sneezing fits, tinitis, and neck, arm, and hand pain.

In the parietal artery of the temple

Applying *tok* to this point, the *curandero* allows only a few drops of blood to escape. In cases of fever the bleeding of this point is accompanied by a vapor bath (to break the fever).

In Chinese medicine the point *sizhukong* (Triple Heater 23—Silken Bamboo Hollow), is located in the lateral depression at the outer end of the eyebrow. The point is used to calm liver wind and eliminate heat. It is indicated in cases of epilepsy, vertigo, inflammations of the eyes, difficult vision, facial tics, toothache, and nausea with vomiting.

Points that form a cross around the fontanel

These points represent the four cardinal directions of the head. They are used most commonly to treat asthma. We are familiar with the case of a child of one-and-a-half years whose occipital and parietal plates in the skull were late in fusing, causing the fontanel to protrude excessively; these points were punctured as part of his treatment.

This combination of points corresponds to: *houding* (Governing Vessel 19—Behind Top), *quianding* (Governing Vessel 21—Before Top) forming the vertical axis of the cross and both points *louoque* (Bladder 8—Decline) forming the horizontal axis.

The function of *houding* is to clear the head and eyes and calm the mind. It is used for madness, headache on the medial and superior aspects of the head, epilepsy, and vertigo. *Quianding* functions to eliminate heat, disperse wind, and to nourish *yin* and pacify *yang*. It is indicated for headache, painful vision, nasal obstruction, epistaxis, and vomiting. The function of *luoque* is to expel wind, clear heat, open the orifices and clear the vision. It is used in cases of dizziness, tinitis, blurred vision and mental disturbances.

On the posterior aspect of the arm, between ulna and radius, near the center of the forearm

This point is used to combat shoulder pain caused by wind. It is said that "the air enters at the elbow and runs towards the shoulder." Although we have not ascertained a systematic understanding, the *curanderos* explain that a sort of canal connects the points, and the wind runs through this canal.

This point on the forearm, *sidu,* or Four Ditch in Chinese acupuncture, is located five *tsun* below the olecranon, between the ulna and radius. It is point nine on the triple heater meridian. Its function is to open the orifices and clear the ears, the brain and the throat. It is used for arm and shoulder pain, rigidity and paralysis in the fingers, painful gums and teeth, and deafness.

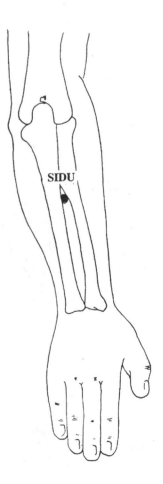

In the internal posterior aspect of the elbow, in a hollow in the cubital bone

This point is used in Mayan medicine to treat rheumatism in the shoulders caused by a cold wind.

It corresponds to Small Intestine 8, *xiaohai* (Small Sea), in the Chinese system. It is located in a hollow in the cubital bone, above the nerve on the interior aspect of the elbow. Its function is to eliminate heat and wind, unite the sense organs, and stimulate the blood. *Xiaohai* is stimulated in cases of pain, arthritis and rheumatism in the elbow, shoulder, arm and neck, torticolis, trismus, spasms, tics, intestinal spasms, diarrhea, gastric ulcer, facial edema, inflammation of the gums, and pain in the upper jaw.

In the hollow between the pinky and the ring finger

This point—the most commonly used of the inter digital points—is used for problems in the hands and pain in the elbow. It is said that this is where the wind in the body is stored.

Triple Heater 2, *yemen* (Fluid's Door), is one of the four *baxie* points—extra points located in the inter digital spaces of the hand. The point is located, with the hand closed in a fist, between the knuckles of ring finger and pinky. Its function is to eliminate heat and wind, and to clear the ears and the eyes. *Yemen* is worked for pain and stiffness in the fingers, hand, and arm, sadness, fear, headache, inflammation of the eyes, amygdalitis, deafness and malaria.

All of the *baxie* points are used to stimulate the nerves of the hand and to rehabilitate and waken the hands from injuries of the nerves, tendons, ligaments, and bones.

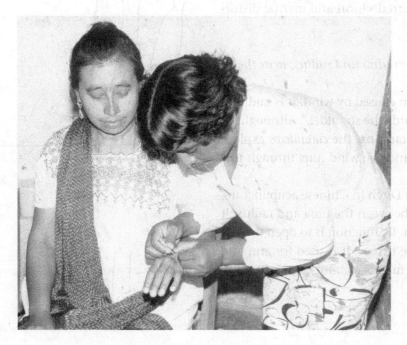

On the dorsal side of the hand between the fourth and fifth metacarpals

This point is also commonly used for pain in the hand and arm (up to the elbow).

It corresponds to *zhongzhou*, Triple Heater 3 (Middle Island), which is located on the back of the hand between the fourth and fifth metacarpals in the depression beside the articulation. It's function is to open the orifices, nourish the intelligence, reduce pathogenic heat, and circulate *chi*.

Zhongzhou is used in cases of arm, elbow, shoulder, and back pain, motor problems in the fingers, headache, red eyes, deafness, ringing in the ears, pharyngitis, and febrile illnesses with sweating.

In the spinal column above the protrusion of the seventh cervical vertebrae

This point is used by some *curanderos* to lower fever *(chokuil)*.

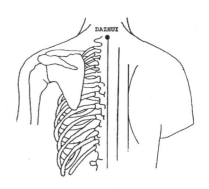

Dazhui or (Big Vertebra) is the fourteenth point on the governing vessel. It is the reunion point of all the *yang* meridians. It functions to disperse heat, eliminate wind, and bring down the *chi* which has tended to move in the opposite direction. It is indicated in cases of fever, heat-related illnesses, malaria, pulmonar tuberculosis, general weakness, asthenia, depression, catarrh, hysteria, sensation of heat in the bones, spasms in the back and arms, and infantile convulsions.

In the back, on either side of the spine, below the fourth lumbar vertebrae

This point is used to treat *manu jana* or "the sounding of indigestion;" it can be stimulated by pinching between the fingers or by using *jup*.

Dachangshu or Bladder 25 (Large Intestine's Hollow), as the name implies, is the *shu* point (point of correspondence) with the large intestine meridian. It's function is to regulate the stomach and colon, harmonize the *chi*, and release stagnant energy. It is used for constipation, abdominal distention, rectal prolapse, hemorrhoids, incontinence, lumbago, and diseases of the colon.

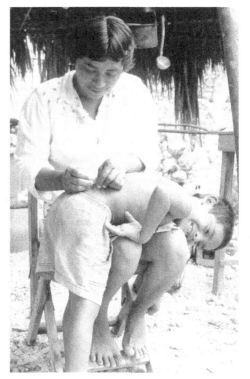

In the leg, on the medial side of the tibia, in a hollow four fingers from the knee

This point is used by some masseuses and *curanderos* to treat swelling of the legs and feet.

This is one of the most recognized and commonly used points in Chinese medicine. It is called *zusanli*, or Three More Miles (Stomach 36), because it renews the body's vigor. It is said that upon the stimulation of this point, a weary traveler can walk three more miles.

The point is found three *tsun* below the kneecap, along the medial side of the tibia. Its function is to regulate the spleen and stomach and to fortify the body's original and protective *chi*. It is the *he*, or sea point on the stomach meridian, meaning that it dominates the meridian and shares *chi* with *he* points of all of the meridians.

It is used to treat pain, exhaustion and weakness in the feet and legs, swelling in the knees, pain in the hips, chronic and acute conditions of all of the internal organs, weight loss, discontent, melancholy, lack of visual acuity, bad digestion due to weak digestive fire, gastric pain, constipation, diarrhea, incontinence, hypertension, and ammenhorrea, among other illnesses.

Two fingers above the knee on the outer aspect of the thigh

This point is used by Mayan doctors for rheumatism and pain in the feet and legs.

Found two *tsun* above the top of the kneecap on the outer aspect of the thigh, *Liangqiu* (Ridge Mound) is point 34 on the stomach meridian. It regulates and harmonizes stomach *chi,* eliminates wind, transforms dampness, relaxes the tendons, and stimulates the circulation. It is used for pain, stiffness and swelling in the knees and the front of the legs and feet, lumbar pain, fear, mastitis, and gastric pain.

In the center of the dorsal aspect of the foot, below the inferior end of the tibia

This point is known by Mayan *curanderos* for facilitating the movement of the toes in treating pain and inflammation of the feet.

It is known in Chinese medicine as *jiexi* (Release Stream), or Stomach 41. It is the tonification point on this meridian. Located on the top of the foot, equidistant from the two maleoli (on top of the common extensor tendon), it is known to fortify the spleen, transform dampness, calm the spirit, and eliminate heat. It is indicated for pain and swelling in the legs, feet, and knees, cramps and paralysis of the lower limbs, headache, weakness, depression, and palpitations.

On the foot, at the root of the second and third toes

The skin between the second and third toes is pinched and pulled to treat pain and inflammation in the foot and toes.

In Chinese medicine, the point between the second and third toes is *neiting,* or Stomach 44 (Inner Court). Its function is to disperse heat, eliminate dampness, and regulate the function of the intestines and the stomach. It is used to combat rheumatic pains in the lower limbs, swelling in the feet, over excitement, nightmares, pains in the pharynx, anginas, gingivitis, toothache, and lack of appetite.

The sublingual veins

The veins on the lower side of the tongue are punctured to prevent attacks of epilepsy and hysteria.

These two sublingual points—extra points known as *jinjin yuye*—are used to treat convulsions, uncontrollable vomiting, aphasia with rigidity of the tongue, edema of the tongue, diarrhea, and diabetes.

JIN JIN YUYE

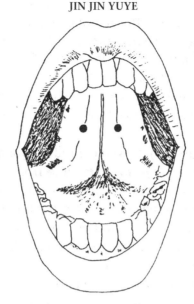

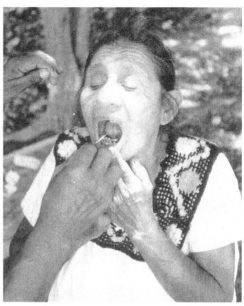

Other points in Mayan medicine for treating pain in the upper extremities which correspond to points in Chinese traditional medicine.

All of the following points are treated in Mayan medicine with massage, poultices, jup, and tok:

Houxi (Small Intestine 3—Back Creek). This point is located on the medial side of the fifth metacarpal, in a depression where the skin color changes from the pale of the palm to the darker skin of the back of the hand. Its functions include eliminating heat and dampness, opening the orifices, and calming the spirit. It is indicated in cases of tics and spasms of the elbow, arms, and fingers, headache, stiff neck, congestion of the eyes, deafness, febrile illnesses, epilepsy, malaria, and night sweats.

Wangu (Small Intestine 4—Wrist Bone). *Wangu* is found on the medial side of the hand, in the depression between the base of the fifth metacarpal and the triangular bone. Its function is to eliminate heat and wind, promote circulation of blood, and release stagnation. It is indicated in cases of finger, arm, and elbow pain, headache, stiff neck, cloudiness in the cornea, pain in the hypochondria, jaundice, febrile illnesses without perspiration, tinitis, and diabetes.

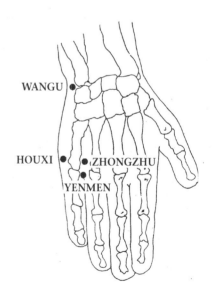

Quchi (Large Intestine 11—Crooked Pool). Located in the elbow (when it is fully flexed) in a hollow at the end of the elbow crease. Its functions are to eliminate heat and wind and regulate blood and *chi*. It is used for arm and elbow pain, motor problems of the upper limbs, scrofula, hives, abdominal pain, nausea, diarrhea, dysentery, febrile illnesses, pain and inflammation in the throat, apoplexy, and hypertension.

Zhouliao (Large Intestine 12—Elbow Seam). On the outer aspect of the humurus, one *tsun* above *quchi*. It is used in cases of swelling, pain, and calcification in the arm and elbow.

Binao (Large Intestine 14—Arm and Scapula). Located on the external aspect of the arm, in the deltoid V, two *tsun* below the axillary crease. Its function is to activate the *chi*, eliminate stagnation and wind, and drain the collaterals. It is indicated in cases of arm and shoulder pain, scrofula, neck tension, and stiffness in the arms.

Points used by Mayan curanderos *for pain in the lower limbs which correspond to points in Chinese traditional medicine*

Yinshi (Stomach 33—Yin's Market). Found three *tsun* above the top of the kneecap on the exterior aspect of the thigh. *Yinshi* functions to bring the meridians into communication, to activate the collaterals, and to eliminate heat and dampness. It is used in cases of swelling, pain, and disorders of the lower limbs.

Dubi (Stomach 35—Eyes of Knee). Located in the articulation of the knee, in a hollow over the tendon. Its function is to eliminate cold and wind. It is indicated for pain, swelling, beriberi, and motor disorders of the knee.

Kunlun (Bladder 60—Kunlun Mountains). Located in the ankle above the heel bone, between the exterior maleolus and the Achilles tendon, on the outer aspect of the foot. Its function is to clear the head and eyes, relax the tendons, and transform phlegm. It is indicated in cases of pain in the heel, back, and head, neck stiffness, pain and spasms in the arm and shoulder, lumbago, blurred vision, nosebleed, epilepsy in children, and difficult labor.

Pushen (Bladder 61—Serve and Consult). Beneath *kunlun* in the depression of the heelbone where the light and dark skins meet. Its function is to reduce inflammation and pain, clear the brain, and wake the spirit. It is used in muscular atrophy and weakness of the lower limbs, pain in the heel, lumbago and motion sickness.

Shenmai (Bladder 62—Extending Vessel). It is just below the external maleolus, in the depression along the edge of the lateral maleolus bone. Its function is to clear heat, dampness, and stagnation. It calms the spirit and regulates blood and *chi*. It is indicated in pain of the lower limbs and back, epilepsy, mental disorders, headache, dizziness, and insomnia.

Qiuxu (Gall Bladder 40—Mound of Ruins). Before and below the external maleolus, in the hollow. Its function is to disperse stagnant liver and gall bladder *chi* and eliminate stagnation. It is used in weakness and pain of the lower limbs, pain and swelling of the ankle joints, motor disorders,

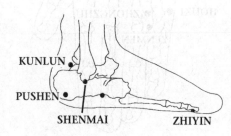

KUNLUN

PUSHEN

SHENMAI   ZHIYIN

neck, chest and hypochondriac pain, swelling in the axillary region, nausea, acid indigestion, muscular atrophy, and malaria.

Points in the hips and waist

Wuli of the femur (Liver 10—Five Measures on the Foot). Found on the interior aspect of the thigh, towards the front, three *tsun* below the upper edge of the pubic bone.

Yinlian (Liver 11—Yin's Modesty). Above *wuli*, two *tsun* below the upper edge of the pubis, on the outer aspect of the large abductor muscle. Its function is to regulate and tonify the kidney and liver and to eliminate heat and dampness. It is used in cases of irregular menstruation, pain in the genitals, thighs, and legs, and leuccorhea.

Jimai (Liver 12—Urgent Pulse). In the inguinal crease, along the same line as *yinlian*. Its function is to tonify and regulate the liver and kidney, to clear heat, and eliminate dampness. It is used for hernia, and pain in the abdominal region and genitals.

Points in the waist used to treat painful growths without abscess

Wushu (Gall Bladder 27—Five Pivots). This point is found above the iliac crest, on a horizontal line one-and-a-half *tsun* below the umbilicus.

Weidao (Gall Bladder 28—Maintain the Way). Over the frontal iliac spine, one-half *tsun* below *wushu*.

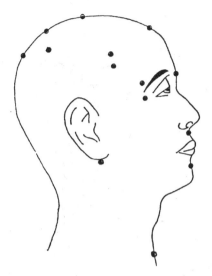

Points in the head and face used by Mayan curanderos and masseuses.

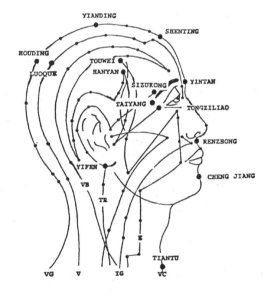

Meridians and points from Traditional Chinese Medicine (large intestine, stomach, small intestine, bladder, triple warmer, gall bladder, and governing vessel).

Therapeutics

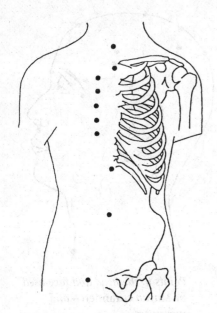

Points on the front of the body used in Mayan traditional medicine.

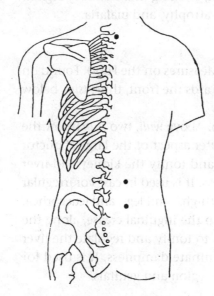

Points on the back used in Mayan traditional medicine.

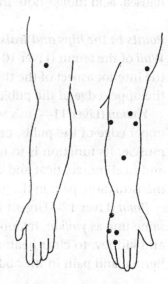

Points on the arms used in Mayan traditional medicine.

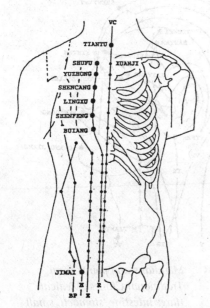

Points and meridians on the front of the body used in Traditional Chinese Medicine (stomach, spleen-pancreas, kidney, liver, lung, and conception vessel).

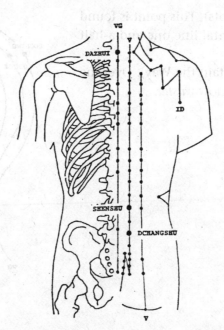

Points and meridians on the back used in Traditional Chinese Medicine (bladder and governing vessel).

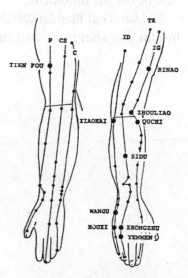

Points and meridians in the arms used in Traditional Chinese Medicine (lung, pericardium, heart, large intestine, triple warmer, and small intestine).

124

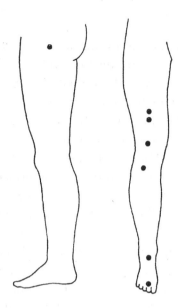

Points on the legs used in Mayan traditional medicine.

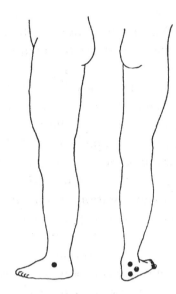

Points in the feet used in Mayan traditional medicine.

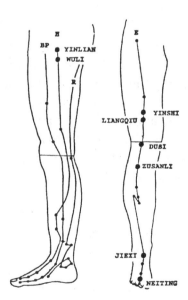

Points and meridians in the legs used in Traditional Chinese Medicine (liver, spleen-pancreas, kidney, and stomach).

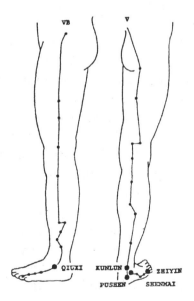

Points in the feet used in Traditional Chinese Medicine (gall bladder and bladder).

125

Wang Xuetai tells of how the first people to appear in the vast territories of China learned to cure themselves of disease and heal wounds. These early medics, he speculates, used sharpened stones to drain abscesses in the skin—which must have been common given the precarious form of life. Since that time, Chinese medicine has been enriched by healing modalities which have been introduced and taken root over the course of centuries of experience and observation. The use of stone needles to open wounds and ulcers might have given rise to the fundamental understanding that "the point to be treated is the point where there is pain." Repeated exploration of sensitive points gradually led to the discovery that certain pressure points have some connection with other parts of the body—that is, that points on the limbs might affect the trunk, and vice versa. By bleeding certain points and stimulating others, disorders that were not ostensibly located in these points could be treated. These points were united among themselves and bore specific relations to the internal organs. The understanding of what is called meridian theory—the idea that pressure points are organized along specific channels or meridians—was supported by seeing that the application of heat and the insertion of needles produced a sensation like an electric shock running in a certain direction.

It was acceptable in China to use human cadavers for medical study. Through empirical study it was learned that the blood vessels bring the distal points of the body into contact, and that the distribution of these vessels had a certain relation with the movement of sensation and energy throughout the body. It was realized that irregularities of the skin and sensitive and painful points might be used as points of entry in the treatment of disease. These points were organized into fourteen lines which crossed the body like a web, similar to the veins and arteries, though less physically apparent.

Through studied observation of the color and movement, dryness or dampness of the tongue, the qualities of the tongue fur, palpation of the body, and reading of the radial pulse, one could discern whether the disease was serious or passing, if it affected only the surface of the body or was deeply rooted, if its cause was heat or cold, if it was located in a particular organ, and if the body was strong enough to recover by itself. It was concluded that changes in the interior of the body manifest in the exterior, in the skin, and that consequently internal illness could be treated at the surface.

The Yellow Emperor's Classic of Medicine describes the formation of the points along fourteen meridians that run the length and breadth of the body, from the surface to the internal organs. Acupuncture—the insertion of needles into these points to stimulate, sedate, and regulate the energy that runs through the channels like water in a stream—is rooted in this notion. It is said that when the *chi* flows there is no pain, but when the *chi* is detained it is like the flow of a river stopped by a dam, and there is pain. Eventually three-hundred seventy-one points were recognized which belonged to the fourteen channels, along with other miscellaneous points which were not on the meridians. There was no general agreement as to the names, functions, and locations of the points until the *Tang* dynasty (618–907 A.D.), when the famous medical doctor Zhenquan ordered a revision of the system. Previously, acupuncture techniques had been passed from father to son or from master to apprentice; during the *Tang* dynasty an imperial college was established to promote the study of acupuncture and moxibustion (see below).

In the year 1026, under the *Song* dynasty, another revision was undertaken to establish the exact function and location of each of the points. A life-size bronze figure was forged which displayed all of the recognized acupuncture points. Over the centuries acupuncture became increasingly specialized, and different types of needles were manufactured for different uses. Needles were made to be inserted to different depths, others to augment or diminish the *chi* in a given point, others for bleeding, others for very light treatment, and still others for special surgery.

Acupuncture is considered a science in China, with complex and varied techniques. The most common technique is that which we discuss here, the stimulation of bodily points with needles to fortify the body and promote healing. One of the many techniques of Chinese acupuncture, that known as *Ci xue liao fa,* involves the puncture of pressure points or superficial veins to extract a small quantity of blood. This technique, developed in the hot and humid zones of the south to draw heat from the body, is sometimes combined with cupping to disperse heat, treat vascular problems, reduce pain, diminish inflammations, draw wind from the meridians, and relax the *chi*. The technique goes back to the ancient roots of acupuncture, and does not always work along the meridians. The principle is to find a point close to where the blood is stagnated and open the point to release stagnation.

Once the point is chosen and cleaned, the skin is pinched between thumb, index, and middle finger, and a sterile three-pointed needle or small lance is inserted. A cup is sometimes placed over the opening to facilitate the bleeding. The cup is left in place between five and fifteen minutes, depending on the amount of blood to be extracted. The quantity of blood desired depends on the illness. For example, in cases of manic schizophrenia, acute skin infection, or trauma of a limb, between 30 and 100 milliliters of blood might be extracted. Obviously too much blood should not be drawn—in general the limit is 200 ml. between all the treated points.

In recent years in China, Japan, France, Germany, the ex-Soviet Union, and other parts of the world investigations have been undertaken to understand the "scientific" basis of Chinese medicine, and acupuncture in particular. From an occidental viewpoint we can look at acupuncture as a phenomenon possessed of a certain physical-electrical reality. The statistical efficiency of acupuncture treatment has been documented, as well as the fact that many of the points treated, when tested with a galvanometer, display less electrical resistance than other parts of the body.

Acupuncture points present particular electrical characteristics which have been widely studied over the past fifty years.[36] The difference in electrical resistance (cutaneous impedance) between the acupuncture points and the rest of the skin is of the order of ten-to-one. It has been shown that at the center of a point the impedance varies between 30,000 and 350,000 ohms, diminishing as the measure is taken further from the point. At one centimeter distance the variation may be between 450,000 and 5 million ohms. It has been shown, as well, that these measurements depend on the hydration of the skin and the condition of the sebaceous film which covers it; the measurement of electrical resistance is confounded by the cleaning of the skin with products like alcohol, ether and acetone. These characteristics have stimulated the development of numerous apparati designed to measure the electrical resistance of different parts of the body.

It has also been demonstrated that the electrical resistance between two points on the same meridian is always weaker than between one of these points and a point on any other meridian—the least electrical resistance is always found between two points on the same meridian. Similarly, investigations in electrometry have demonstrated that a halo of electrons appears around an acupuncture point in need of treatment, and disperses when treatment is applied.

The discovery of electromagnetic fields which surround the body has been examined, in China, by the use of the Kirlian camera. Coming in contact with a determined electromagnetic frequency, the camera revealed hundreds of points in the energetic field with colors more brilliant than the general field itself. These points coincide, to an extraordinary degree, with the points of Chinese acupuncture.

PLASTERS AND POULTICES IN MAYAN MEDICINE

In Mayan medicine poultices and plasters are commonly used, as is the application of heat in the form of burning charcoal, to warm and stimulate points on the body and treat surface pain. Poultices can be of animal, vegetable, or mineral origin, and can be made from herbs, fat, or clay. The material applied depends on its thermal nature—whether the poultice is being used to heat or cool the affected area. In some cases the poultice material may be parboiled to augment its warmth.

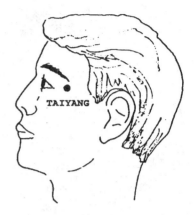

The following is a partial look at points which are specifically treated with poultices by Mayan healers:

The temples

Poultices of cold-natured plants are often applied to refresh the head and ease the pain of some types of headache.

This treatment coincides with the point *taiyang* in Chinese traditional medicine. It is an extra point located in the depression midway between the end of the eyebrow and the midline of the angle of the eye. The point is used to treat migraines, general headaches, eye pain, common cold, neuralgia, and ocular illnesses.

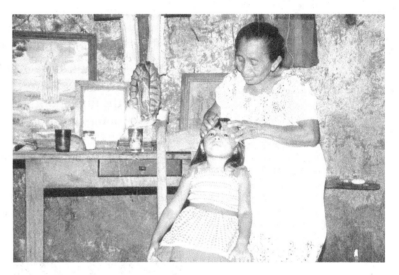

The external aspect of the tip of the small toe

Some midwives, when a woman is experiencing difficult labor, crush a clove of garlic and rub the tip of the small toe with it, believing it helps to intensify the contractions. Others, in addition, place a clove of garlic on the tongue, saying that it facilitates labor. It is said that the garlic helps to provoke birth "because it is hot, like chili, and it has its own poison which helps the child come out; it burns so the child runs from it."

In Chinese medicine this point is known as *zhiyin* (Bladder 67—End of Yin). Its function is to regulate the blood vessels, eliminate wind, regulate *chi*, clear vision, disperse heat, and coordinate the meridians. The point is generally known to ease labor. It is indicated in the retention of placenta, bad positioning of the fetus, difficult labor, stuffed or bloody nose,

Therapeutics

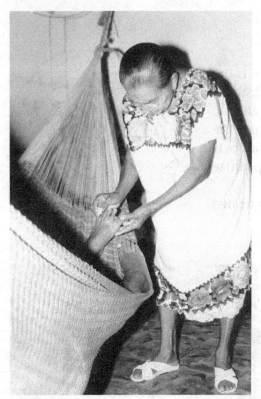

headache, pain or heat in the soles of the feet, spermatorrhea, difficult urination, swollen feet, and itching.

In the chapter on unusual illnesses, the *Neijing Suwen* says: "The collaterals of the uterus are connected to the kidneys."[37] If the *chi* of the kidney is deficient, the uterus is also deficient, making it difficult to maintain the normal position of the fetus; if the resistance is weak, *chi* and blood are weak and there is no strength for giving birth; if a woman has a weak constitution from birth, labor will be lengthy and difficult, causing increasing loss of energy and blood and diminishing the force to expel the placentá.

The point *zhiyin* of the foot joins with the *shaoyin* (kidney) channel. Based on the idea that "*yin* is calm and *yang* movement, if *yang* grows *yin* develops," heating or applying moxa to *zhiyin* will fortify the kidney, increase its essence, and strengthen its blood. Sufficient *chi* and blood will strengthen the uterus allowing an easy and healthy birth.

This point can be punctured and bled, but generally during the final month of labor it is treated daily with fifteen minutes of moxibustion.

In the back, three finger widths from the spine, below the second lumbar vertebra

Poultices of warm-natured plants are applied to this point in cases of women who are infertile due to "cold in the womb." Some midwives recommend burning charcoal placed immediately below the hips of a patient sleeping in a hammock.

This point is *shensu*, or Bladder 23 (Kidney's Hollow), in Chinese medicine—the *shu* point (point of correspondence) with the kidney.

The kidney meridian rules not only the kidney but also the sexual organs (uterus, ovaries, testicles, and urethra). It has important actions regarding sexuality, mental energy, and willpower. When stimulated adequately, the kidney meridian functions to nourish water and strengthen fire.

The stimulation of *shensu* is indicated in cases of lack of energy, feminine infertility, dismenorrhea, metritis, vaginal discharge, inflammation of the urethra, urethritis, diabetes, premature ejaculation, impotence, lumbago, and sciatica. It affects, as well, the glands around the kidney. The point, associated with diminished *yang* of the kidney, is often treated with moxibustion.

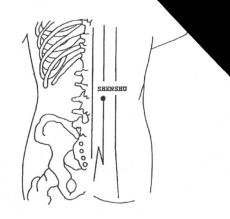

MOXIBUSTION AND POULTICES IN CHINESE MEDICINE

Moxibustion, which developed alongside acupuncture, is the application of heat to the skin through the burning of mugwort *(Artemisa sinensis)*. In China moxibustion is called *zhen jiu,* which means "needle and fire," or "needle and *moxa.*" Moxibustion was developed in the north of China where intense cold gave rise to the need for heat treatments, but over the centuries it spread throughout China. The word moxa comes from the Japanese *mogusa,* referring to the dried and ground herb used in the treatment. When dried and ground, mugwort maintains a cotton-like consistency.

In Mexico, moxibustion can be performed using the leaves of *estafiate.* The dry leaf material is removed from the veins and ground to the consistency of cotton. A pinch of the herb is rolled between the fingers into a cone shape, placed over the point and treated in a variety of ways. The most common way is to place it over a needle that is inserted in the point and burn it. The herb will burn slowly and the process should be repeated various times. Another option is to burn a cone of mugwort placed on a fine slice of garlic or ginger on the point to be treated. If it becomes too hot it should be removed. Another option is to roll the herb into the form of a cigar and burn it, moving the burning tip in slow circles above the point.

For numerous illnesses the application of moxibustion is said to be more effective than needles. It is used especially in cases where the application of needles would not have a direct or rapid effect—chronic cases and cases of *yin* deficiency and pathogenic cold, for example. It is applied frequently in cases of rheumatic pains, pains in the joints, asthma, asthenia (weakness), cough, bronchitis, ulcerous colitis, and general weight loss.

Many points are treated with poultices and plasters made from animal fat, herbs and minerals to produce *yin* or *yang* effects on the surface of the skin.

Therapeutics

Mayan Incantations and Limpiezas

Incantations (Petz')

Incantations *(petz')* are orations and spells which are used to invoke the gods, to offer treatment of the ill, ask permission for curing, and ask the

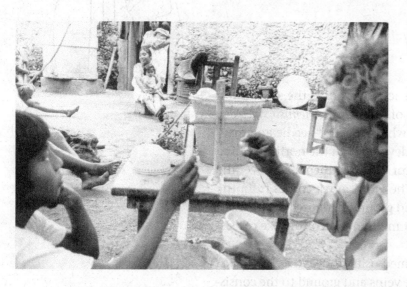

divinities to lift evil winds and diseases. Some orations are quite common, while others are used only on specific occasions.

In beginning any cure, Mayan *curanderos* generally invoke the protection of the Father *(nojoch bil)*, the Son *(mejen bil)*, and the Holy Ghost *(santo iik')*. Besides these invocations, a *curandero* might on occasion ask for the intervention of specific saints or Mayan deities. It is believed that the cure is performed by God, and that, if the *curandero* forgets this essential fact, even the strongest of medicinal plants may have no effect.

The ancient incantations, like those compiled in the book *Ritual of the Bacabes* are of the nature of symbolic, ritualistic poetry, that reveals the unity of medical, magical, and religious concepts. In these orations each disease is referred to by the moment of its birth during the creation of the universe—the animals, plants and objects associated with it are mentioned, as well as the cardinal points and the colors. The symptoms are announced by way of complex verbal games, as are the names of the gods who brought the illness, their place of habitation, and the site of final battle against the disease.

Contemporary Mayan orations have been passed down through generations of families or from *curandero* to *curandero,* and, although they retain some of their ancient characteristics, they have undergone vast changes. While there are many variations within the incantations, we have observed the consistency of particular structural elements. As an ancient rite, the holy trinity is invoked, as well as the help of the spirits of heaven and earth, and the *bacabes* who hold up the four pillars of the world. Through prayer the *curandero* asks the forces of nature—related with the four directions—and the gods or saints to come and "lift" the evil from the sick person. In other cases the *curandero* directly orders the evil influence to leave the body of the diseased, to let him or her free. The incantations are often related to orations used in agricultural rituals, which are recited in order to cure illnesses directly involved with the cycles of the earth.

When some of the *curanderos* perform their orations in Spanish traces of medieval Christian psalms and prayers are evident. One *curandero* in the region owns several ancient books—including the writings of Saint Ciprian (from the year 1001) and a collection of spells and psalms sent as a gift in 1740 from the Pope Leon Magnus to the Emperor Charles Magnus—and he uses orations and charms to accompany medical treatment.

MAYAN ORATION IN CURRENT PRACTICE

Jalal in t'aal	*From the water place I come*
tu k'aba bacan	*in the name of Bacan*
tu kantis ka'an	*in the four points of Heaven*
tu kamal in t'aal	*twice they circle*
tu kana ya'ab in lu'um	*high over the Earth*
Kin talin in tan kex	*I come to speak to you*
Tin káchiik t'ik tech	*I am tying you to the wind*
yum a'ximbalex kotenex	*Let the passing spirits come here*
tia'a uam k'oom	*to help us*
alutzik' le kojani	*to relieve the illness*
tiauala balche'o	*of your servant*
Ah kalan ch'aak	*You, drunken rain!*
ah ximbal k'aax	*You who pass by the wild places!*
ah jo'ya'ka'ax	*Water the wild places!*
ah Dios yumbilo'ob	*God of the spirits of wild places!*
ah Dios yumbil ak lak'in	*God spirit of the East!*
ah Dios yumbil xaman yumtzil	*God powerful spirit of the North!*
ah Dios yumbil chikin yumtzil	*God powerful spirit of the West!*
ah Dios yumbil ah nojol yumtzil	*God powerful spirit of the South!*

CLEANSINGS (LU'USA' K'EEBAAN)

Cleansings *(lu'usa' k'eebaan)* include a variety of ritual activities to expel evil winds from the body. Mayan *curanderos* understand evil wind to be a harmful or pernicious influence that arises from air, water, or food, and is transmitted by living beings or by the gods and spirits.

The *j'meen* treats those ill with evil wind with cleansings. Reciting prayers, laying hands on the body, and sweeping the air around the body with various plants, the *j'meen* seeks to expel the wind from the body and balance the thermal condition. In the ritual cleansing called *k'ej,* or "change," the patient arrives with an animal, plant, egg, or other object and the *curandero,* passing the evil wind into the object or animal, leaves the patient free of the illness. Several eggs may be used if the evil wind is very strong. The eggs are opened into a cup with a small amount of water and are read to see what sort of damage is being caused by the evil wind. The *curandero,* sweeping the head, arms, and legs of the patient towards the four direction, invokes God the Father, the Son, and the Holy Ghost. Some *curanderos* also invoke Santiago

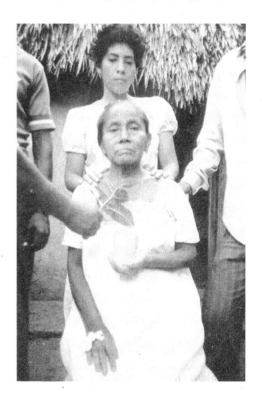

Therapeutics

Caballero and the Sacred Heart of Jesus. After the cleansing, the animal dies, the plant changes color and dries out, and the eggs go bad and are thrown away.

Among a group of Mayan *curanderos* speaking of the cleansing of evil winds we witnessed the following scene: one of the *j'meenob* said to the others, "you can perform an experiment. I have done it many times to prove that it works. You take a bundle of branches that you've just used and put them in a glass of water with another bunch that you haven't used, and see which goes bad first. This experiment never fails."

We asked if this might simply be caused by the shaking of the branches used in the cleansing, and he told us, "well, shake the clean branches over a healthy person or a strong and healthy tree, and you will still see the difference. Just don't shake it over the bed of the sick person, because it could pick up some of the evil wind. When the cleansing is complete the plant always changes color."

Another *curandero* present added, "for plants to pick up the evil wind the work of the *curandero* is necessary; the *curandero* uses spells to push the wind to where the plant can suck it up. And we always burn the plants when we finish, to avoid doing any harm."

We asked if it made a difference that the plants had their origins in other countries, like rue and basil which were brought by the Spaniards. "It doesn't matter as long as they pick up the evil wind," we were told. "We prefer to use *tzipche'* (Bunchosia schwartziana, Gr.) and *chalche'* (Pluchea odorata, L.). *Tzipche'* smells like mahogany and has yellow flowers and red fruit. *Chalché* has a strong anis scent. The odor repels the bad winds, and the colors red and yellow, which are warm, attract cold air and draw the wind from the body."

The plants used in cleansings are considered to have strong balancing properties. The most commonly used plants combine strong scent with warm colors like yellow and red. After the cleansing, to complete the process of eliminating wind, the patient is recommended a diet based on the thermal nature of his body and illness. If the wind is cold, for example, warm foods are recommended.

All of the objects, whether they be of living or inert origin, are gathered up and burned far from where people pass so as to do no harm. The animals used die in the course

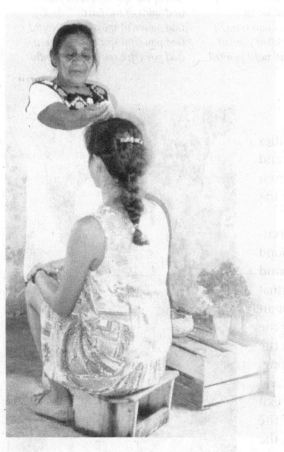

Spirit cleansing with an egg.

of the cleansing; afterward the corpse may be opened and the insides examined to find where the evil resided.

The rites of the *j'meen* are sometimes carried out in the shade of the *yaaxche'*, ceiba *(Ceiba pentandra)*, a tree central to Maya symbology and possessed of its own spirit. Other trees recognized as having distinct spirits include *pich, tzacan,* and *bacalche'* (walnut). In some places the *j'meen* will hug the tree as part of the ritual.

In Nunkiní, municipality of Calkiní in the state of Campeche, a collective cleansing ritual is performed. This is the same

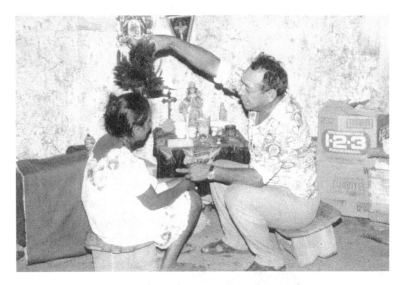

Spirit cleansing with a chicken.

community where the *Ritual of the Bacabes* is supposed to have been written. The cleansing ritual is carried out twice a year—on the 18th of April (in honor of San Diego de Alcalá), and on the 12th of November. These celebrations witness the ritual of the burning of the *u dzuli k'aak'*, or Horse of Fire. The story goes that in the middle of the seventh century the population of Nunkiní was exploited by the *dzules* (the rich). In punishment, the town was stricken by an outbreak of smallpox, which decimated the population. A *curandero,* after having a revelation, suggested that an effigy be made from old rags which would represent the rich, who were responsible for the plague. A ceremony was held in which all of the sick people touched the effigy to pass their illness into it. It was later burned. According to the story, the disease miraculously vanished. The ritual is repeated every year to continue protecting the population from illness and evil winds. There is a special society which organizes the event. Every day during the celebration, they bring out the figure and carry it from house to house for all to touch. Later, on the 18th of April and the 12th of November, the figure is carried to the plaza, where a long wick and rosary of fireworks is attached to it. The combination of bonfire and explosions creates a tremendous spectacle—it is this fire which destroys the evil wind and banishes it from the community for the time being.

The figure, previously made simply from grain sacks in the form of a human being, is now dressed in the fine clothes that its rich condition dictates. Since 1993 it has been accompanied by a *xunan,*

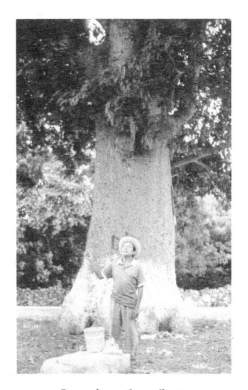

Prayer beneath a ceiba tree.

Therapeutics

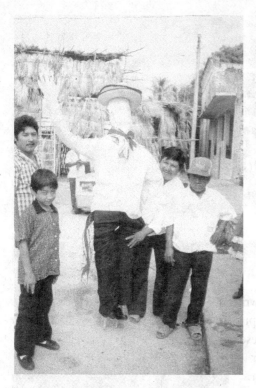

The dzuli k'aak'.

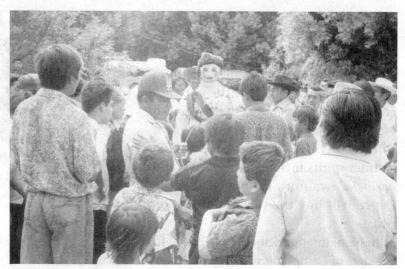

The xunan k'aak'.

or rich woman, dressed similarly in fancy clothes and fake jewelry. It is said that the company of the *xunan k'aak'*, the wife of the original figure, wards off the new threat of illness that was first perceived during an outbreak of cholera here in 1992.

CHI KUNG IN CHINESE PRACTICE

The word *chi,* (life energy), combined with the word *gong, gung* or *kung* (art, work, or practice), describes the art of developing, balancing, and circulating *chi* throughout the body. By means of the art of *chi kung,* health is preserved and developed—bringing as a consequence the prevention and control of illnesses and the prolongation of life. *Chi kung* is also used to reestablish the equilibrium of a body recovering from disease. It is an art and a healing practice integral to the Chinese medical system—a series of activities with a basis in spirituality whose goal is the perfection of balance in the body and the spirit.

Chi kung brings to bear three modes of action—known as the three basic factors of *chi kung.*

1. Tuning the breath to obtain *vital* or *essential chi.* This includes different exercises in inhaling, exhaling, deep breathing, blowing, and holding the breath. The theory of *chi kung* affirms that, by way of the breath, one

can regulate the function of the autonomic nervous system and control disorders such as hypertension, gastric ulcer and neurasthenia, as well as diminish internal secretions, lower cholesterol, and improve cardiovascular health.

2. Establishing a state of mental tranquility by way of concentration and relaxation exercises which "sharpen the light of the heart-mind" (the mental *daoyin)*. This is achieved by concentrating on a specific object to relax the cerebral cortex. This mental state can reverse mental pathologies and aid in the treatment of chronic illnesses of the heart, liver, lung, and spleen as well as systemic illnesses such as cancer and neurosis.

3. Maintaining harmony among the organs by "configuring the body" through movement techniques and exercises. It is said that by way of the dual action of movement and repose the secretion of bile is balanced—thereby regulating the digestive function.

Chi kung methods taught in Chinese schools are often interrelated with other similar principles in medicine and spiritual practice in Taoism, Buddhism, Confucianism and other traditional Chinese philosophies.

Chi kung stimulates the internal *chi* flow by draining the meridians to allow circulation and dispersing negative or pernicious *chi*. The expulsion of rotten or stagnant elements in the body—the obtaining of "pure *yang*"—is achieved through *chi kung*. The essential *chi* is tonified and invigorated by the healthy circulation of fluids through the body and by balancing *yin* and *yang* energies. When the *chi* is adequate it works to protect the body from all pernicious influences and external toxins.

There are various types of medical *chi kung*. One of them is *tai chi ch'uan*, a series of exercises designed to balance the body and spirit and thus prevent illness. Another method used specifically as a therapy for ill people takes the form of a series of exercises designed to strengthen organs and meridians. In a third form known as external chi healing a therapist—by way of a series of concentration and breathing exercises—can project her own energy into her hands. Sweeping the patient's body with her hands, she stimulates circulation, balances the body's energies, and expels pernicious influences.

Medical *chi kung* is relatively unknown in the West because of its incompatibility with occidental science and because its secrets have been carefully guarded in China. With philosophical roots common to both medicine and ancient religious practice, *chi kung* can be considered the element of Chinese medicine with the closest affinity to spiritual undertaking. Though current Chinese medicine is practiced separately from religion, in *chi kung* we can trace the ancient roots of the modern practice back to early Taoist and Buddhist meditations.

Religious *chi kung* exists to the present day through Taoist, Buddhist, and Confucian currents. In these schools the movements of the body are combined with orations and, at times, with *yi* (divination). The goal is to obtain "pure *yang*" and to reach physical and spiritual perfection, manifested as radiant health.

Recently, in China and other parts of the world, investigations have been undertaken to explain the "scientific" basis of the phenomena of *chi kung*. The exercises of *chi kung* have been shown to lower the lactic acid content of the blood and diminish the activity of the peripheral nervous system and of rennin—a secretion of the kidneys involved in regulating blood pressure. The density of prolactin in the plasma is incremented and the secretion of cortisone falls to close to 50%; these hormonal changes can explain the retardation of the aging process and the strengthening of the immune system which are some benefits of *chi kung*.

It has been demonstrated with an electroencephalogram that a practitioner of *chi kung* emits low frequency vibrations three times higher than a non-practitioner—suggesting that *chi kung* helps to build the electromagnetic activity of the brain, thus augmenting cerebral function.[38] Similarly, researchers Lu Zuyin and Wang Yaolan have discovered that the field of energy generated around the practitioners during the exercises of *chi kung* can be registered with a detector of thermoluminescence.[39]

Researchers have also studied the projection of energy known as external chi healing—the form of medical *chi kung* in which a therapist generates a field of energy and lays hands on the patient. The majority of these studies investigate the physical characteristics of the *chi* emitted. The results have been surprising and fascinating. It has been observed, for example, that the energy emitted by a *chi kung* therapist can stop the discharging process between the two poles of a Van de Graff generator and that the energy emitted in *chi kung* can be registered on a Geiger counter.

CHAPTER 6

TRADITIONAL HEALTH WORKERS

TRADITIONAL
MAYAN HEALERS

TRADITIONAL MAYAN medicine embodies a range of practices performed by shamans *(j'meenob),* herbalists, midwives, masseuses, bone setters, and other skilled practitioners. Researchers often tend to identify the different indigenous medical practitioners with occidental medical specialists, explaining, for example, that "the herbalist would be the general practitioner; the midwife the gynecologist, the bone setter the trauma specialist; and the *curandero* the psychiatrist." This analogy is overly reductive and has little bearing in reality. For the Mayan people, conceptions about the work of curing are fundamentally different from occidental ideas. All curing agents typically perform the role of doctor, psychiatrist, and priest.

Practically all medical workers know something of herbology, and all invoke God the Father and the diverse gods in beginning their work of healing. Many have a profound intuitive and empirical knowledge of the human spirit. They understand the problems of their communities and are capable of producing a strong emotional impact in their patients. Treatment of the patient is familiar and friendly, and illnesses are understood within the context of the social life and history of the patient. Often the patient's family is present for the consultation, and it is not infrequent that a collective cure will be performed. It is notable, as well, that the majority of traditional healers belong to the same social class as their patients.

The traditional doctor puts the holistic conception of health and illness into practice. Disease is never viewed as an isolated problem; no illness of the body will be treated without regard to the spirit. The toxic influence that can surge from the environment is widely taken as the root of illness. Microbiological factors are unknown; rather, toxic influences come about as the result of the rupture of harmony in one's own body, in the family, in society, in nature, or among the divine beings.

There exist among the Maya other specialized medical practitioners: there are specialists in fright, in *dzibolal* (desire), and in *manu jana'* (collapse of the crown). There is, as well, a propensity towards specializing in more than one practice—so we find masseuse midwives, midwife *j'meenob*, midwife herbalists, and herbalist masseuse midwife *j'meenob*, for example. Thus, rather than thinking of traditional health workers as "doctors" with all of the specialization and accreditation implied, we might think of them as "healers" in a very broad sense.

Another problem that is posed for the Westerner when looking at Mayan traditional medicine is that there is no fine line between a *curandero* and

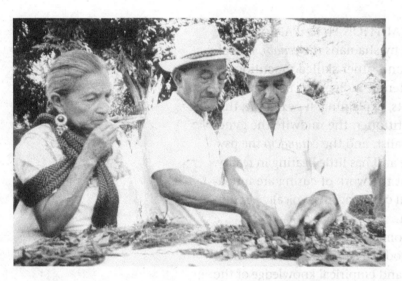

a lay person; there exists no clear difference, in practice, between "domestic medicine" and "traditional medicine." A blacksmith may gain fame as a bone setter; an old man who doesn't consider himself a *curandero* in the least might be considered by his community to be the local authority on *dzibolal,* the disease of desire. It is very common for women, notably grandmothers and older women, to have elaborate knowledge of acupuncture techniques which they practice on their children, grandchildren, and perhaps the children of their neighbors. Some of these "lay people" might take up further study, develop a more extensive practice, and learn from other *curanderos* until they become known as healers among their community.

The formation of each *curandero* is as unique as her or his individual teachers, inspiration, and experience. Although the cosmovision underlying systematic treatment is generally held in common, the handling of particular diseases varies greatly among traditional health workers. There is no school which organizes a curriculum of study and certifies that a healer is, indeed, a healer (as exist in both occidental and Chinese traditions). For this reason, although we recognize that many individuals possess a set of medical understandings, the title "traditional doctor" is often inappropriate to a community healer, lay herbalist, or grandmother who cures with her hands.

In occidental culture there are many people who have extensive medical knowledge (nurses, pharmacists, masseuses, interns and clinic attendants, as well as chronically ill individuals who have come to understand the dynamics of disease and treatment). Although they may be called upon at times to resolve problems regarding health, society in general understands that these people are not doctors and that their knowledge and skills are limited (although, at the same time, there are certified doctors of medicine who perhaps should not be given the responsibility of healing). These qualifications do not apply when looking at "traditional healers." The category of healer or *curandero* is one which often goes unrecognized in the community. A woman who is considered an expert in *dzibolal* is not nec-

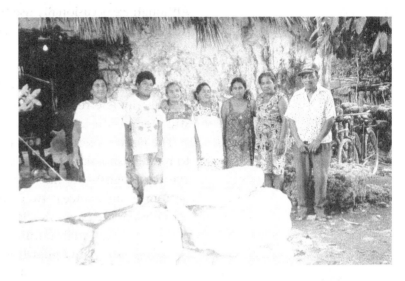

essarily an indigenous medic or doctor, and may not be considered a *curandera* or healer; she is simply someone who knows about *dzibolal.*

The economics of healing—how healers charge for their services—is another subject which has no uniform rules or recognizable standards. Many *curanders* are *campesinos*—subsistence farmers who rely on their own agricultural labor—or make their living at some other profession (like masonry or carpentry). In general healing service is rendered for little or no fee. In other cases, being a *curandero* or midwife may be an individual's only way of earning a living, and he or she may not be able to afford the luxury of working for free. This is common among older people who can no longer work in the *milpa* or exercise their other skills. In other instances, the fee may be charged in kind, or the patient may be asked to give what he can beyond the price of the materials.

The payment may, of course, depend on the type of treatment offered. The same fee will not be charged for the prescription of herbs as for a *limpieza,* which generally commands a higher price. Prices will often differ for an indigenous patient and for a *mestizo* with money. The majority of *curanderos* where we worked ask, for a simple consultation, between five and fifteen *pesos* (roughly seventy cents to two dollars at the time of this writing), although there are cases of *curanderos* who, for a spirit cleansing against witchcraft, will charge as much as 500 *pesos* (roughly seventy dollars).

THE ROLE OF THE J'MEEN

Although we occasionally use the word *curandero* to refer to all traditional healers, the title most commonly used on the Yucatán Peninsula is *j'meen*. Among the Tzeltal and Tzotzil Maya in the state of Chiapas the role of *j'meen* is differentiated into two categories: the *ilol* (pulsetaker), and the *x'oponej witz* (he-who-prays-in-the-hills). In some communities the *j'meen* is generally referred to (in Spanish), as *yerbatero* (herbalist), which lends still more confusion to the assigning of roles and titles.

The *j'meen* is not simply a traditional doctor. He or she has the power to reestablish balance in those suffering from diseases of the spirit (evil eye, loss, fright)—for having violated some natural or supernatural law—or from an imbalance between cold and hot energies—produced by foods, activities, or the patient's relation with others. He or she is responsible for

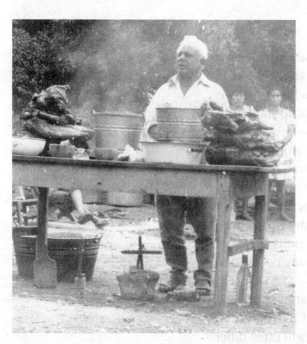

maintaining the internal cohesion of the community and guarding the traditions of the people. The social function of the *j'meen* is to maintain equilibrium among the spiritual and supernatural forces that surround the Mayan community and are manifested on both an individual and collective level. The *j'meen* is a spiritual leader trusted by the people.

The primordial role of the *j'meen* is associated with agriculture; in the centrality of the *milpa* to Mayan health and social life we find the root of the *j'meen's* role as both overseer of the agricultural cycle and healer. The relationship of the *milpa* to the supernatural forces of the gods and *aluxob* has repercussions in the health of the entire community, and the *j'meen* mediates between the community and these forces. The role of the *j'meen* is, above all, preventive. He is in charge of establishing and maintaining a good relation between the community and the spirits of wild places. This activity is realized by way of a number of rituals: *ch'a chak* (praying for rain), *maan chak* (buying rain) *jets' lu'un* (nourishing the earth), *jani kool* (feeding the *aluxob*), *wajil kool* (giving thanks for the harvest), *jo'olche* (the offering of the first corn), and *lu'usa' k'eebaan*.

There is one major difference between the role of the *j'meen* and the other healers. Bone setters, herbalists and midwives might learn their skills and their personal practice in an apprenticeship or an extended course of study and practice, as one learns to be a carpenter or a parent. The skills of the *j'meen,* however, in establishing relations with the spirit world and curing diseases of the soul, are said to be a gift of the gods. This gift includes the power to control the winds and currents of air, the spirits, the helpers of the divinities, and the divinities themselves. It is not required that the *j'meen* have a will to study or learn. It is a divine gift that is perfected with practice.

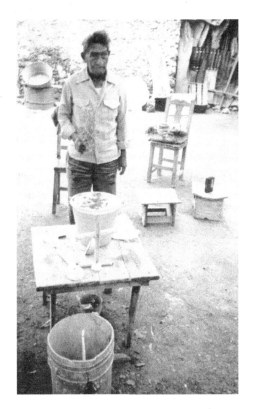

There are different ways by which the divinities choose their apprentice; it might happen at birth, in the strike of a lightning bolt or other natural sign, or it might be revealed in a dream. The traditional authorities and the community will recognize the initiate, who may be sent to the traditional healers for her or his formation. Those who are born with this gift and who begin to exercise it upon reaching the age of eighteen are called "illuminated." Other *j'meenob* are disciples of the illuminated, and undergo twenty or thirty years of apprenticeship.

It is common for one who is going to be a *j'meen* to go into the hills for three days to fast "in direct contact with the spirits." In this period the apprentice acquires the potential energy and the knowledge that will be developed later; it is also in this time that the *sastún* is found. If the initiate does not find a *sastún* during his journey, on returning to the community he will not become a *j'meen.*

One may also become a *j'meen* by simply finding a *sastún* in the hills. One then proceeds to a consultation with a *j'meen,* who "reads the luck" of the initiate and reveals the spiritual design.

Each *j'meen* is distinguished by his *sastún.* The number of *sastúnob* in the possession of a *j'meen* is the measure of his skills and power. If a thief steals a *sastún,* it is said that he will be attacked by an evil wind which will bring illness and possibly death. Some *j'meenob* refer to series of dreams in which they discover the properties of plants. At a certain age the *j'meen* proposes a successor and, three days before turning over his power, he returns his *sastún* to the Earth.

Jup and *tok,* the most common techniques for expelling evil winds, are commonly practiced by *j'meenob* more than by other healers. It is not uncommon for a *j'meen* to perform a *limpia* as a diagnostic looking for the evil wind, and to then apply *jup* and *tok* to expel the wind from the body.

Besides being in charge of agrarian rituals and cleansings, *j'meenob* are also responsible for performing ceremonial rituals like *jetzmek* and *yook ja'* (types of baptisms), *uxiibtaal paal* (the rite of passage in which youth of thirteen or fourteen years of age are presented to the community), and *k'amnicte* (the marriage ceremony).

At the present moment the tradition of the *j'meen* is in crisis. The majority are of a very advanced age, and there are very few youth undergoing apprenticeships. Many communities currently lack a *j'meen*, and their inhabitants are forced to go long distances to ask for a ritual or a curing. The absence of *j'meenob* is common in recently formed communities with settlers from other ethnic regions. This crisis is accompanied by disorganization, loss of values, and community disputes. In many cases the lack of initiates and general inattention to the culture of the *j'meen* is due to the work of Protestant sects. These sects attack traditional medicine, modes of dress, traditional celebrations, and Mayan languages as "fountains of sin and idolatry," continuing the opposition to indigenous values that began with the conquest. The strongest influence working against the practice of the *j'meen*, however, is the dominant local, national, and international ideology. Ancient values and the knowledge of past generations is dicarded in favor of everything modern. In the modern economy the *j'meen* has no price, and therefore no value.

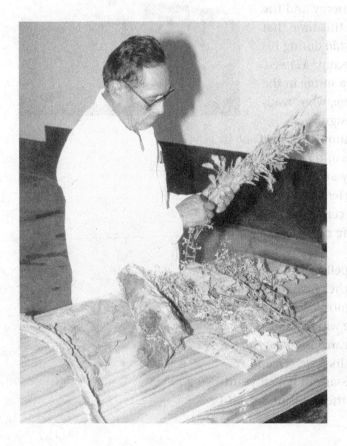

HERBALISTS OR TZAK XIU

Tzak xiu are traditional health agents who are experts in the use of medicinal plants. A recognized herbalist will be familiar with the applications of over 200 plants. Many herbalists are, at the same time, *j'meenob*, or have some of the marks and the training of the *j'meen*.

Due to the politics of state institutions such as the National Indigenous Institute (INI) and various private groups there is a tendency for Mayan herbalists to become simple herb sellers. A distinction is made in Spanish between "*yerberos,*" (herb sellers), and "*yerbateros,*" (herbalists). *Yerberos* elaborate medicines from plant bases and sell them, without necessarily giving a consultation first; the role approaches that of pharmacist rather than healer. In this way, the work of the herbalist meets the logic of the market and becomes at once more visible and less effective—a spectacle which gives rise to deep misunderstandings of the traditional culture.

Masseuses and Bone Setters

Masseuse and bone setter are two distinct categories of traditional medical specializations, although bone setters often perform both functions. They are often people with no special experience or training who realize that they have a special touch in their hands which comforts the ill. The skill of the masseuse and bone setter is generally considered to be an innate quality of the individual.

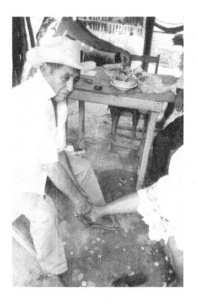

Masseuses (*sobadores* in Spanish) are those who perform *talladas* (rubbings) in their various forms; they heal with their hands. They can detect, with great precision, irregularities in the tendons and muscles, and they understand the treatment of rheumatoid illnesses, pain from tension, trauma, "the opening of the hips," the *cirro*, etcetera.

Mayan masseuses are commonly experts in diseases of the skin, and their area of knowledge encompasses muscles, tendons, and bones—the entire supporting structure and surface of the body. The skill of the masseuse involves intense observation and practice. Many of them prepare their own salves for common illnesses like rheumatism, wind, pimples, heat rash, scabies, and other surface infections. Masseuses are often well-versed in *jup* and *tok*. A simple, localized massage treatment will cost around five *pesos* (less than a dollar), and a whole body massage may cost twice that.

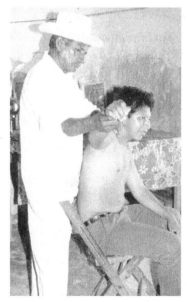

Bone setters, besides practicing rubbings, *jup* and *tok,* know how to set broken bones and fractures. Considering the absence of x-ray technology, Mayan bone setters are remarkably efficient at their craft. They commonly use various species of plants to aid the reconstruction of bone tissue and speed the healing process.

Midwives

Midwives are responsible for illnesses in women, care and treatment during pregnancy, the overseeing of labor and birth, and treatment of infantile diseases. Generally they are practitioners of massage who often practice *jup* and *tok* as well. They are familiar with the array of medicinal plants for women with problems in pregnancy, labor, or recovery. The majority of midwives attend an average of one to four births each month.

Until a few years ago, the midwife in a Mayan community was known as the *gaan champal* or *nojoch mam*, "the mother of the village." Everyone greeted the midwife with respect, recognizing in her the force that brought them into the world. Recently, however, the Mayan name of "the mother

Traditional Health Workers

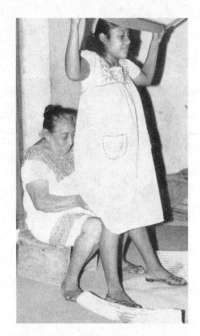

A midwife attending a traditional birth.

of all people" has been left behind in favor of the Spanish *partera*—meaning, simply, "midwife."

The majority of midwives currently are of an advanced age, and are poor. The youngest that we have met is forty-five years old, the oldest, seventy-three. Of twenty midwives in Campeche that we know, the average age is 63 years. The length of their practice varies between eight and thirty years, averaging about eighteen. It is notable that the majority began the practice of midwifery later in life. Some are self-taught, beginning with the experience of their own labor, while others are initiated by their mother, grandmother, mother-in-law, an aunt, or a friend. The majority of the midwives that we know have children already married, leaving them free to practice and attend births. Others live alone, are widows, or have sympathetic husbands who support their work without complaint. The role of the midwife, though not as prestigious as in the past, is recognized by the community and midwives are generally treated with an esteem that is not given to other women. In this way they achieve a greater social role than most women.

Midwifery in Campeche is subject to rigorous control by official institutions like the Department of Social Security and the National Indigenous Institute. Many midwives participate in a monthly course offered by the Department of Social Security. The general content of the courses is dictated by the State and covers family planning, infant nutrition, vaccinations, and general medicine. Currently, all of the midwives who participate in these courses are paid forty *pesos* (about five dollars) a month.

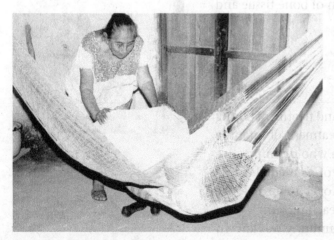

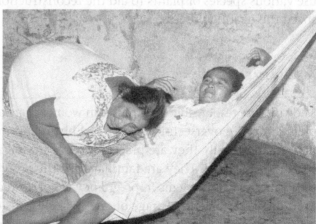

Above: A midwife attending a birth in a hammock. Right: A midwife using medical instruments.

TRADITIONAL HEALTH WORKERS IN CHINESE MEDICINE

Chinese history has seen the appearance of countless types of medical therapies. Roberto González,[40] citing the *Shuoyuan* of Lin Xian, comments that medicine began with the magical techniques of the *wuren* (shamans) who gradually began to use alcohol, plants, and other medicinal products to perform cures. In another Chinese text, the *Shang Hai Jing*, it is said that on Mount Lin—the mountain of the spirit—there were ten groups of shamans,

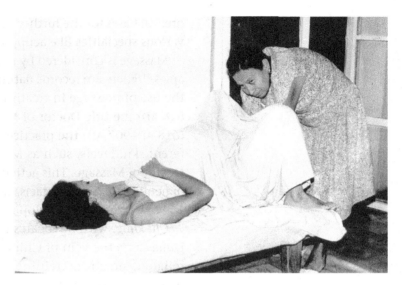

A midwife attending a modern-style birth.

including the *wuxian* (universal shamans) and the *wupeng* (old shamans) who collected wild medicinal plants. The *wupeng* were probably the first to use the herbal pharmacopoeia during the *Shang* dynasty (16th century BC –1066 BC).

During the Eastern *Zhou* dynasty a strong pragmatic tendency became prevalent which rejected metaphysical concepts. In this period came about the separation of the functions of the *wu* and the *yi*. The *wu* could be considered a sort of shaman or witch whose healing work is involved with spiritual and magical practices. Generally these shamans, besides practicing magic, had a strong knowledge of herbs. The *yi* would be the medical doctor in the more familiar sense, whose practice became formalized and regulated by the Chinese nobility. These doctors made wide use of the pharmacopoeia, and prepared medicinal liqueurs. Their knowledge was systematized in textbooks and taught in schools throughout China. These two strains of medical laborers have existed throughout Chinese history. Among these strains fine divisions have formed. Since ancient times the *yi* have been differentiated into four specific groups:

- the *yi*, who work with nutrition and general health;
- the *shi ji yi* who deal in internal medicine;
- the *yang yi*, in charge of the study and treatment of tumors, ulcers and fractures;
- the *shou yi*, in charge of veterinary medicine.

Further on, philosophic and religious thought had a determined influence on the evolution of medicine; Taoism and Confucianism formed the-

Traditional Health Workers

oretical bases for the further development of traditional medicine and the various specialties like acupuncture, herbology, and massage.

Massage is considered by many to be the oldest of the traditional therapies.[41] There are records dating back 2500 years which make reference to the use of massage in treating illness. During the *Sui* Dynasty (581 AD–618 AD) the title Doctor of Massage appeared, and in the *T'ang* Dynasty (618 AD–907 AD) the practice of massage was classified according to different skill levels, such as Massage Technician, Master of Massage, and Doctor of Massage. This activity was linked to herbology through the use of poultices, creams, extracts, and liniments. In the *Ming* Dynasty (1368 AD–1644 AD) came the development of child and infant massage.

Chi kung, with advocates in various sects of Buddhism, Taoism and Lamaism is the vein of Chinese medicine with the strongest element of religious practice. Training in *chi kung,* both as a sport and a medical therapy, can begin at a very young age. In the case of medical *chi kung* it is important that the therapy continue over the course of years if it is to be truly effective.

Herbalists and acupuncturists are other groups of traditional healers with roots going back thousands of years. Their work, derived from the traditions of the *wuren,* is typified by study and practice of herbalism, or more specifically, of the *ben cao,* which combines the use of plants with the use of substances of animal and mineral origin (as discussed in chapter five). In hospitals to this day medicinal plants are used in treatments in specific fields such as neurology, gastroenterology and gynecology, and detailed work is undertaken by pharmacists in preparing botanical medicines.

Within the practice of acupuncture there are professionals who specialize in the use of a specific instrument or technique such as the plum-blossom needle (an instrument combining a number of needles on the head of a small hammer), electric acupuncture, or laser acupuncture. There are special techniques like *mang zhen* (long needle), used by relatively few acupuncturists. Others specialize in bleeding techniques or specific groups of illnesses, like those who work with vascular cerebral trauma—whose training includes studies of neurology, internal medicine, and the English language.

Another important branch of acupuncture, relatively unknown outside of China, is anesthesiology. Applied alone or in conjunction with topical anesthetics or muscle relaxants this discipline has achieved great success. Acupunctural anesthesia is commonly used in the performance of Cesarean sections.

The more common formal medical practices currently studied in China include, among others, herbology, traditional pharmacology, acupuncture, massage and *chi kung*. Each of these specialties is practiced in the field and in clinics and hospitals that specialize in traditional medicine. Often acupuncture, massage, *chi kung,* and the use of herbs are combined in the treatment of a single case. Each specialist in the various fields studies for four or five years to achieve license in her or his practice. The different disciplines begin from the common trunk of traditional medical theory and then branch off into the particular practices; at the same time, courses are given in Western medical theory which complement the study of the Chinese system. Doctors with Western medical training can study for Master's Degrees in acupuncture or other fields like *chi kung*—whose course of study lasts six years.

The traditional doctor in China, like other professionals who work for a government institution, receives relatively low pay. The saying goes, "it is better to work the outside of the head than the inside," referring to the fact that a barber may earn more than twice as much as a neurosurgeon.

There is currently a strong movement among traditional Chinese doctors to do research in various branches of Western medical science in order to deepen their understanding of occidental physiology. Researchers also work towards the reconstruction and interpretation of their own history and traditional knowledge using ancient texts, recovering their content through clinical investigations in accordance with present health care needs.

CHAPTER 7

THE EVOLUTION
OF TRADITIONAL MEDICINE

MAYAN TRADITION
AND WESTERN
MEDICINE

WE BELIEVE THAT, before the arrival of the Spanish in the beginning of the sixteenth century, there were two general forms or levels of indigenous medicine—a popular medicine and a medicine reserved for the practice of studied elites.

On the elite level highly trained healers formed part of a social class which had access to the written word and systematized information. This medicine had a great deal to do with astrology; it was important for the healer to know facts such as the patient's date of birth (which had great influence on the rest of her or his life and propensity towards particular patterns of disease). Knowledge of astrology, writing, herbology and surgical technique are a few examples of the kind of specialized information in which the elite healer would be trained.

On the popular level knowledge was less specialized and less systematized, though it must have been inscribed by the same cosmovision and understanding of health and disease as the elite medicine. The most notable traditions would have been the herbal pharmacopoeia and the rituals which affirmed the relation of personal health to the agricultural cycle and to natural and supernatural forces.

The Classic period of Mayan civilization had long passed by the time the Spanish *conquistadores* arrived. With the conquest of the indigenous nations by the Spanish the loss of formalized medicine—and all of its representatives and technologies—was completed. On the Yucatán Peninsula this loss is due to the unfortunately celebrated Friar Diego de Landa, who banished to oblivion innumerable writings and codices which took as their subjects the sciences, art, religion, and the civic and political life of the pre-conquest Maya.

In Campeche and Yucatán many concepts were lost, such as the relation of disease to the calendar and the patient's astrological assignation (although this knowledge continues to be practiced to varying degrees in some regions of Guatemala and Chiapas).

The more popular understandings and practices have not suffered such a devastating loss. In many cases the fundament of the traditional concepts was preserved and assimilated with concepts and practices from colonial Spanish medicine (like the introduction of plants of European origin). It is important to note that the fundamental mechanism of reproduction of these concepts was (and still is) the oral tradition—which, upon losing the conceptual systematization of the more elite medicine, began losing richness and cohesion, transforming generation by generation into a different medicine altogether. The loss of knowledge and customs differed according to the origin of each practice; this differentiation explains why some practices were lost completely while others were conserved. The concepts and practices that were not lost in the violent shock of the meeting of the two cultures entered into a process of defense and syncretism with colonial Spanish medicine, African medicine (by way of the slave trade), and, more recently, modern occidental medicine.

Like any cultural system, traditional medicine undergoes constant change. As it encounters new factors, it replaces ancient Mayan concepts with conceptions and words from the Spanish colonial era or from modern medicine, incorporating them into the cosmovision.

Mayan illnesses can be classified into four groups:

- Organic illnesses
- Illnesses produced by contact with other people
- Illnesses of divine origin brought about by supernatural forces
- Illnesses related to the individual's astrology (the role of destiny)

Many of the organic illnesses recognized presently by the Maya have their counterparts in occidental medicine. In workshops with *curanderos* we have noted the following correspondences in terms that denote known and recognized illnesses:

- *Wach' k'aja'al, wach' it*—common diarrhea
- *Taki'ik*—dysentery
- *Tu chokui tu choche*—intestinal fever
- *Chuu kal*—sourness in the stomach
- *K'an chik'in*—disease of the spleen
- *Se'en*—catarrh
- *K'alwix*—water retention

- *Chujuk wix*—diabetes
- *Sapu' k'ab uyim*—lack of milk after birthing
- *Sak wech*—scabies

For all of these illnesses the traditional healer uses herbal therapy more than anything else. In the treatment of these illnesses we see strong competition between herbalists and Western doctors. In many areas people are accepting technological change, and, although they continue preparing their household medicines with the same plants, they stop consulting with herbalists. The difference in cost for examination and treatment ensures that a significant part of the population continues consulting with traditional healers, and traditional medicine still dominates the field in the area of midwifery and in cases where massage is clearly indicated. At the same time there exists a series of organic and supernatural illnesses which have no counterpart in occidental medicine—which the Western doctor can neither recognize nor treat. For this reason the services of traditional healers remain in demand. Some of these illnesses, which are unrecognized by Western terminology, include:

- *Tipté*—fall of the *cirro*, untied *cirro*, tight *cirro*
- *Xaka taa*—nocturnal defecation which leaves the umbilicus chilled
- *Tzan nu yaal*—collapse of the crown
- *Manu jana'*—swelling in the abdomen
- *Minana nu yool, ma ool*—collapse of the *ool*, collapse of the spirit
- *Al kaximba*—corrimiento, "running"
- *Xoco ola'*—heat
- *Ju naaki*—*pasmo;* astonishment, or chill (a sort of cramp related to blood stagnation or wind in the body)
- *Je'k'a'*—opening of the hips

There exists as well a series of spiritual illnesses which are treated with simple blessings. These illnesses generally require the attention of a *j'meen.* These spiritual illnesses include:

- *Tu menta ojo, ojo chambal*—evil eye
- *Chup yo'lal dzibolal*—swelling caused by the envy of seeing another satiate his hunger; desire for food
- *Xak olal*—fright in infants (from birth to two years old)
- *Sa'kil*—fright in older children
- *Uiik, K'ak'asiik*—evil wind borne by children from birth
- *K'ak'as iik'*—evil wind in general

- *Iikal xoch*—wind of the owl, a disease of newborn infants
- *Iikal alux*—wind of the *alux*
- *Tu jentan ta iik al mozon*—whirlwind
- *K'akal iik*—wind from the *cuyos* (the ancestral burial mounds)

Besides the existence of traditional illnesses that are untreatable by Western methods, there are other factors which favor the pragmatic use of traditional medical practices. In many areas the *curanderos*, because of the social role that they play, continue to be treat organic illnesses. The herbalist is the traditional healer of the poor. Because of their distribution throughout the population and the type and cost of their prescribed remedies and services, herbalists are more accessible to the rural poor population and present a practical alternative for many illnesses—especially in areas where medical attention and health services are scarce. We must also look at the relation between the healer and the patient. The traditional health worker and the patient are generally of the same social class and culture, favoring a more sympathetic relationship than that between the rural, poor indigenous and the urban-trained *mestizo*.

For spiritual illnesses, whether they be of human or divine origin, modern medicine presents no alternative. In these cases people generally continue consulting with *curanderos*, unless some pressure, (often brought to bear by the conflict with modern medicine), causes them to do otherwise. But many cases will be brought to a Western doctor unless only the touch of a *curandero* can do the job. People often will not hesitate to take advantage of both types of medicine. According to a certain sector of the population, traditional medicine can easily be complemented by modern medicine to achieve stronger results; some *curanderos* use Western pharmaceutical medicines in conjunction with traditional remedies. This line of reasoning is not reciprocated by many occidental doctors or health professionals.

Since the conquest an attack has been leveled against traditional Mexican medicine. The attack is currently led by forces in favor of the occidental corporate medical establishment—specifically private and institutional medical services, most notably the Mexican Secretary of Health. In the last decade we have seen the beginning of a process of recognition of Mexican indigenous medicine by some official institutions. The National Indigenous Institute and the Mexican Institute of Social Security, for example, have come to accept the herbal pharmacopoeia though they continue to deny the efficacy and denigrate the use of other traditional indigenous medical practices.

The Evolution
of Traditional Medicine

Though there now exists an open discussion about the advantages of traditional medicine within the halls of state institutions, a strong discrimination continues at all levels. The traditional medicine, lacking the methods and the aura of science, is subordinated to institutional medicine. Continued attempts are made to "Westernize" the *curanderos*. Without the slightest attempt to open a dialogue, they are given training in the values and concepts of occidental medicine in order to give them official medical status. Generally speaking, institutional doctors do not study and understand the traditional medicine; far less do they make use of its values and concepts in their practice.

Constant attacks are leveled against the *curanderos* by Western doctors, who tell the ill in the communities that the attention of a traditional healer will only cause them harm and worsen their condition. At times the attack of occidental medicine and dominant (institutional) ideology against the indigenous population weakens their confidence in their own traditions. Vain attempts are made to make modern concepts fill the spaces left in traditional culture and praxis. In many cases, however, the aggression of the institutional doctor is turned against him, generating a rejection of outside physicians.

Nevertheless, in many parts of Mexico (and specifically in the case of the Yucatán Peninsula), we are witnessing the appearance of groups of Western doctors who are beginning to value the traditional medicine, to respect and learn from it, to support its (re)systematization, and to reaffirm its understandings and practices.

CHINESE TRADITION AND WESTERN MEDICINE

A look at the long relation between traditional Chinese medicine and occidental medicine can help us to understand the dynamic that exists between traditional and modern medicines in Mesoamerica.

Traditional medicine, dominant in China from several thousand years before the time of Christ, continued developing under the stewardship of the emperor until the *Ching* dynasty (1644 AD–1911 AD). In this period the Manchu government developed a more open relation with the occident—especially with the English, who brought to bear strong economic and political pressure in favor of industrial development, especially in the last century.

In this last century occidental medicine was introduced by force and the traditional medicine was criticized as it was in Latin America—with the argument that acupuncture was an obsolete and superstitious practice and that the needles were instruments of torture. Acupuncture was excluded from official study and finally, after the Opium War, its practice was altogether prohibited. This prohibition, however, remained more theoretical than practical, as the small number of health professionals with Western training were able to treat less than an estimated ten percent of the urban population. In reality, traditional practitioners continued developing, practicing and teaching their art. Nevertheless, the Western influence had a tremendous effect and traditional Chinese medicine fell into a long period of stagnation. In this period, many healers and health professionals gathered together to defend and develop the legacy of traditional medicine. They founded associations, published books and journals, and taught correspondence courses in acupuncture. It was in this period that the first attempts were made to explain the theory of acupuncture according to the norms of Western medical science. Since 1899 regular studies have been developed around acupuncture and the combination of acupuncture with Western techniques. In 1934 the technique of electroacupuncture was introduced in China.

In 1955, with the formation of the People's Republic, the government officially recognized the traditional medicine and allowed it to exist alongside occidental medicine. This official recognition brought about the synthesis of the two medicines. This synthesis was fostered by the development of two strategies. On one hand the systematization of all the diverse wisdom of traditional medicine was stimulated (an official work which lasted over twenty years); on the other hand the collaboration between traditional doctors, clinical researchers, and Western-style health professionals was officially solicited. Traditional schools of acupuncture were formalized and incorporated into universities where traditional therapies were complemented by materials from Western medicine. Hospitals opened their doors to the traditional medicine, including some which became exclusively devoted to the ancient practices. In other hospitals, according to their specialty, traditional therapists shared the treatment with Western specialists, treating diseases with both therapeutic instruments and combining ancient diagnostic theory with the best of modern laboratory research.

In the research centers medical teams using various methods of investigation verified the efficacy of the traditional Chinese meridian system. These investigations included the comparison of the action of acupuncture with the action of diverse pharmaceutical medications and the testing of different types of handling and manipulation of the needles (some recommended in the ancient texts). Physiopathological experiments were carried out in order to understand the therapeutic actions of acupuncture treatment. It is important to note the level of seriousness of the Chinese researchers, their zeal for discovery and invention, and particularly, their interest in couching the investigation within the norms of modern science. Much, however remains to be done.

The results, fascinating as they are, are little-known in the West. The research of the Chinese health professionals and clinicians has served to stimulate various branches of modern occidental science, whose development was, and continues to be, limited in its own sphere. Upon studying and attempting to understand the mechanisms of traditional medicine with Western concepts, somatic processes and neurochemical phenomena have been discovered which, until recently, were entirely unknown or dismissed by Western science.

In the West in general the medical establishment has begun to accept the effectiveness of traditional Chinese medicine, especially certain acupuncture techniques for the control of pain; other elements of Chinese medicine, such as *yin/yang* theory, five element theory, and the efficacy of *chi kung* are often rejected out of hand, in part due to the difficulty faced by the Western mind in understanding these processes. Similarly, a prejudice against anything "unscientific" makes it difficult to open a space for understanding concepts so radically different from those whose fundament is in the West.

CHAPTER 8

CONCLUSIONS

GENERAL OBSERVATIONS

THE UNDERSTANDINGS of Chinese traditional medicine, extraordinary in depth and richness, are not based on a biological and microbiological order (as is occidental knowledge), but this does not make them any less rational or "scientific." The explanations found in Chinese medicine—responding to meticulous and systematized observations of nature and the human body and woven together to form an intricate and efficient system—allow us to see that conceptual systems other than the "scientific" occidental system can be possessed of great rationality and expressions of truth. By examining other cultural systems, we open new vistas upon our world. Looking with new eyes, we can detect our profound interconnection with the cosmos, the natural world, and each other. Observing with eyes opened by an understanding of the Chinese medical tradition, we are given the insight to understand and interpret Mayan medicine and other traditional medical systems from Mesoamerica.

In the preceding chapters we have presented a small bit of information concerning Mayan medicine; some of this information was already known and familiar outside of the villages, while other bits of local knowledge we compiled with the help of *curanderos*. This information speaks to us of a system of thought bearing great richness in its knowledge and practices. The usefulness of concepts from Chinese medicine in embracing the majority of practices and ideas from Mayan medicine seems to us exceptional, and so we have used the visions of Chinese medicine to begin a deeper search into little-known concepts of Mayan and other Mesoamerican traditions.

It is clear that the different categories of Chinese medicine help us to see the elements of Mayan medical thought as parts of an intricate system— a system which possesses a logic and perception of the world very different from its occidental counterpart, a system which is based in a body of mystical philosophic thought integrated by a series of profound understandings of the natural and human worlds.

Although there are many similarities between the two medical systems there are also many differences. There is certainly not a complete and horizontal equivalence between the two systems in any manner of speaking. When Western doctors such as ourselves approach the study of Chinese medicine, there is a distinct difficulty in understanding and assimilating its concepts and categories. Many Westerners find it necessary to try to Westernize the concepts, to give them a basis in our own rationality. Often this study has been accompanied by an anxious feeling that the rug is being pulled out from under us. We are presented with a vision of the world that shakes the foundations we have so carefully and determinedly laid. In explaining Chinese acupuncture and moxibustion to the Mayan *curanderos*, we have been surprised by the ease with which they understand and assimilate the meanings, without a sense that embracing the new concepts must lead them to reject their own. On the contrary, their traditional understandings seem to be reinforced by the new and complementary knowledge. This immediate pedagogical experience reaffirms our belief that the two systems share a certain conceptual ground.

The similarity between the Chinese and Mayan conceptions has helped us to understand and reconstruct some Mayan concepts which are currently fragmented, lost, or deeply misunderstood. This analysis calls for the efforts of other enthusiastic researchers who can see the possibilities for understanding permitted by this comparative approach. In the end, the importance of this analysis comes not from a deeper knowledge obtained from Mayan medicine, but from the possibility of understanding this other world in its entirety—of appreciating it from a point of view that is profound, ordered, complex, and not simply folkloric. We believe that this understanding can open doors towards the understanding of other traditional American medical systems.

Some specialists in this field have raised the point that we must take into account the possibility of migrations from China to the Yucatán Peninsula that have occurred in the past few centuries, and that, in some way, Mayan medicine has been informed and enriched by resulting cultural encounters. This is certainly one possibility among many which might be added to the explanations we present here; of course such a possibility would require decisive investigations in order to determine its degree of influence.

Following, we present a summary of the major themes of this book.

THE COSMOS

The Mayan cosmovision, as a system of concepts, is derived largely from the productive relation of these rural people with their natural surroundings. Mayan medicine has been integrally formed by and with cosmic and natural forces. A relation with the natural world derived from agricultural production explains at least in part the similarities between the indigenous and traditional medical systems of the Maya and other Mesoamerican peoples and those of cultures in other parts of the world. These rural people depend for their living on an understanding of natural phenomena; they must know, among other things, when is the best time to plant and to harvest, when certain plagues will affect their crops, and what signs anticipate drought. This brings them to study in great detail the changes of the seasons (solstices and equinoxes), and demands a precise knowledge of the movements of the stars and planets.[42]

The ancient Maya were a patient and observant people with a great ability to document and systematize information. Unfortunately, with the deterioration of the splendor of Mayan civilization and the further destruction brought about by the Spanish conquest, these technologies have been lost.

The most important relation between the traditional medicines of China and Mesoamerica are found in the conceptualization of nature and its influence on human life in terms of health and disease. Chinese culture understands that in great or small measure, all natural phenomena have a direct influence on the behavior and attitudes of human beings. At the same time, human attitudes and actions have a direct influence on the cosmos. If a man acts in accordance with the laws of the natural world, a balance is established between himself and his environment—a balance that brings as a consequence health and harmony. If he violates these laws, he breaks the balance and invites trouble. From this understanding, the Chinese arrived at the conclusion that they could maintain and even improve their health if they respected the natural world, adapted to its changes, and came to a rational understanding of how to use its resources.

In the Mayan vision the same understanding is established—though it is expressed in another form and charged with other symbols.

An important conceptual difference between the cosmic visions of Mayan culture and Chinese culture is the pragmatic character that marks the latter, where explanations of nature and the human body tend to lose their mystical component in favor of a certain rationalist objectivity. Over the centuries this tendency has been lightened by the Buddhist influence.

Conclusions

Meanwhile, it seems, Mayan culture continued in the opposite direction, elaborating a series of metaphysical concepts integrated with rational explanations of the workings of the natural world.

For both Mayan and Chinese cultures, nature more than society is determinative in shaping human lives. For this reason the forces of nature are deified and venerated by the Mayan people (and by the Chinese roughly until the *Zhou* dynasty). In both cultures many mechanisms are recognized which demonstrate the influence of the environment and the cosmos on human life, and which explain the workings of the body in terms of the larger bodies of the universe. This basic conception explains many of the similarities between their mythologies, religions, and astronomical systems—from the dual conception of the physical world to the specifics of the calendar and the meanings of the four directions. This similarity of vision is apparent in their medical systems—from their diagnostics to their therapeutic practice. The *yin-yang* theory of China allows us to examine, in a more dynamic and complex way, the concepts of heat and cold among the Maya; it gives us a theoretical basis for understanding the phenomenon—a framework with which to view it as more than a random factor or a folkloric, magical, or symbolic conception.

Both the Chinese and the Mayan people have established, through long observation and systematization, that the forces of nature act differently and display different patterns according to the time of day and the time of year, and that these patterns can affect the health of an individual. The Chinese discovered seasonal patterns of energy flow and discovered that these patterns are replicated in the energy of the individual. Similarly, the Maya developed a complex understanding of the affects of the times of day and year on the human body and mind, and this knowledge is circumscribed in their cosmovision. Recently the new scientific discipline known as chronobiology studies the action of biological rhythms on the physiology of the organs.[43] Again, we see contemporary advances in science replicating the understandings of ancient cultures.

THE BODY

The holistic thought that results from this close observation of the cosmos has had great influence on other concepts present in the two cultures, including the relation between body and soul, between all the parts and organs within the body, the body's thermal and temporal relations, and the understanding of the vital principals in the conceptualization of illness as imbalance. Other apparent commonalties might be attributed, simply, to the discovery of certain "universal truths"—truths which are reinforced when we look at them in their cross-cultural context. This view applies to the use of the herbal pharmacopoeia, the bodily points, and the method of healing through working with thermal qualities.

In ancient traditional Chinese medicine the perfection of the body and soul were desired goals. The body-mind is viewed as a united, indivisible entity. It was affirmed that if the body fell ill, the spirit would receive the illness, and if the spirit fell ill, the body would be affected. For the Maya the concept is similar. The work of curing is understood to be an integral treatment of the body and the *"alma—ool"* (the soul)—which explains the existence of practices working in both directions (body/spirit and spirit/body) and causes Mayan medical practice to appear charged with supernatural forces and "magic."

Chinese medicine gives special importance to parts of the body understood to be reservoirs of energy (such as the *dan tian*) or key points in the trajectory of *chi*. Chinese doctors recognize the circulation of energy across the skin and internal organs by way of channels which connect points on the surface to the interior of the organism. By way of these points one part of the body is directly connected to another; thus the manipulation of one part of the body has a therapeutic effect on another.

In Mayan medicine as well certain zones of the body are recognized for the role they play in the concentration of vital forces (the umbilicus, the *tipté,* the heart, and the head). The joints are recognized as areas where disease is likely to enter the body. Also recognized are channels through which wind circulates between one joint and the next in the extremities or along the back. This phenomenon is well-known by masseuses and *j'meenob*. Channels recognized by the Maya are fewer and shorter than their Chinese counterparts, and the Chinese system recognizes a more complex relationship between the points and their particular functions; still, what is significant is that therapeutic effects can be produced along these channels and that these therapeutic effects are similar in Mexico and in China.

The various traditional Mayan therapies also recognize a series of points on the body whose treatment through puncture or bleeding produces therapeutic effects in nearby zones (the head, back, and extremities), and through which the wind in the body can be manipulated. There are also points used to treat distal zones of the body—such as the points in the back used to treat indigestion and cold in the womb, and the point in the foot that is commonly used to facilitate labor. For contemporary Mayan *curanderos,* these points, except those which run between two extremes of a "wind canal," connecting one articulation to the next, are not connected among each other.

For the Mayan people there exists a vital principle in the body—the *ool*—which was ignored and scorned by Christianity and later by academic researchers, being confused with the soul (which for the Maya is the *pixán*). The *ool,* considered the "air of life," possesses characteristics which lend it a real or metaphorical relationship with wind. For the Chinese the *chi* is a principle of life energy which is considered, equally, to have the quality of "air" or the "breath of life." Again, we can say that the *chi* is encompassed by a much more complex system of understanding.

In Chinese medicine there exists a system of relations between the organs and tissues and the emotions and vital principles, that is, a direct correspondence between emotional state and health. In Mayan medicine these relations are not as systemetized, although considerable importance is given to states like anger, sadness, worry, and fear, and we see direct relations between anxiety and headaches, fear and the diseases of the *ool,* to name a few examples. For the Chinese, the heart—the storehouse of the spirit *(shen)*—is the emperor of the organs. Although emotional stimuli influence all of the organs, they affect the heart first. In Mayan culture the heart is the storehouse of *ool*—that force which is responsible for the spirit and will in its course through the body.

CAUSALITY

In studying the entirety of the causes of disease understood by Mayan medicine we discover a rich system—one arguably more complete and complex than its occidental counterpart. In Mayan medicine physical imbalance can be produced by the organism itself, the family or community, events in the natural world, or by the various divinities. Acting against these elements or showing lack of respect and thus breaking the balance that exists within the family, society, nature, the cosmos, and the gods can generate harmful forces which, in their turn, affect the individual's physical balance and result in ill-health. Health is therefore the result of living according to the laws of nature and society; illness is the result of the transgression of these laws.

In Mayan medicine some of the chief causes of an imbalance between hot and cold elements in the body include eating disorders, bad posture and sudden movements, excessive work, dirtiness, weakness, changes in the *ool* caused by winds, and voluntary or involuntary actions by other beings. In Chinese medicine causality in general is systematized and divided into internal and external factors—including (as in Mayan medicine) eating disorders, excessive work and excessive rest, sexual activity, parasites, trauma, pestilence, and emotional and environmental pathogens.

For the Chinese, climatic factors are typified by wind, cold, heat, damp, dryness, and fire. The differentiation and complex understanding of climatic factors responds to the cycle of seasons, whose changes in China are very marked. On the Yucatán Peninsula the predominant climatic factor is extreme heat. The region, exposed to lashing winds, maintains a constant level of humidity. This explains the importance given to the winds and the hot-cold polarity, as well as the absence of other factors like dryness and dampness.

Currently, official Chinese medicine is presented with an aseptic logic in regard to "the supernatural." This posture is fruit of the pragmatism which, beginning centuries ago, influenced the division between "medicine" and "shamanism" (the latter having become allied strictly with religion). This division was accentuated by the systematization undertaken during the anti-religious regime of Mao Tse Tung and the People's Republic of China. Nevertheless, manifestations of a religious medicine still persist in China, bound with the practices of Buddhism and Confucianism, in which procedures very much like *limpias* or exorcisms are carried out and the treatment of spiritual ills is undertaken using orations and incantations.

In Chinese medicine it is understood that the rupture of internal balance is responsible for the body's susceptibility to external causes of illness. This is a transcendent concept; although in China today microbiology is well known and accepted, the earlier conception maintains its importance in both diagnosis and treatment.

Mayan concepts of causality and the mechanisms of diagnostics are similar to those of the Chinese. In favor of a diagnosis based on bodily imbalance, little importance is given to nosological diagnostics (diagnosis based on a typology of diseases). The Mayan clinician will be interested more in signs of "heat," "cold," and "wind" than in what occidental thinking would recognize as "standard symptoms." This way of understanding illness is not as fully systematized and explicit as in the Chinese system, and it is currently subject to a synthesis with elements of other medical systems which have distorted its ancient qualities.

DIAGNOSTICS

In an attempt to understand the patient as a human being with a determined history in a specific social and geographic environment, Chinese medicine (in contrast to occidental medicine) gives importance to climatic, seasonal, geographic, social, and emotional factors. The emphasis is on the person, not the illness. Mayan traditional medicine, in a form similar to Chinese medicine, considers it necessary to investigate, on performing the diagnosis, factors related to the patient's social environment, lifestyle, diet, activities, emotional state, personal relations, exposure to climatic factors, adherence to tradition, and relationship with divinity. This speaks to us of a holistic conception of health and disease which establishes a diagnosis taking into account physical, mental, spiritual, and environmental aspects. This diagnosis isn't simply a formulation of what is wrong with the body, as happens in occidental medicine. Rather it composes an analysis of a person's life and how the health is affected by her or his general habits, tendencies, and constitution.

The two medicines possess some diagnostic principles in common, like the taking of the pulse and the observation of signs of wind and thermal imbalance; in Chinese medicine these principles have reached a high level of refinement. The system of pulse-taking is extremely developed, as are other methods that have no direct counterpart in Mayan medicine, such as tongue diagnosis.

Mayan medicine assigns an important role to methods of divination, "illumination," and physical diagnosis. Contemporary Chinese diagnostics has abandoned divination along with every vestige of spirituality or belief in the supernatural—though branches of medicine aligned with Buddhism and Confucianism continue to have currency.

THERAPEUTICS

Herbology

In Mayan herbology *(tzak xiu)* the salient characteristics of medicinal plants are their thermal nature and their effectiveness in easing and expelling winds from the body. Although animal and mineral elements are used as well, there is no separate classification for them. Plants are prescribed taking into account not only the current illness, but also the patient's previous illnesses, personality, state of strength or weakness, and the time of year.

The Chinese *materia medica* is based on similar concepts, and others whose development is not mirrored by contemporary Mayan medicine. The Chinese have developed a study of the interaction of diverse remedies—classifying them as king, minister, or subject. They have developed classifications based on energetics (light plants which ascend and float and heavy ones which descend and sink, for example), the five flavors, and the thermal natures of the plants. All remedies are considered to possess *yin* and *yang* properties, and to direct their healing properties towards specific organs.

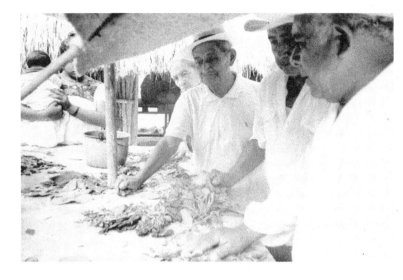

Massage

It is curious that despite its role in traditional American medicines, attention from researchers and investigators has not been given to massage. Researchers generally report practices which seem frankly strange, not to say folkloric, and gloss over the rest. To touch where it hurts is one of the most ancient approaches to illness. It is logical to think that this simple and direct intervention would give birth to complex systems of massage, especially in cultures which do not deny the body its role as the storehouse of human potential.

The various massage techniques in Mayan culture partake of a logic which is profoundly embedded in the cosmovision of the people. In our studies, we have distinguished rubbings, accomodations, stimulation of points, suction, and *apretadas* (the massage performed by midwives on women recovering from childbirth), among others. Mayan massage is applied in both curative and preventive forms for a multitude of illnesses, external and internal, with great frequency. It is common in Mayan communities to turn to *talladas,* or rubbings, for both localized pain and more complex internal conditions. While in China the conceptual base of massage is more complex and profound than that which we witness in present-day Mayan communities, many theories and techniques in Mayan and Chinese massage coincide—among them friction, the stimulation and pinching of points, the manipulation of articulations, and the "capturing of the winds," or cupping.

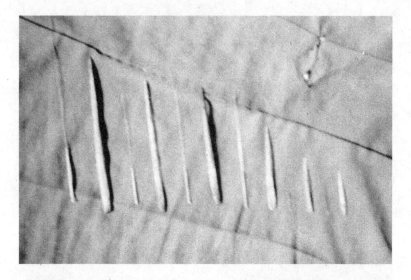

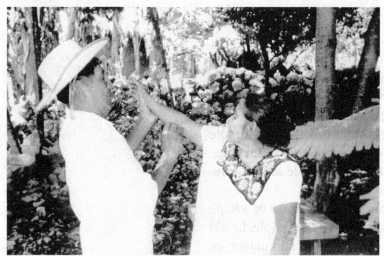

Acupuncture

It seems to us frankly paradoxical that so little written information exists regarding Mayan *tok* and *jup,* while the therapeutic development of these systems and their application is actually quite extensive. This may be due to the fact that many researchers give these practices a character more symbolic than real, and see them as elements which merely reaffirm the "primitive" character of Mayan culture. Without devaluing or discarding the symbolic or mystical value borne by these practices, we consider that they possess an important therapeutic application based on observations of the body's functions and the results of its manipulation. These understandings coincide largely with the findings of the Chinese.

The majority of the Mayan points we have identified correspond with Chinese points. The therapeutic use of the Mayan points is also startlingly similar to that of the Chinese points—specifically in their local effects. We have identified nearly fifty points, although few practitioners of *tok* and *jup* work them all. This quantity, compared with the nearly two thousand recognized in Chinese traditional acupuncture, may sound slight, but it speaks of a common logic and of a therapeutic system which, had it been allowed to develop further, would undoubtedly have continued to increase in breadth and sophistication.

Poultices and the Application of Heat

The Chinese use plants, animal products, and various types of clay to make their poultices. In Mayan medicine plasters and poultices are made chiefly with plants, though there is some use of animal and mineral products in their preparation as well. The principle in both systems is to apply poultices with thermal properties which relate to the illness being treated.

In China, preparations of warm-natured plants are rarely used, as there exist more efficient techniques such as moxibustion, which applies heat directly to the area of concern. The Mayans have a practice very similar to Chinese moxibustion in which heat is applied by holding charcoal embers above the desired point.

Cleansings or Limpias

Cleansing embodies a series of practices used by Mayan *curanderos* to expel evil winds from the body of a patient.
The therapy involves applying certain plants, animals, eggs, or other objects which absorb the wind. The *curandero* attempts to corner the wind and facilitate its expulsion by praying to different divinities whose participation makes the treatment possible.

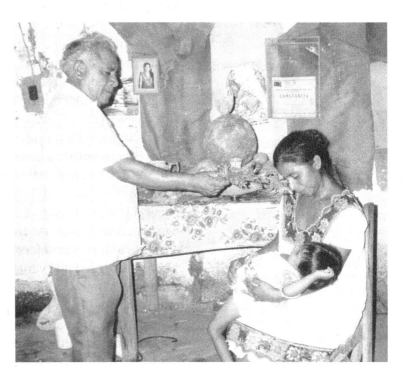

Chinese *chi kung,* one branch of traditional medicine with its roots in Taoism and Buddhism, embodies both the search for energetic balance in the meridians and the expulsion of pernicious influences; the first is realized by way of breathing exercises, concentration, and movement, which bring about the awakening of stagnant energies and the balance of the bodily flow; the second involves treatment in which a practitioner projects energy through the hands over the body of the patient. Through this therapy the energy in the meridians is stimulated, pushing the stagnant and negative influences out of the body and increasing the flow of *chi.*

MAYAN DISEASE CLASSIFICATION

The workshops in which we participated, designed to lead us to an understanding of Mayan disease typology, introduced us to a large list of organic and spiritual illnesses and allowed us to begin the work of typifying and systematizing these illnesses according to their nature. This list can be

Conclusions

found in the appendix on disease classification. The list includes many occidental diseases, along with others which present no clear equivalence with Western illnesses. Some might be recognized as what some doctors call "diseases of conscience." Others, like fright, the evil eye, and the various wind-related illnesses, can be explained to some degree in terms of "energetics," as is suggested by Chinese disease classification.

GENERAL CONCLUSIONS

The current system of traditional Mayan medicine practiced in the states of Campeche and Yucatán is fragmented and recomposed of elements from other medical models and cultures foreign to the prehispanic Maya. It is practiced under multiple limitations and severe ideological pressure, with access to scarce resources. To complicate matters, it is dependent on an oral culture which is unable to establish a uniform theoretical understanding among the various health workers in the region.

In spite of its great deficiencies, Mayan traditional medicine surprises us with its richness and depth of understanding, its ability to maintain a practical body of therapies and its flexibility in dynamically incorporating new modalities. Over the course of years of contact with traditional Mayan health practitioners empirical evidence has assured us of its efficacy in treating a wide variety of illnesses, including cases in which occidental medicine was not a viable alternative or presented unsatisfactory results. In other cases we have witnessed the opposite—failures and significant errors in treatment.

As with any medical system, Mayan medicine possesses valuable qualities as well as serious limitations. Occasionally a *curandero* will have great skill and wide knowledge, appearing to have been gifted with the ability to heal. These individuals are admittedly rare. Generally the healing arts are practiced by therapists with good intentions and varying degrees of training and skill. Each practitioner will have some degree of specialization—illnesses he treats with greater skill than others. And of course there is no lack of charlatans who practice a mixture of Mayan and occidental medicine without proper understanding, bringing great risk to their patients and their communities.

Five-hundred years after the arrival of European concepts, the ancient agricultural systems and intimate relation with the natural world have persisted to varying degrees. The persistence of these systems explains the survival of Mayan medicine. But in recent years rural productive systems have been subject to deep and rapid change bringing with them significant transformation in the practice of traditional medicine.

Traditional indigenous medicine is a complex system of knowledge and practices which transcends the simple effects of any one of its elements viewed in isolation. In order to deepen our understanding of this medicine we must study it in all its complexity, rather than reduce it to an exclusive understanding of its botanical *materia medica* or its symbolic effects. We believe that gathering together all of the elements which make up traditional medicine and indigenous culture can give us a wider vision of our own history and culture, and afford us a better understanding of ourselves as a people. We hope that the comparative approach we have used in this study will contribute to a deeper understanding and, over time, to a reconstruction of the medical knowledge of indigenous Mesoamerica.

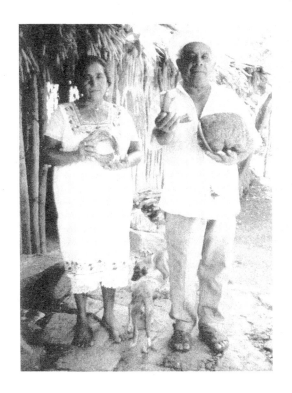

APPENDIX

DISEASE CLASSIFICATION

THE STUDY OF TRADITIONAL DISEASE CLASSIFICATION

THE TYPOLOGY AND CLASSIFICATION OF ILLNESS is as ancient as consciousness itself and responds to the need to explain the origins, mechanisms, and ways of controlling illness. Each culture has a particular way of approaching phenomena of health and disease, determined by its relation with the natural world, the advance of "scientific" or empirical investigation, and the culture's conceptual-religious way of understanding the world. In occidental scientific medicine we have a way of classifying disease known as nosology, which distinguishes between signs, symptoms, syndromes, and diseases. Its form of diagnosis is based on the scientific method, occidental rationality, the advances of technology, and a series of norms based on the classification structure itself—what symptoms belong to what syndromes, etcetera.[44] It is assumed in the West that only modern medical science can establish the true bases of medicine, and that the medical classification established in the West is the only methodological instrument capable of approaching an understanding of disease. Practices of identification and classification of disease established outside of this system are considered unscientific and invalid and will be judged not merely irresponsible, but illegal.

In the eighteenth and nineteenth centuries there was a great debate between ontology and physiology over how to classify disease. Ontology conceived of illness as a "thing" which arrived from outside to damage the organism, and which was governed by specific laws of formation, growth, and development. Physiology sustained that illness was caused by alterations in the normal functioning of the body, and therefore was not an element apart from, but rather a condition of, the body itself. Disease is the physiology of the diseased body. After long disagreement, a system of typology was established which synthesized the discrepancies and disagreements of the past.[45] As a schematics and abstraction of reality this system has found itself plagued by internal limitations when put into actual practice; it encounters, time and again, medical conditions which it can neither understand nor adequately treat according to its rules.[46] Aside from these primary limitations, the focus of this system on biological understanding leaves no room for psychological, social, or cultural interpretations. This influences in turn the structure of medical practice, the teaching of medicine, and the politics of health.

A vacuum exists between the reductionist explanations of official medicine regarding health and disease and the manner in which the Mexican population with its various popular sectors (*campesino,* indigenous, suburban, urban) understands the problem and intends to resolve it. In general the medicines known as "traditional" and "indigenous" come closer to a complete view of illness, integrating social, cultural, psychological, and historical factors while at the same time developing an understanding of the patterns of particular diseases.

With its reductionist logic, the incapacity of the dominant medical model to understand Mexican popular culture gives rise to the need to understand the thought of the various peoples that populate the nation. It is important to take into account epidemiological profiles which include traditional illnesses and an understanding of the social groups to which they correspond in order to facilitate the design of programs which will be integral to given regions.

In this section we hope to approach an understanding of the traditional Mayan disease classification of the states of Campeche and Yucatán, using the results that we established in our workshops with *curanderos* there in 1991 and 1992. From there we hope to present an epidemiology based on the actual cosmovision, attempting to understand phenomena of health and disease as they are understood by the culture itself.

In these workshops we followed a guide for the collection of information regarding recognized illnesses, making large charts as we went. With the help of translators, we filled out the guide according to the ideas proposed by the *curanderos.* This is the guide we worked from:

- Definition
- Variants and types of the illness
- Causality
- Signs and symptoms
- Diagnostics
- Differential diagnostics

- Ethnophysiopathology
- Seasonal variation
- Distribution in the population
- Frequency
- Seriousness
- Treatments
- Complications
- Prevention
- Relations with other medical models

The information regarding disease classification in this appendix comes basically from the workshops, with changes made during personal work with the *curanderos*. The majority of discussions took place in the Mayan language. In translating the text every effort has been made to preserve the original sense.

MAYAN DISEASE CLASSIFICATION

Illnesses in the traditional Mayan world are divided generally into two large groups—organic or terrestrial illnesses *(luum kabil)* and illnesses which are considered "spiritual," "supernatural," or which are caused by the wind *(ik naal)*. This second class of illnesses can have their origins in living beings or can be provoked directly by supernatural beings (gods, saints, spirits, *aluxob,* etcetera), by way of the winds.

ORGANIC ILLNESSES

These are illnesses which affect the physical body and whose causes are natural or *luum kabil*—"here on the earth this happened." These illnesses are called *"kojani tzu u tzik"* by some *curanderos*—that is to say the illness comes to be "just like that." Some illnesses in this list are named in Spanish rather than Maya; these will be indicated with an asterisk.

Mayan Disease Name	Translation
Wach' k'aja'al, cursus, k'axi	Diarrhea
X-ak'a taa, cheche taa, jub nak, x-aka patio	Nocturnal defecation leaving a chill in the umbilical region
Tzan nu yaal, emu yaal, lubu lu yaal, jalk'ajaan u yaal	Collapse of the crown
Kiik naak, dunta	White dysentery
Ta'k'i'ik', tu mansi k'iik'	Red dysentery
Tipté, cirro, kan tipte	Fall of the *cirro*, loosening of the *cirro*
Manu jana', je jet ki, titi ki, chup naak	Indigestion
Chi'ibal naak', ya' u naak, k'inan naak	Stomach ache
K'asa'an naak, pu naak	Chill in the stomach, weak digestion
Chotnaak, tzot naal	Colic
Tu chokui tu choche, chokui to jone' chokui tu jobon	Intestinal fever
X-kan chokuil	Typhoid
U k'o janil chambal taantu sijile'	Crying and vomiting in newborns
Chu'kal	Stomach acidity
Ele' naak'	Gastritis
K'an chik'in, u peki lu naak'	Excess bile
Chujuk wix, tzujuk wix	Diabetes
Yaya' wix, ele wix, k'inan wix	Bladder infection
K'alwix, ch'a ch'a wix	Urine retention
Sipit ka'ak	Inflammation of the point of the penis in young boys
Se'en	Catarrh, flu
Tikin se'en	Dry cough

Mayan Disease Name	Translation
K'iinan xikin, chiba xikin	Ear infection
Sasak kal, tz'atz'a'kal	Cough, bronchitis
Jeesbal se'en	Asthma
X-tuus ik se'en, lodt o kab, tus ik, tzana kaap u chalate, ya'ya se'en	Whooping cough
Tuul k'i'ik' iini, u ch'ak paja', u venasilu'ni	Nasal hemorrhage
Chiba pool	Frontal headache
Kinan poo	Generalized headache
Jiit a jool, kinan pach ka'	Pain in the neck and shoulders
Al jool, x-jolon aal	Post-partum headache
Al kaximba', al kaxinba' kaak', Corrimiento	"Running," "Running of the Blood," "Running of the Wind"
Aak'ab k'ilkab	Night sweats
Chokuil	Fever
Minana nu yool, ma ool, ma utz ola'	Lack of will, depression
Choco ola', kina' ola'	*"Caluroso"*—a state of imbalance produced by heat
U po'o, tu mesankil, tu yiku' p'oo	Alterations in menstruation
Yu chu k'as, uch lob ti'	Miscarriage
Sak mancha	Vaginal discharge
Chak mancha	Vaginal hemorrhage
Pasmo de sangre (Chill in the blood)	Sterility
X-jul im nul im, ya' im, x-jolab aali	Pain in the breasts
Ma'jok'u k'abu yim	Absence of mother's milk
Sa'pu' k'ab uyim, tij u kabu yim', sal ka u yim, sa'p u k'aab u yim	Mother's milk dries up

Mayan Disease Name	Translation
K'al ta'-kaltal winik	Alcoholism
Chiich naak	Depression in single women
Kikilan ka a winkil	Nerves, shivering
Kasan u tuku	Dementia
Ma' tioo ani'	Mental retardation
Pa-o', paoo, choko ola', kina ola'	Heat from the *xaman kan*—an evil wind from the northeast—that produces rash, itching and pain, possibly accompanied by asthma
Chakmukla'	Rash, skin eruption caused by heat
Wirich	Hypersensitive skin
K'ulen siis	Skin lesions that look like lashings, caused by heat
Sak wech	White scabies
Ax	Warts
Mal del atrevido (Insolent disease)	Dermatitis in the legs and pubic region
Bo'o ray winkilil	Skin blotches
Chup tu'ux ku taa	Piles
*X-kubenba' ka'a'ak, cancer**	Skin ulcers
Lukción	Skin ulcers
Xa'ayak u chi	Ulcers and cracks in the mouth
Yzakan ak	Mouth ulcers
Xuk ka'ak	Herpes
Chu'u chun	Tumor or abscess of the skin
Chup u k'al, chup k'al	Mumps
Xa'a chi	Drooling

Mayan Disease Name	Translation
Buy	Swelling, abnormal growth in the eyes
Xo'oy oox piích	Chalazion
Ti'ich ma'ak, nube* (Clouds)	Cataracts
Kan kan winkil	Yellow skin, jaundice
Kinan bakelob, kinan winkilob	Pain in the bones
Saya' siis, tzak ba winkil	Chill in the extremities, rheumatism
X-tunk uy siis	Chill in the heel of the foot
Je'k'a, je'ka u tuchne'	Opening of the hips
Kam pach, ya' pach	Back pain
Kinan putzikaal, ki'ina puksi'ik	Pain in the heart

SPIRITUAL AND WIND-BORNE ILLNESSES

These illnesses can be provoked by winds originating from people, animals, plants, objects, or supernatural beings.

Mayan Disease Name	Translation
EE'K ICH TABI, TU MENTA OJO	*EVIL EYE*
• Ojoy maak	• *Eye of a man*
• Ojoy kalan	• *Eye of a drunk*
• Ojoy xion kolee	• *Eye of a pregnant woman*
• Ojoy balche'	• *Eye of an animal*
A k'an	*Cry of the newborn*
Jo'ko k'iik tu tuch	*Umbilical hemhorrage in newborns*
U xu'uy pool	*Whirlwind in the head*

177

Mayan Disease Name	Translation
CHUP YO'LAL DZIBOLAL, KU BEN BA', PUL BAJ, TZIBOLA', XKU'U BENBA	*DESIRE*
Chupul yo'ola poch	Desire for food
Chupul yo'ola xi wak koole	Desire for a man or a woman
MEYA K'AS	*WITCHCRAFT*
Men bi k'ini de jambi	Bewitching of the food
Men bi k'imi yeteliik	Bewitching by wind and spells
Men bi kasti solar	Bewitching of the fields
Men bi kasti naal	Bewitching of the house
Men bi kas yola, ek ta nech	Bewitching caused by envy
JAK'OLAL, XAK OLAL, SA'KIL	*FRIGHT, FEAR*
Jak'iool	Fright originating in the womb
Jak'ola	Fright of the mother, which passes to the child
Jasa ool	Fright passed to the child in the mother's milk
Xpak'i	Fright in children and newborns
Sa'kil	Fright caused by fear of older children
Pask'il	Chronic fright in children
Xa'k'ool	Susceptibility to fright
Lubawool	Loss of will, listlessness
Mak tzil	Restlessness of the spirit
K'AK' AS IK'	*EVIL WIND*
Tu jentan ta iik'al mozón	Whirlwind
Mozón k'an	Evil whirlwind, wind of the snake

Mayan Disease Name	Translation
Xkaban mozón	Whirlwind of the hummingbird
Sujuy mozón	Small whirlwind in the street
Mozón ibel	"The most dangerous"— Putting on a hat, a snake appears
Sujuy ximbal iik', sujuyte' ximbal iik'	Small whirlwind
Alkab ximbal t'up iik'	Tiny whirlwinds that pass without growing larger; small two-headed snakes that pass below the hammock or in the street when you're not looking
*Mozón grande**	Large whirlwind

EVIL WIND RELATED TO ANIMALS

Iikal xoch	Wind of the owl
Iikaĺ koos	Wind of the witch bird —white wind, from the east —black wind, from the west —red wind, from the south —yellow wind, from the north
Chak dzi dzib alkab iik	Wind brought by the cardinal; looked at through the trees the color of his eyes affects the body
Chapat' iik'	Wind of the centipede, a hot wind that bites
Chimes iik'	Wind from the fat, yellow centipede
Ooch iik'	Wind of the ant

Mayan Disease Name	Translation
Alkab k'ok' ob iik'	Illness caused by the shock of seeing a snake or green iguana that talks and laughs like a woman
Sxjitjits' beji	Wind produced by a little jumping field mouse
Viento del raton chó'	The children don't sleep at night—if they sleep they may be stolen from the house
Juantul wakax ik'	Air produced by cattle, producing chill and shivers
Iik'a eki pol kejo'	Wind produced when a wasps' nest lodges in the antlers of a deer
Iik'al (yik'al) keej	Wind of the deer—very high fevers leading to death
Kamaya' iik	Wind produced by a black cat conjured by witchcraft
Xtus (alkab) iik'	Evil wind from the grave. Poisonous gases are produced by the earth. It comes from a little lizard which breathes the air near a grave; when it breathes out this air it produces asphyxia

OTHER ANIMALS RELATED TO WIND

Xchiwol alkab iik'	Wind tarantula: it comes out at sunrise, 6 AM or at 12 midnight. It acquires its venom from a witch or by being bitten by a poisonous snake

Mayan Disease Name	Translation
Sinaan ximbal iik'	Wind scorpion. It has the same characteristics as the wind tarantula
Xko'ch'iich'alkab iik (xcooch'ich)	Bird of the evil wind; people go crazy after this bird flies over them
Tzaa kin (tzai kin)	A small insect with a shrill cry that can be heard very far away, and which announces the wind; after its cry the rain comes
Cho'lin	If it chirps by day it means it will be sunny; if by night it means it will rain; if the chirping is short it means sun; if it is long, rain

EVIL WIND CAUSED BY SPIRITS
OF PARTICULAR PLACES

K'akal iik'	Wind of the burial mounds
Iik k'aja'	Wind of the water, of rain
Rekai muyal	Disease of the red cloud
K'ojani kabak iik'	Wind produced by the *aluxob* that live in the foothills. This wind causes insomnia, hallucinations and nausea. To cure it the *aluxob* must be offered food.
Iikal alux	Wind of the *alux*

WINDS FROM THE FOUR
DIRECTIONS

Chikin iik', k'an chik'in	West wind: "Red cloud," causes asthma. Wind of bile, affecting the will

181

Mayan Disease Name	Translation
Nojol iik'	South wind. Beneficent wind
Lakin' iik	East wind. Good for the burning season, when the fields are cleared for planting
Xaman iik', xamankan	North wind. Causes or complicates asthma, diseases of the eyes, fever, and headache

WINDS RELATED TO THE INCOMPLETION OF A PROMISE

Xlu muk, xk'amuk ool	When a promise is not fulfilled, this is the punishment: the spirit becomes weak, exhausted. When the promise is fulfilled, the person's will returns
Jik'al janli kol	Wind of the food of the *milpa* produced by incompletion of a promise, causing headache, fever and dejection

EYES OF THE WIND

Ojoy k'a'am	Wind of the cloudy sky
Ojoy luum	Eye of the earthly wind
Ojoy yi ka ja'	Eye of the water
Ojoy kiin	Eye of the sun
Ojoy mama uuj	Eye of the moon
Ojoy aluz	Eye of the *alux*
Ojoy balam	Eye of the spirit of wild places

WINDS RELATED TO CURANDEROS

Jalach pach ik'	Wind left by witches when they pass in the road

Mayan Disease Name	Translation
WINDS THAT ATTACK SPECIFIC PARTS OF THE BODY	
Jole ali	Air of the head
Zipit k'aak	Air of the genitals
Estérico	Wind in the breast
OTHER WINDS	
Chakiikal	Air of pregnant women
Kubemba	Evil wind, insolent wind
Xpap (chi, ximbal) iik	Wind which circulates around the body and stings like chili peppers

WORKSHOPS IN TRADITIONAL MEDICINE

The Principal Mayan Diseases

Following, we present a list of the illnesses discussed in a series of workshops carried on in Calkiní, Campeche in 1991 and 1992. In the various workshops each group of *curanderos* chose the most important or representative illnesses that they regularly attended. The results were reviewed by other *curanderos* who added additional comments. Later the information was ordered, with the intention of respecting its original sense and the original language used in the description.

Organic Illnesses
WACH' K'AJA'AL

A syndrome marked by diarrhea, also known in the region as *cursus, k'axi* and *junaaki*. There are various causes of *wach k'aja'al:*

Hot-cold conflicts:

- Drinking ice water or eating cold food while the stomach is in a warm state, or after eating hot foods
- When the mother in a hot condition breastfeeds her child

Eating disorders:

- Eating to excess.
- Refusal to eat (common in children).
- Eating at the wrong hour.
- When a mother eats heavy foods and breastfeeds her baby.

Relation with winds:

- Going out into the wind without preparing for the chill.
- The "Wind of Water" and the "Wind of Rain" *(Iik k'aja')*.
- When the mother breastfeeds her child after coming from the forest.
- Evil wind *(xaman kan* and *chikin ik)* in children (common in summer).

Caused by emotional complications:

- When a mother argues with her husband or neighbors.

Caused by "dirtiness":

- Eating unclean or raw foods, drinking untreated water, drinking raw milk, not washing plates before serving a meal, eating dirt (common among children).

Caused by bad posture and brusque movement:

- Sitting a long time in an uncomfortable position.
- Carrying a child for a long time.
- Lifting heavy objects.

As a symptom of other illnesses—*wach' k'aja'al* may be symptomatic of:

- Fall of the *cirro (tipté)*.
- Collapse of the crown *(tzan nu yaal)*.
- Indigestion *(k'an chi k'in* or *manu jana')*.
- Evil eye.
- Intestinal worms.

Others causes:

- When a person cured with rue sees a child.

A person ill with *wach' k'aja'al* passes liquid without warning and experiences stomach cramps, thirst, lack of appetite, weakness, and exhaustion. The eyes appear sad and sunken. There may be nausea and fever accompanied by itching and chills; the patient may lose vision, hearing, and speech abilities; the teeth and bones are loose and the throat may become blocked. Heavy thirst is caused by heat in the stomach, especially in cases of *tu chokui tu choche* (intestinal fever).

In diagnosing this illness the radial pulse is taken and the head and lungs are palpated. The abdomen is palpated for gas and the feet are checked for stiffness or weakness.

To verify the cause of *wach'j'aja'al* the following examinations are undertaken:

- The color and odor of the stool; green or whitish are indications of evil eye.
- Palpation of the abdomen to check for inflammation or parasites.
- Palpation of the belly and back for signs of coldness.
- Palpation of the *cirro.*

To evaluate the seriousness of the condition, the following should be checked:

- The color of the body, and the ears and hands in particular.
- Signs of *jeesbal* or labored breathing.

Wach' k'aja'al is easily confused with *xaka taa, kiik naak'* and *x-ju naal',* indigestion, parasites, and intestinal fever.

Wach' k'aja'al appears most frequently in July and August, during the height of summer when insects appear which can bring the illness. The evil winds of this season complicate the illness. It also appears, though less frequently, in October, November and December, along with *xaman kan* and *chikin ik.*

Wach' k'aja'al is the most common cause of death in children between six months and two-and-a-half years old. In the height of summer, however, it attacks without regard to age or sex. It becomes fatal when there is evacuation of bile and blood accompanied by vomiting and weakness; the patient's body grows thin, swollen and pale, the blood thins, spots appear on the face and body, and there is fainting and dizziness possibly followed by death.

Treatments

- For children, the root of *chi ke' (Chrysophyllum mexicanum)* is parboiled in a quarter of a liter of water. One spoonful is taken three times a day for three days. This may be accompanied by *atole (choko sakan)* (a beverage of ground corn and water). The effect of this treatment is very rapid.
- In a quarter liter of water parboil two pieces of *chi ke' (Chrysophyllum mexicanum),* ground anis *(Pimpinellis anisum,* L.*),* three orange leaves

(*Citrus sinensis*), 3 leaves from a lime tree (*Citrus aurantifolia*) to be taken thrice daily for three days. *Atole* and cold water are administered, but first a small dose of olive oil is administered to purge and clean the stomach.

- If *chi ke'* is unavailable the rind of sapodilla (*Manilkara zapota*, L.) or *chi abal* plum (*Spondias purpurea*) can be used. Root of the orange tree (*Citrus sinensis*) or guava fruit (*Psidium guajava*) can be substituted as well. Another treatment can be done with green banana cooked in a half-liter of water.

- A bit of sapodilla bark (*Manilkara zapota*, L.) is boiled along with bark of the *chi abal* plum (*Spondias purpurea*) in a half-liter of water. Half a glass is taken twice a day for two days; on the third day the treatment is complete.

- The flower and growth tip of the tree *ich juj* (*Eugenia axillaris*, Schwartz) are mashed and mixed with a half-spoonful of honey in a glass of water. The mixture is strained and given to a child a little at a time. For adults a quarter kilo of cabbage heart is boiled with three liters of water, and taken as desired.

- Leaves of *x'tokaban* (*Calea urticifolia*, M, D.C.) (with a white flower) and *sinanche'* (*Zanthoxylum cuneata*, L.*) (with a purple flower) are mashed with a cup of boiled water and taken in two doses. *Sinanche'* is a shrub with small leaves (like a plum tree) and a penetrating odor. The male plant has more spines than the female, and only the female bears fruit. If the patient is a boy, leaves of the female plant are given, and if a girl, leaves of the male. The effect is instant. Children should be given five leaves of *x'tokaban* and three of *sinanche'*, and adults double this quantity, three times a day.

- A handful of *x'puk'im* (*Callicarpa acuminata*) fruit is mashed in a liter of boiled water. Adults take it for one day, half a liter in the morning and half a liter at night. For children a quarter of a liter is prepared, given half in the morning and half at night. *X'puk'im* is a shrub with white flowers and fruits that grow in clusters. The mature fruit is purple; it looks and smells like guava, but is not eaten.

- Mash a handful of *sinanche'* (*Zanthoxylum cuneata*) and a handful of *xkakaltún* (*Ocimun micránthum*, L.) with two leaves of *xoltexnuk* (*Limpia umbellata* or *Hyptis pectinata*) in a liter of boiled water. Strain and divide in thirds to be administered three times a day for one day to adults. For children, prepare half the number of leaves in a half-liter of water.

- A handful of leaves from *tanlos che'* (*Zanthoxylum fagara*, L.) and *sinanche'* (*Zanthoxylum cuneata*) are mashed in a liter of boiled water. Strain and administer to the patient in three doses over the course of one day.

- One branch of rosemary *(Rosmarinus officinalis, L.)*, a pinch of *alucema*, star anis, and anis seed *(Pimpinella anisum, L.)* are boiled in a liter of water, given one spoonful an hour for three days. This is taken for common diarrhea.
- For adults the bark of *guaco* or *ek (Aristolochia pentandra), chibo che*, and *tinto ek (Haesatoxylon campechianus,* L.) are used. *Guaco* and *chibo che* are boiled together. Once boiled, the *tinto* is added. The preparation is taken in three doses over two days.
- A handful each of *po' pox (Urera baccifera,* L.) and lemon grass *(Cymbopogon nardus* R.) are boiled together in a liter of water. A handful of *tinto ek (Haesatoxylon campechianus,* L.) is added. Half a cup is taken before meals and half after. This treatment is only for adults.
- The patient takes the medicine known as "Spirit of a little girl": eighteen branches of rue are placed in a pomander or jar and two heaping spoonfuls are taken under the noon sun.
- The first water of a rainfall is collected in a tub and a handful of leaves of *payche (Petiveria alliacea)* are added. The patient bathes in the cold infusion water beneath a chicken coop. The chickens take on the illness, leaving the patient's body healthy.
- *Sinanche' (Zanthoxylum cuneata,* L.) *pichich'e (Psidium yucatanense)*, *xkakaltún (Ocimum micranthum, L.)*, and *xpukim (Calicarpa acuminata)* are boiled together in a quarter liter of water and the infusion taken in two doses.
- Young fruit and bark of guava *(Psidium guajava)* are boiled with leaves of *pichiche' (Psidium yucatanensis)*, a small coconut, and bits of cinnamon, and the infusion is taken fresh.
- Scrapings from the root of *tipte'ak*, four leaves of mint *(Mentha piperita,* L.) four leaves of *Cedronella mexicana*, and one each of allspice *(Pimienta officinalis)*, *alucema*, and rosemary are parboiled in a liter of water. It is taken cold. Adults take the liter in four doses, children in eight.
- Two pieces of the root of *x-kambalhan (Dorstenia contrayerva,* L.), a handful of wild oregano *(Lipiia graveolens)* and two pieces of the bark of *k'ok'obche' (Pilocarpus racemosis)* are boiled in a liter of water and taken in three doses over the course of one day.
- Several leaves of mint are boiled with *poleo (Mentha pulegium,* L.) in a small amount of water; three spoonfuls a day are taken three times a day for two days.
- Two leaves of *tzitzin* (mugwort) *(Artemisia vulgaris, L.)*, nine leaves of "lemon tea" *(Cymbopogon citratus)* and two pieces of lemon grass *(Cym-*

Disease Classification

bopogon nardus, R.) are boiled in 300 ml. of water and taken three times a day. The infusion is repeated for three days.

- The *pica pica* fruit is mixed with *atole* and a quarter of a liter of sugar and taken cold in one dose for intestinal worms.
- Of the following plants, five stems are infused in 250 milliliters of water and taken four times a day. The plants can be used separately or together: *K'ak' ilxiu* (mint), *poleo (Mentha pulegium,* L.), plantain *(Plantago major,* L.), *tzitzin* (mugwort) *(Artemisia vulgaris,* L.), verbena *(Buchea* spp.), *Cedronella mexicana, putxiu (lentejilla) (Lepidium virginicum,* L.), *xik'inpek* or *xikin (Calea zacatechich),* lemon grass *(Cymbopogon nardus), x'puk'im (Calubrina greggii,* W.), *xhalalnal (Calosia virgata,* Jacq.), *sinanche' (Xanthozylum cuneata,* L.), *pichí* (guava) *(Psidium guajava,* L.), *xtok'abal (Eupatorium odoratum,* L.), *chocuil xiu, pasmoxiu* or *claudiosa (Capraria biflora,* L.).
- Of the following plants, 20 cm. of the mashed root or bark is infused in a half liter of water and taken in two doses: *mul och (Triumphetta semitriloba,* Jacq.), *mak che (Ximenia americana,* L.), *chukum* or *chimay (Pitecollobium albicans,* K.) in a half-liter of water, taken in two doses for a day.
- Infusion of a handful of *peteltún (Cissimpelos graveolens)* in 400 ml. of water, repeated several times.
- Mashed leaves of oregano *(Lippia graveolens,* H.M. et K.) soaked in water for several hours. The water is drunk at the patient's discretion.
- Ten lime leaves *(Citrus aurantifolia,* Ch.) and a pinch of anis seed *(Pimpinella anisum,* L.) are infused in a quarter of a liter of water with a teaspoon of bicarbonate of soda, to be taken repeatedly.
- Three burnt tortillas, 30 grams of unwashed corn mash, 400 ml. of water and a young, peeled banana, mashed together and taken at the patient's discretion.
- *Guaco kaax (Aristolochia pentandra)* infused in 100 ml. of water taken in one dose.
- *Lukum xiu* (epazote) *(Chenopodium ambrosioides,* L.). The whole plant is infused in a half liter of water. Contraindicated during pregnancy.
- Ten cm. of bark of *x'pichiche' pach* or *pach chi'* or *pach abal* or *pach pichi' (Psidium yucatanense)* mashed into 200 ml. of water and taken in two doses.
- A clay pack made of *kan kab lu'um*—red clay—applied three times to the abdomen.
- Nine hearts of *xpuk'ím (Calubrina greggii,* W.) infused in 300 ml. of water is taken in two doses accompanied by incantation.

- Nine leaves of *oox "Ramón" (Brisimum alicastrum, Trophis racemosa)* are boiled in 250 ml. of water.
- A piece of the bark of *x-tún che (Chiococca alba,* L.*)* taken in a half glass of water. Avoid hot foods.
- Make an infusion of burnt tortillas. Results are apparent in an hour-and-a-half.
- Infusion of *sinanche' (Zanthoxylum cuneata,* L.*), xoltexnu (Lippia umbellata)* and *x'kakaltún (Ocimum micranthum,* L.*),* taken only once.

Prevention
- For newborns: the mother administers a tea of chamomile and *alucema* three days after birth and doesn't expose herself or the child to harmful winds *(saman kan* or *chikín ik)* during these days.
- Put the child's clothes on backwards and give the child a necklace of deer's eye (a type of seed resembling the eye of a deer) to ward off evil eye; kiss the child and smudge her with charcoal; rub her with rue *(Ruta graveolens)* on the forehead and nape of the neck and put rue in her clothes.
- Avoid giving heavy foods to children, elders, or those recently cured of illness.
- Do not lift heavy objects.
- Make sure all food is clean and free of flies. Wash hands before eating and boil water before drinking. Do not allow animals to live in the house with the family.
- Regularly eat guava fruit and drink lemonade.

Relations With Other Medical Models
- In Western allopathic medicine the illness *wach' k'aja' al* corresponds to various globally recognized syndromes recognized as common diarrhea. The causes of this syndrome include infections, parasites, allergies, immune deficiencies, malnutrition, bad circulation, toxicity, and tumors. Diarrheas of a greenish coloration consisting of abundant, greasy feces are due to ferment in the small intestine. In small children these bowel movements will be due to the presence of excess sugars. Fermentation of food in the intestines generates gases which are reabsorbed into the blood, temporarily slowing the cellular exchange of gases in the plasma. This explains the generalized symptoms. There is a type of parasitic or giardic diarrhea which causes duodenitis with inflammation of the mucosa and which bears the aforementioned symptoms; it is caused by malnutrition and accompanying atrophy of the duodenum.

- In Chinese traditional medicine this illness might correspond to a syndrome of excess due to a conflict of heat and cold. Cold is an external agent capable of entering the body by way of foods, cold water, or cold air (entering the lungs by way of the skin). When cold settles in the spleen or middle burner, the organs lose their ability to transport and transform foods and liquids. Nutrients are unable to rise and nourish the rest of the body, stagnating in the intestines and causing diarrhea. Diarrhea caused by a cold syndrome is characterized clinically by its liquidity and lack of color and odor; when the illness is not serious the stools are loose; in more serious cases there will be undigested foods present. These signs are accompanied by abdominal pain which is relieved by hot compresses or massage. There will be aversion to cold, coldness in the limbs, pale face, thin tongue with white coating, and a deep and slow pulse.

Heat is an external agent which can enter the organism by way of hot foods, hot water or warm air (entering the lungs by way of the skin). When heat becomes concentrated in the middle burner (the digestive organs) it can damage these organs. The stomach loses its fermenting function and the intestine loses its ability to transport foods, causing foods to putrefy and transform into a yellow, fetid mass. Defecation is difficult and painful. There is strong thirst and possible fever; when the stomach fails in its descending function, the energy tends to rise in the form of nausea and vomit. The urine is bright yellow, the tongue is red and the pulse rapid.

Eating Disorders
When one eats to excess the functions of stomach and intestines are challenged, the stomach loses its ability to descend the energy, there are acid regurgitations and a replete sensation in the abdomen and thorax; when the intestine fails in its function there is frequent, fetid flatulence; the stools are thick and watery, the tongue is yellow and the pulse is slippery.

Relations With the Wind (Syndrome of Excess)
The Maya speak of "the wind of water," a cold, wet wind that attacks when "the mother comes from the forest." This wind penetrates the lung channel by way of the skin and travels through the middle burner to chill the spleen. The thermal conflict causes diarrhea.

Emotional Changes
When one is angered the first organ affected is the liver, which concentrates energy in its interior; this energy transfoms into fire; fire damages

the spleen, which then fails to exercise its function of transforming and transporting foods; foods stagnate in the intestines causing diarrhea. The characteristic of this diarrhea is that it appears immediately after one becomes angered; there is pain in the abdomen and the ribs, a sensation of abdominal fullness and thoracic tightness, belching, and loss of appetite. After evacuation the pain vanishes. The tongue is thin with a thin coating, and the pulse is tense and deep.

The clinical description of *wach'k'a'ajal* given by the *curanderos* is similar to a state of dampness. For the spleen to do its work efficiently it should be "dry." Dampness in the spleen causes the organ to fail in its job of transforming and moving foods and the dampness stagnates there resulting in the non-separation of clear and turbid liquids and the inability of nutrients to rise and feed the organism. These liquids fill the intestine resulting in abdominal distention, frequent evacuations, weakness and heaviness in the legs, and labored breathing. There is a lack of appetite, thin tongue, and weak, soft pulse.

XAKA TA'A

This is a state of dirtiness and cold in the stomach. There are various causes of *xaka ta'a*:

- Worms, caused by dirty dishes or bad meat.
- When unsupervised children eat hot foods accompanied by cold liquids, or when they eat hot limes.
- Worry and preoccupation.

The patient suffers from nocturnal defecation leaving chill in the stomach. There may be dizziness, loss of appetite, inflammation of the cheeks and feet, pale face, blurred vision, excessive worry, and irritability.

Diagnosis involves taking the pulse, palpating the abdomen, and noting tightness in the jaw and blurriness in the eyes. Diagnosis can also be done using the *sastún*.

Xaka ta'a can be easily confused with *cirro, ele wix* and *maan u janal*.

Xaka ta'a is spontaneous, appearing in any season and in any individual. In an advanced state the illness may last only twenty-four hours before the patient dies of chills.

Treatments

- Scrape a spoonful of the bark of *guaco (Aristolochia pentandra)*, add a teaspoon of leaves of *ko' ko' che'* and lemon tea *(Cymbopogon citratus)*, lime leaf *(Citrus aurantifolia)*, five leaves of Santa Cruz rue, a bit of cinnamon, nine peduncles of bitter orange *(Citrus aurantium, L.)*, and a pinch of baking soda. Boil these ingredients in ten large spoonfuls of water. Adults take two spoonfuls every half-hour, children one-half spoonful every half-hour.
- One hundred grams of the leaves of *chi kee (Chrysophyllum mexicanum)*, four leaves of lime, a pinch of anis seed, four leaves of mugwort, a piece of *"bonete" (kuhche') (Pseudobombax ellipticum* H.B. et K.*)* and a slice of the rind of sapodilla *(Manilkara zapota, L.)* are boiled in a quarter-liter of water. Children take a spoonful every two hours.
- One young ginger plant *(Zingiber officinalis)*, four pieces of star anis, a spoonful of Nescafe, a small piece of *x'kabachi (Buchnera pusilla)*, and fourteen drops of *incienso maravilloso* are boiled in one liter of water. Children take one quarter of a glass, adults a full glass, every four hours.
- Three young plants of *po'pox (Urera baccifera, L.)*, three young plants of epazote *(Chenopodium ambrosioides, L.)*, nine leaves of lime *(Citrus aurantifolia)*, and nine leaves of young bitter orange *(Citrus aurantium, L.)* are boiled together in a liter of water. Nine pieces of charcoal are added when done, and the infusion is taken three times a day.

Prevention:

- Don't allow children to put just anything in their mouths.
- Keep dishes and utensils clean.

Relations with Other Medical Models:

For occidental medicine nocturnal or morning diarrhea can be caused by a hypertransit in the small intestine. This is common in diabetics and people infested with ascaris (an intestinal parasite). Often it is chronic but does not occur by day.

Traditional Chinese medicine would explain this syndrome as a weakness of the spleen-kidney which destabilizes the liver. If the kidney is weak it cannot warm the spleen; a weak spleen cannot nourish the kidney. The weakness of both brings about a weakness of the general energy, manifesting as cold throughout the body. Weakness of kidney *yang* causes an over stimulus to kidney *yin* which can manifest as alterations in liquid metabolism, like edema; if the spleen is weak the organ cannot adequately transport fluids and the legs become swollen.

A general state of weakness interrupts the transformation and passage of liquids in the bladder. "The water does not find its path" and it may rise to the upper extremities, causing facial swelling. Weakness of the spleen manifests as bodily exhaustion, fatigue, pale face, lack of appetite, and diarrhea. In the chill of night the spleen is not heated and so diarrhea appears at night, especially in the early morning hours.

Similarly, a weak spleen cannot nourish the liver and the liver *chi* becomes stuck; having nowhere to go it turns to fire; liver-spleen imbalance explains the patient's irritability.

TZAN NU YAAL

This is another diarrhea-related illness, known in Spanish as *caída de mollera* or fall of the crown, and in Maya as *emu yaal, lubu lu yaal* and *jalk'ajaan u yaal*. It is caused when a child falls, is thrown in the air during play, or is moved brusquely and forcefully. It has little to do with the child's overall constitution.

The diarrhea is a greenish paste; there is inflammation in the throat and infants find it difficult to suckle. There may be fever, nausea, exhaustion, and paleness.

To establish the diagnosis, the head of the child is observed. They say that in *tzan nu yaal* a sunken spot appears in the crown of the head, slightly different from the sunken spot present in dehydration. The diagnostic is confirmed when, after treatment, the crown has returned to normal.

This illness is easily confused with *wach' kaja'al* and evil eye.

Tzan nu yaal is common in children from three months to three years of age. It is not very frequent, but it can be fatal if not promptly attended.

Treatments
- The hollow in the crown, or *yaal,* can be raised by sucking on it through a fine fabric. Two quick breaths are often sufficient; the illness is quickly cured this way.
- Sometimes, to reinforce the above treatment, a finger is inserted in the mouth to raise the palate. This is commonly done by midwives. Also the child may be held upside down and hit on the feet.

Prevention
- Be careful to not play too brusquely with the child.
- Watch over children playing with their older siblings.

Disease Classification

Relations With Other Medical Models

In occidental medicine there is no disease which corresponds entirely, though intestinal ailments with respiratory complications are well-known by pediatricians: bronchopneumonia often manifests with abdominal pain; diarrhea with infection in the respiratory canal.

KIIK NAAK' OR TA'KI'IK

This is an illness of the stomach and intestine characterized by liquid evacuations with mucus, blood, and stomach cramps *(chot naak')*. It is also known as dysentery. There are three types of dysentery: simple dysentery, dysentery from heat, and white dysentery *(dunta)*.

This illness is due to:

- Eating food with excess grease and spices, overindulging, or going a long time without eating.
- Eating cold foods with a hot stomach.
- Getting too much sun.
- Eating rotten foods.
- Not washing hands, plates, or utensils before eating.
- Dust, flies, and parasites.
- Excess stress on the back.
- Indulgence in alcohol.

Signs and Symptoms

This illness is characterized by diarrhea with blood and mucus. In the beginning there is simple mucus, and later there is blood. The patient experiences pain in the abdomen, cramps, fever, and lack of appetite *(kul o'lal)*. There may be nausea and vomiting, headache, backache, pain in the coccyx, inflammation of the abdomen *(chup naak)*, and nocturnal defecation *(xaka taa)*. The face of the patient has a weak aspect with dark rings below the eyes and general physical discomfort. There is constant yawning; the patient oversleeps; in children there are crying fits.

The diagnosis is undertaken by symptoms: the *curandero* looks for signs of blood and mucus in the stool or painful evacuation, fever, headache, *xu o'lal*, and general weakness in the abdomen. The stomach is palpated to see if it feels hot or spongy; the temples are palpated for a strong pulse; the tongue is examined for inflamed veins. Some *curanderos* take the pulse and use cards or a *sastún* to establish a diagnosis.

This illness is commonly confused with *xju-naak* and *k'asa'a naak*

Kiik naak' can occur at any time of year but is most common between June and September, due to rains which bring insects and microbes. The disease can affect anyone regardless of age and sex. It is not very frequent. On average a *curandero* will treat four or five patients a month during the height of *kiik naak'* season.

Kiik naak' is fatal if not attended in time; if a complete treatment is not undergone the illness will resurface. In serious cases the illness can become cancer and death can occur in eight-to-twelve days.

Treatments

- In a liter of water boil bark of the *chulul* tree (*Apoplanesia paniculata*, Presl.), leaves of *sinanche'* (*Zanthoxylum cuneata*, L.), anis seed, *tzitzin* (mugwort), and four handfuls of sapodilla bark (*Manilkara zapota*, L.). The liter should last all day, one swallow an hour. The dosage is reduced gradually until the medicine disappears, but the patient continues receiving consultations and orations on Tuesdays and Fridays.

- *Jabín (Piscidia piscipula*, L.) (Jamaican Dogwood). Infusion of 20 cm. of the root in a half-liter of water, sweetened with sugar and taken in two doses in the morning.

- *Xpuk'im* or *Tzulubmay (Colubrina gregii*, S.W.). Infusion of 10 cm. of bark in a half-liter of water taken in two doses in the morning.

- *Pixoy (Buazuma ulmifolia*, L.). Infusion of 30 grams of bark in a half-liter of water taken at discretion.

- *X'peteltunak' (Cissampelos pareira*, L.). Infusion of 13 leaves in a half-liter of water, with three drops of the resin, taken in three doses per day.

- *Kakaltún* or basil *(Ocimum* spp.). Infusion of a small stem with flowers in 300 ml. of water taken twice in the morning.

- Of the following plants, an infusion of 20 cm. of the root in a half-liter of water is taken repeatedly throughout the day: *oop* (cherimoya) *(Annona cherimola)*, *nemax (Heliotropum parviflorum*, L.), *chakmoltmuul (Gomphrena dispersa*, St.), *chi*, *k'anibinché* or *nance (Malpighia glabra*, L.), *x'paxak'il (Simarouba glauca*, B.C.), *ya* (sapodilla) *(Manilkara zapota*, L), *ek'* (palo tinto) *(Heamatoxylum campechanium*, L.), *kolokmaax (Craxaeva tapia*, L.), *tsinché* or *tsuiché (Pithecolobiumunguis cati*, L.), *caimito (Chrysophyllum cainito*, L.).

- Plantain *(Plantago major*, L.). Infusion of a handful in a half-liter of water taken repeatedly throughout the day.

- *Chichibé (Sida acuta*, B.). Infusion of a handful in a half-liter of water taken repeatedly throughout the day.

195

Disease Classification

- *X'tunché (Chiococca alba*, L.*)*. Infusion of 30 cm. of the root in a half-liter of water taken as an enema three times a day for two days.
- *Pomolché (Jathropa gaumera*, G.*)*. A handful of the crushed plant in a half-liter of water, with the plant resin, taken as an enema; it is toxic if taken orally.

Prevention
- Eat regularly.
- Avoid excess grease and spices.
- Avoid alcohol.
- Frequent massage of the back.
- Boil drinking water and wash vegetables before eating.
- Take olive oil to clean the stomach.

Relations with Other Medical Models
For Western medicine the signs and symptoms of *kiik naak* correspond to amebic dysentery, although it may also correspond to some cases of bacterial dysentery (shigellosis).

Irritating foods can cause the presence of blood in the stool in cases of chronic, non-specific ulcerated colon (rare) and in cases of hemorrhoids (more common). Cancer of the rectum or prostate can also cause the presence of blood and mucus accompanied by pain.

For Chinese medicine these symptoms correspond to a syndrome of excess due to damp heat or damp cold. This can be acquired by a pernicious dampness accompanied by cold or heat which penetrates the organism by way of the lungs (and the skin), becoming concentrated in the middle burner.

When the dampness is warm this same heat evaporates the dampness, disturbing the collateral channels, causing stagnation of *chi* and blood. This stagnation occurs mostly on an intestinal level; the abundance of dampness makes the diarrhea mucous; if there is not much blood the dysentery will be white; when heat predominates there will be more blood; the two factors are generally combined.

Due to the blockage of *chi* the patient will feel the need to evacuate but will not be able to, causing damage to the spleen and stomach. The stomach loses its descending function and there is nausea, vomiting, weakness of the spleen, pale face, and loss of appetite. Damp cold brings about a white mucous stool.

CIRRO

The name *cirro* denotes an organ called *tipté* in Maya which is located in the area of the *tuch* (umbilicus). The *cirro* can be detected by its palpitation and is understood to be part of the umbilicus. It is said to store the power of the individual and have a strong influence on its neighboring organs. The word *"cirro"* also refers to illness in this organ. The illness is understood as the destabilization of the normal state of the *cirro*, as if it moves out of its proper place—it drops or becomes "tightened" or "untied."

A fallen *cirro* is caused by brusque movements or a fall. An untied or loose *cirro* is brought on by brusque movements or exerting force after eating. A tightened *cirro* is due to excessive hunger or eating at the wrong hour, which causes weakness in the *cirro*. Eating a heavy meal after not eating for some time can bruise the *cirro*, causing it to contract and tighten.

Signs and symptoms include: diarrhea with undigested food, lumbar pain, weakness, abdominal inflammation, nausea, loss of appetite, and abdominal pain, notably in the sides of the ribcage after eating.

Diagnosis is done through palpation of the abdomen—from the navel to the top of the stomach—to see if the *cirro* palpitates, and if so, how and in what part. The thumb is placed directly over the *tuch* (navel), while the other fingers palpate for a beat. A strong palpitation should be felt halfway between the navel and the mouth of the stomach. If the rhythm isn't felt clearly it signals that the *cirro* is tight. If it is exceptionally strong, this means the *cirro* is loose or untied. It can also be out of place, up, down, to the right or to the left.

This illness can be confused with illnesses of the gall bladder, kidney, and bladder, as well as with hernia.

Diseases of the *cirro* appear mostly in adults, equally in men and in women according to the type of work they do, and these illnesses can appear at any time of year. The patient who has suffered it once has a greater chance of contracting it again. It is not grave unless it goes unattended for a long time, leading to complications.

Treatments
- When the *tipté* is tight, an abdominal massage is given with the knuckle of the index finger, pressing inward and turning the hand counterclockwise. After two or three times it should begin to normalize.
- When it is loose the massage is given in the opposite direction. Some therapists tie off the abdomen with a kerchief to keep the area tight.

- When the *tipté* is out of place, a rubbing is given in a counterclockwise direction.
- The plant *tipté ak* or *tipté ché (Jacquinia auriantiaca,* Aiton*)* can be prescribed; a piece of the stem is parboiled in a half-liter of water and taken for a day. Cold water should be avoided over the course of three days.

Prevention
- Eat in good quantity and at regular hours.
- Don't work immediately after eating. Squat when lifting heavy objects.

Relations With Other Medical Models
For Western medicine this syndrome is very difficult to interpret. By the location, we might think of searching for anatomical relations with the structures present in the abdomen: the residual umbilical cord, the mesentery, the small intestine, the descending aorta, and other vessels. In terms of the location and its appearance in adults it could be something like a hernia on the midline.

Because of the appearance of the illness after brusque movements and the presence of nausea and abdominal pain, we might associate *cirro* with non-specific mesenteric lymphadenitis, which causes sharp pains in the umbilical region.

For Chinese medicine this syndrome might be read as a severe debility of the spleen. When the spleen is very weak, food is not fermented or transformed into nutrients; the "looseness" of the spleen allows food to enter the intestines practically whole, causing liquid diarrhea. Lack of appetite is accompanied by abdominal distention and weakness; the stomach fails in its descending function leading to nausea and vomiting.

CHI'IBAL NAAK'

This is a stomach ache marked by strong abdominal pain. It is caused by eating heavy foods that strain the stomach and by eating very hot or cold foods. The patient feels an intermittent pain in the stomach, occasional vomiting, sleepiness, and possible trembling of the arms and body due to strong pain.

In making the diagnosis, the therapist looks for a rapid pulse. The pulse in the temples is accelerated, the veins inflamed, and the face is flushed.

This illness attacks adults, both men and women, at any time of the year.

Treatments
- Several leaves of sour orange *(Citrus aurantium, L.)*, several leaves of lime *(Citrus aurantifolia)*, along with *tu bux* (ginger) are boiled in a liter of water and then chilled. One cup every three hours for three days, or until the medicine is used up. It is very important to monitor the patient's progress.
- If the treatment is not working it is important to change it: boil one seed of *bálsamo*, one piece of *guaco* root *(Aristolochia pentandra)* and one piece of lime root *(Citrus aurantifolia)* in a half-liter of water. Allow it to cool and administer six times a day until the medicine is used up.

Prevention
- Boil water before drinking and keep eating utensils clean.

Relations With Other Medical Models
For traditional allopathic medicine a cramp or pain caused by a specific type of food is read more as a symptom than as a disease unto itself. It may be parasitic, ulcerous, or infectious, among other possibilities.

For Chinese traditional medicine, eating foods that are extremely hot or cold can damage the *chi* of the spleen and stomach. Cold causes stomach energy to stagnate, causing pain; if the food is heavy and damages the stomach, the spleen can be affected, losing its function of transforming and transporting, and this manifests as diarrhea and pain. When the stomach fails in its descending function there is vomiting. If the food is extremely cold, this stagnates the spleen converting to phlegm which blocks the clarity of *yang*, causing drowsiness.

TU KEE

This is an illness characterized by sour stomach and gas. It is caused by:

- Contamination in the stomach from dirtiness of food and dishes.
- "Stunning" the food by drinking cold water after eating.
- When a dog licks the kitchen utensils.
- When pre-refrigerated meat is bought at the market.

The patient has a sad aspect, constantly strokes the stomach, has no appetite, has sour breath, yellow in the eyes, swollen belly, tiredness and listlessness, vomiting and cramps in the feet.

The diagnosis is undergone symptomatically. Also, the fingers are placed over the belly and thumped to check for inflammation.

Tu kee can appear in any season. It appears more commonly in children but is passed by them to adults. It is not extremely common; a *curandero* might attend to one or two cases a month. If it goes untreated the belly can continue bloating until the patient dies from the gases trapped there.

Treatments

- Heat three stones red-hot and use them to heat a quantity of urine with cedar bark *(Cedrella mexicana,* M.*)*, nine leaves of *payche (Petiveria alliacea,* L.*)* and a bit of animal feed. Use this formula to treat several leaves of *x-k'o'och* (Castor) *(Ricinus communis,* L.*)* and tie them to the patient's abdomen.

- Infuse a piece of orange root *(Citrus sinensis),* lime root *(Citrus aurantifolia)* and a little baking soda in a half-liter of water. Take a half-cup before eating and the rest after. The treatment should last nine days. The patient should avoid eating lime, as well as fatty foods; rice and crackers are recommended. Considering that the medicine is of a warm nature, the patient should not go out in the night air. The treatment is accompanied by incantations.

Prevention

- Take olive oil, one swallow every eight hours; boil a handful of leaves of epazote in a half-liter of water and drink three times a day.

Relations With Other Medical Models

For occidental medicine an illness characterized by sourness and gas, in which the patient lacks appetite, has stomach pain, pale skin, and sulfur breath can be attributed to a fermentative dyspepsia, occasioned by parasites (tricomoniasis, giardiasis, ascaridiasis), exacerbated by food of poor quality (refrigerated meat). In adults fermentative dyspepsia is related to the insufficiency of digestive processing, an inadequate diet, intestinal atrophy due to gastritis, and insufficient pancreatic exocrine.

For Chinese traditional medicine the syndrome described by the Mayas as *tu kee* is considered a syndrome of excess; cold or heavy foods cause the spleen, stomach and intestines to lose the capacity of movement and transformation. The vital energy is not fluid and stagnates in the middle burner causing abdominal distention, pain, weakness in the spleen, and lack of appetite.

The face is pale and the patient feels listless and unresponsive. Stagnant food in the stomach causes the energy to concentrate here and later to transform into heat, "cooking" the fluids in the stomach. Since the stomach has lost its descending capacity there will be acidic regurgitations and sourness (from the rising liquids in the stomach) smelling like sulfur or rotten eggs. The cramps are due to the spleen's inability to process nutrients and send them out to the muscles.

K'AN CHI K'IN

This is a malfunction of the gall bladder caused by fear, anger, or other strong emotions, as well as by lack of care in the diet. When the stomach is dirty, phlegm accumulates there, produced by the gall bladder.

The patient shows a lack of appetite, bitterness in the mouth, headache *(kinan pool)*, nausea, yellow stool, inflammation of the stomach, yellowness in the eyes, dirty tongue, and bad breath.

The diagnosis is according to the symptoms; this illness is easily confused with gastritis.

K'an chi k'in is most common in the dry season *(xaxk'in)*, and in adults, both men and women. It is very common in people who drink alcohol, and can be grave if not adequately treated. If it is not treated well it can become complicated, with gallstones, cirrhosis of the liver, hepatitis, and nerve damage.

Treatments
- Ten grams of boldo *(Peumus boldus)* in one liter of water.
- Five grams of powder of jalapa root *(Convulvulus jalapa* or *Ipomoea purga,* W.L.)* in a glass of boiled water, diluted.
- Boil a handful of senna leaves in a quarter-liter of water, and take on an empty stomach. Do not eat until four or five hours after.

Prevention
- Undertake an annual stomach purge.
- Drink orange juice regularly.

Relations With Other Medical Models
- For Western medicine this syndrome relates to dyspepsia and complications in the gall bladder, possibly due to nerve disorders caused by stress.

- For Chinese medicine this syndrome corresponds to damp-heat in the liver and gall-bladder or simply to liver heat.

When damp heat becomes concentrated in the liver and gall-bladder the liver loses its function of dispersion of vital energy and this energy stagnates in these organs. This can damage the stomach which then fails in its function of descending *chi*. There is vomiting and nausea, sourness, and bad breath. Stagnant energy causes abdominal distention and the energy of the spleen ascends in the form of regurgitations and bitter flavor in the mouth. The liver and gall bladder channels will funnel the bile causing headaches and yellow eyes; damp heat passes to the intestines causing the stool to become yellow.

Liver heat can be caused by anger that "represses the energy of the liver," stagnating it and heating it, causing the above symptoms.

CHUJUK WIX, CH'UJUK K'IIK (SWEET URINE)

This is when the blood sugar level rises due to fear, disgust, weakness, heredity, or a high-sugar diet. The patient urinates often, drinks excessive amounts of water, loses weight, the vision becomes blurry, and there is pain in the stomach. The patient becomes moody, pensive, stubborn, easily disgusted, depressed, and tearful, with rheumatic pain, inflamed belly, swollen knees, loss of hair, loosening of teeth and fingernails; skin wounds do not heal. The vision becomes blurred and the patient craves sugar. He or she becomes unable to walk due to "the wind of diabetes."

The diagnosis involves palpating the temples and taking the pulse, checking the tongue, observing the symptoms, analyzing the urine. A jar of the patient's urine is left exposed to the air, and if flies gather around the jar the illness is confirmed. Similarly, a bit of paper may be wet with urine and left near an ant nest to see if ants gather. The urine may be tasted for sugar, or left to dry to observe the residual sugar content.

A diagnosis by divination may be undertaken by throwing grains of corn or by reading cards, the insides of animals, or the *sastún*.

Chujuk wix can be confused with rheumatism and anemia. It can manifest in any season in people over fifteen years of age, and more commonly in adults over thirty. A *curandero* in Campeche attends about two cases a month. If treatment fails, the patient becomes unable to function, undergoes great suffering, and may die. The body dries up little by little, sometimes very rapidly. Some cases last up to ten or twelve years.

Treatments

- *X'kaba-chichibé (Buchnera pusilla*, H.B. et K.*)*. Small pieces of the bark and a cup of leaves are cooked in a half-liter of water. This is taken over the course of a day.
- *Sakxiu (Abutilan lignosum*, G. Don.*)*. Infusion of a handful of leaves to be taken repeatedly.
- *Xpuk'im (Calicarpa acuminata*, H.B. et K.*)*. Infusion of ten cm. of the root in 250 ml. of water taken daily while fasting.
- Of the following plants, an infusion of 30 grams of bark in 250 ml. of water is taken daily while fasting: *xpichiché pach (Psidium yucatanensis,* Lundell*)*, *x'sakchac (Bursera aff simaruba*, L.*)*, *x'tabentún (Pittiera grandiflora*, Rose*)*, *x'tokabán (Calea urticifolea*, Mill, spp.*)*.
- Aloe Vera *(Aloe vulgaris*, L.*)*. 300 grams of the juice taken daily while fasting.
- *X'pechuki (Porophylum punctatum*, Miller.*)*. Infusion of a handful of flowers in a half-liter of water, taken daily while fasting.
- *K'alxixlooch, k'oochllé* or *guarumbo (Cecropia obtusifolia*, L.*)*. Infusion of bits of the bark and root in a half-liter of water, taken daily at the patient's discretion.
- *Vicaria* or periwinkle *(Vinca rosea)*. Infusion of bits of the root and ten red flowers in 250 ml. of water, taken while fasting.
- *Kanlol* or *tronadera (Tecoma stans.*, L.*)*. Infusion of a handful of the plant in a half-liter of water taken throughout the day.
- 200 grams of *nopal* (prickly pear) *(Opuntia cochenillifera*, L.*)*, half a fruit of *k'uum* (squash) *(Cucurbita* spp.*)*, and five green tomatoes *(Physalis ixocarpa*, B.*)*. Wash the fruits and let them soak in 300 ml. of water overnight to take while fasting.
- Infusion in one liter of water of 10 cm. of the root of *tankasché (Zanthoxylum fagar*, L.*)*, six leaves of *guaco (Aristolochia pentandra*, Jacq.*)*, three leaves of *on* (avocado) *(Persea americana*, M.*)*, three leaves of *takoob* or *guanábana (Annona muricata*, L.*)*, six grains of allspice *(Pimenta officinallis*, Lindill.*)* and a pinch of star anis *(Pimpinella anisum*, L.*)*. Drink a small glass three times a day.
- Boil a liter of water with two inches of the root of *te a'k* (bitter medicine). Take after each meal for nine days.
- Bury nine sections of *pa'aken* (wild *nopal*, or prickly pear) *(Opuntia cochenillifera*, L.*)* in hot ashes for an hour. Unbury them and press out the

juice; add two cups of white rum and a pinch of salt and set to boil. When done, put in a jar. Allow to cool and take one cup before each meal. Take a cup of olive oil in the morning before taking the medicine and avoid soft drinks.

- Blend or cook nine sections of prickly pear *(Opuntia cochenillifera, L.)* and take for three days. Avoid soft drinks and fast, taking only fruits like sweet oranges *(Citrus sinensis)*. Take good care for thirty days until the illness passes.

- In a liter of water parboil thirteen leaves of guanábana *(Annona muricata, L.)*, thirteen of avocado, thirteen of *chaya (Cnidoscolus chayamansa)*, eighteen grains of allspice, a strip of *pitaya (Cereus donkelarii)*, a pinch of rosemary *(Rosmarinus officinalis, L.)*, a strip of sour orange *(Citrus aurantium, L.)*, nine leaves of lime *(Citrus aurantifolia)* and thirteen leaves of *Citrus limetta*. Drink at room temperature for thirty days. After a month take tomato juice and hibiscus tea without sugar.

- In a half-liter of water boil two sections of chopped prickly pear, the juice of one lime, five lime leaves, and five leaves of sweet orange. Let cool and take a half-cup before eating three times a week.

- This is a cure involving the use of several plants in a series: first *guayacán (Guaiacum sanctum, L.)*, then *nopal*, then *x'pechwukil (Porophyllum puneatatum)* and finally *pitaya (Cereus donkelarii)*, one a day, parboiled. After six months the cure will be complete.

- Prepare *lon tzu tzuy* : a light meal with a pinch of salt, cilantro, tomato, and vegetable or olive oil (avoid animal fat).

- In a half-liter of water prepare the vine *café ak,* and take repeatedly over the course of a month.

- The indigenous people of Campeche and Yucatán make regular use of aloe *(Aloe vulgaris, L.)*, guarumbo *(Cecropia obtusifolia, L.)*, xtokabán *(Calea urticifolia,* Mill, spp.*)*, xsacchak *(Bursera aff simaruba, L.)*, xpukín *(Calicarpa acuminata,* H.B. et K.*)*, sac xiu *(Abutilan lignosum,* G. Don*)*, and *x kabá chichibé (Buchnera pusilla,* H.B. et K*)*. With the exception of aloe, whose juice is taken while fasting, the rest are taken principally as infusions of the leaves. Accompanied by a careful diet low in sugars, these botanical therapies seem to work; the results are encouraging.

Prevention
- Avoid bottled, sweetened drinks in favor of fruits and fruit juices, and exercise. Avoid coffee and take salt regularly.

Relations With Other Medical Models

- For occidental medicine, this syndrome corresponds to Diabetes Mellitus, the sixth most-common cause of death on the Yucatán Peninsula.
- For Chinese traditional medicine this clinical description corresponds to a deficiency of *yin* of the lungs, stomach, and kidney and manifests when there is excessive intake of heat-producing or greasy foods, when the emotions are repressed causing the energy to turn to fire, and when excessive sexual activity depletes the kidney *yin*.

These factors cause *yin* debility and overabundance of *yang*. Due to this the lung cannot properly distribute fluids, causing thirst and descent of liquids in the body resulting in frequent and abundant urination. This is due as well to the inability of the kidney to control the liquid balance. Weak kidney *yin* causes the patient to appear weak and tired; deficiency of stomach *yin* causes excess heat in this organ and excessive hunger; the spleen is implicated as well, unable to extract the nutrients from food, resulting in weight loss and weakness. Without the capacity to control fluids, they are badly distributed, causing edema, especially in the feet.

YAYA WIX

This is a disease of the kidneys characterized by painful urination. It is caused by:

- The ingestion of heavily spiced (hot) foods.
- The accumulation of residues from the liquids one drinks.
- Lack of personal care and failure to undergo an annual cleansing.

The patient experiences painful urination, pain in the lower back and waist, pain and inflammation in the knees, parched and cracked skin in the heels, and pain in the stomach. There is frequent urination and general weakness.

The diagnostic cues are painful and frequent urination. An observation is done where a urine sample is left to repose; the accumulation of a sort of sandy grit establishes this as the illness.

This illness in women can be confused with inflammation of the ovaries with rheumatism and fever pain. It generally appears at any time of year, though more frequently during the hot months. Anyone is susceptible, but it has been noted that it occurs with more frequency in office workers. If the treatment is not completed, the illness can return regularly. Complication of the illness can result in urinary tract infection, kidney stones, and renal hemhorrage. These complications can eventually lead to death.

Treatments

- Six seeds of sapodilla *(Manilkara zapota, L.)*, ground and mixed in 100 ml. of water, taken three times a day.
- Six cm. of the root of *elemuy (Malmea depressa)* parboiled in a quarter of a liter of water. Take cold on an empty stomach for three weeks.
- Twenty cm. of the root of *"palo warumbo" (Cecropia peltata)*, taken from the west side of the tree. Parboil in one liter of water, sweeten with sugar, and take at room temperature.
- Two 20 cm. pieces of the root and nine leaves of *"chaya de monte" (Cnidoscolus aconitifolius,* Miller). Parboil in one liter of water and take over the course of three weeks.
- A handful of the grass known as *"pata de gallo"* or *"grama"* (Bermuda grass) *(Cynodon dactylon)*, is boiled in one liter of water and taken cold.
- Of the following plants an infusion is made of the leaves or the whole plant in a liter of water. It is taken repeatedly in the morning, daily for one or two weeks: *much kok* or *doradilla (Orobanche,* spp.), *x'bobtun (Anthurium,* spp.), *xik'inchaac (Nymphaea ampla,* Salisb.), *x'cha* or *chaya (Cnidoscolus chayamansa,* Mc.V.), *xikinburro (Calea urticifolia,* Mill.), *kuché (Cedrella mexicana,* M.), *x'pechukil (Porophyllum punctatum,* Miller), *abal* (plum) *(Spondias,* spp.), *jolol* or *cañotio (Bellotia campbelli,* S.), *x'chinto (Krugiodendrum ferreum,* Vah.).
- *Koochlé* or *kallchilxlooch (guarumbo) (Cecropia obtusifolia,* L.). Infusion of 30 cm. of bark and 30 cm. of the root in a liter of water to be taken daily in the morning for one or two weeks.
- *X'pixton (Phyllantus glaucescens,* H.B. et K.). Infusion of 20 cm. of the root in a liter of water to be taken daily in the morning for one or two weeks.
- *Tsuluktok* or *saksulubtok (Baughinia divaricata,* L.). Infusion of 20 cm. of the root in a liter of water to be taken daily in the morning for one or two weeks.
- Coconut *(Cocos nucifera,* L.). Milk and meat, taken repeatedly every day for one or two weeks.
- *Chakuoob* or *pitaya (Cereus undatus,* Haw.). Soak the fruits in water to make a drink which is taken several times a day for one or two weeks.
- Infusion of three 20 cm. bits of the root of *X'tok'abán (Calea urticifolia,* Mill.), of *sak-elemuy (Malmea depressa,* Baillon.), *box-elemuy* and *x'kat (Parmentiera edulis,* DC.). Infusion of three bits of 20 cm. of the root

each in a liter of water to be taken daily in the morning for one or two weeks.

- Chop a red potato and parboil in a liter of water; drink at room temperature.

Prevention
- Take a regular purge of castor oil.
- Take a regular tea of pearl barley or a tea of horsetail *(Equisetum fluviatilis, L.)*.
- Drink regular doses of lemonade or orange juice, as well as tea of corn-silk *(Zea mays)*.

Relations With Other Medical Models
For Western medicine, this syndrome is known by the general population (in Mexico) as *"mal de orín"* or painful urination. In allopathic medicine this is a symptom and not an illness, and can be included under the rubric of various illnesses, determined by other symptoms and signs such as the presence of pus, blood, grit, and their frequency and quantity, the presence of fever and lumbar pain, as well as by the age and sex of the patient. The syndrome may correspond to gonococcal or other types of urethritis, chronic or acute cystitis, urinary tract infection, vesical litiasis, prostatitis, pyelonephritis, hypertrophy, and prostate cancer.

For Chinese traditional medicine this corresponds to a syndrome of heat in the bladder or damp heat from heat-producing foods. The heat concentrates in the bladder and tries to escape by the urinary duct, producing painful urination. If the heat is very intense it can cause bleeding (by heat damage to the collateral channels). The energy in the bladder stagnates producing painful urination; the heat and stagnation of bladder energy move into the bladder meridian causing lower back pain. The stagnant energy will also affect the kidney channel (kidney and bladder run together internally and externally). Pain and swelling in the knees may be caused by blocked energy in the kidney channel, as may the cracked skin in the heels, which implies a drying-out of this area.

SE'EN

This is an illness of the respiratory system caused by:

- Being hot and bathing in cold water. This can cause the blood to have trouble circulating.
- Bathing in lukewarm water and stepping out into the air.
- Eating sweet oranges, which have a hot thermal nature.
- Contact with dust.
- Contagion from infected people.
- Contact with *iik k'aja'*—the wind of water.

The patient exhibits runny nose—watery at first turning to yellowish—and pain in the throat, head, eyes, and lungs, scratchy throat, teary eyes, agitation *(jeesbal se'en)* and possible pain in the ears. The patient is weak, listless, and without appetite.

The diagnosis is by symptoms. This illness can be confused with asthma, bronchitis, amigdalytis, pharyngitis, tuberculosis, and whooping cough.

Se'en is most common in cold, rainy weather (October, November and December) but can appear at any time. Age and sex are not factors. It is a very common illness. Complications can turn it into a chronic condition—chronic cough, bronchitis, pneumonia, or asthma—which may lead to death.

Treatments

- Parboil the flower of *ciricote (Cordia dodecandra*, D.C.), hearts of *jabín (Piscidia piscipula)*, nine ants from the ant acacia *(Acacia collinsii)*, a handful of leaves of *misib kob (Turnera diffusa*, Willd.), a plant of *much kok (doradilla) (Orobanche*, spp.), and a spoonful of sugar in a liter of water. This is taken for three days.
- Parboil *sak mul ("amor seco") (Althernathera ramosissima*, M.), *xtus* of *jabín (Piscidia piscipula)*, cumin, *ramón (Brosimum alicastrum* or *Trophis racemosa)* and the above-ground roots of *jícara* or *luuch (Crescentia cujete)* together in a liter of water, to be taken at room temperature for four days.
- Parboil two hearts of *sak ak'*, basil *(Ocimum*, spp.), *frijolillo (Lepidium intermedium)*, leaves of *x'tujuyche' (Plumeria pudica*, Jacq.) (when the flowers are just opening), the bark of *kuyché (Cedrella odorata*, L.), a bit of the root of *xkan lol (Tecoma mollis)*, a plant of *much k'ok (Orobanche*, spp.), the heart of *pereskúts* and two tablespoons of honey in a liter of

water. Take at room temperature every four hours. At night gargle with the tea, and keep the throat covered for three days.

- Half a lime *(Citrus aurantifolia)* with three tablespoons of honey. Boil and administer before bed. The next day take only boiled water.
- Parboil six leaves of *Brosimum alicastrum* or *Trophis racemosa* with a quarter of a liter of water, sweeten, and drink.
- Parboil the bark of *anacahuita (Cordia dodecandra*, D.C.*), much kok (Orobanche*, spp.*)*, and leaves of avocado *(Persea americana*, M.*)* in a quarter of a liter of water with a handful of salt. Take lukewarm. Keep a towel around the patient's neck to protect it from wind.
- Oregano *(Lipiia graveolens)*. Dry roast the leaves, press, and take the juice.
- Parboil and drink nine avocado leaves and 20 cm. of the root of *pay che' (Petiveria alliacea)*.
- Make an infusion in 300 ml. of water of twelve leaves of *orozús* or licorice *(Glycyrriza glabra*, L.*)*, twelve leaves of *beek' (Eheretia tinifolia)*, twelve leaves of *pasmoxiu* or *claudiosa (Capraria biflora*, L.*)*, twelve leaves of *k'uché*, (cedar) *(Cedrella mexicana*, M.*)*, twelve leaves of lime, and twelve leaves of orange. Sweeten with honey and drink warm.
- Boil the red flowers of bougainvillea with a handful of avocado leaves in a quarter of a liter of water; sweeten with honey and take repeatedly.

Prevention
- Bathe children early in the afternoon.
- Close the doors when it is cold or cloudy.
- Drink a lot of lemonade.
- Take a spoonful of honey every day.

Relations With Other Medical Models
- In Western medicine this syndrome corresponds to catarrh or flu.
- In Chinese medicine this is a syndrome of excess related to wind or cold. These factors enter through the lungs (by way of the skin) or stomach and cause the energy in these organs to become blocked. If the invading factor is cold, the patient will exhibit a clear nasal fluid in the beginning; later, due to blockage, the cold will turn to heat and the mucus will become yellowish. The lung and stomach meridians, being invaded and blocked in their trajectory towards the head, cause pain in the throat and eyes. This explains the chills, fever, and general discomfort.

CHIBA POOL

This is a headache affecting the front and sides of the head.

Chiba pool denotes headaches in general as well; but these are divided into several specific syndromes: *k'inan pool* (pain throughout the head), *jit a jool* (neck pain), and *jolon al* (postpartum headache). Here we describe the *chiba pool* which is specifically frontal and parietal headache.

Chiba pool is provoked by:

- Heat or wind around the head *(jax u jool tumen ik,* "the wind hits you in the head").
- When one is in the *milpa* or in the sun and a mist falls (if it is a strong rain it does not cause a headache because the temperature of the entire body drops).
- When one has a cough and takes a bath, or when one is weak in general.

The cause is a cold wind around the head when the head is warm, especially when the blood is just waking and the circulation is slow. Air enters the head and causes the blood to become dark and stagnant. Due to stagnancy, there is an excess of blood in the head. There is pain in the front and sides of the head and the eyes, the vision is blurred, there may be dizziness, laziness, and imbalance as if drunk. The head becomes hot and sometimes there is fever.

The diagnosis begins with the *curandero* asking what part of the head hurts. The parietal vein is palpated to see if it beats normally or with excessive force; the eyes might be swollen and there may be inflammation of the temples. Tapping on the head may make a hollow sound due to the air trapped inside. Some *curanderos* use cards to make a diagnosis.

Treatments
Tok is done above the temples and along the hairline (the point is *in tan* in Chinese acupuncture). The head is tapped after *tok* is performed to see if the sound has become more acute and less tympanic. Sometimes when the spot is punctured the sound of air escapes along with a few drops of dark blood.

Prevention
It is easy to treat *chiba pool* if one rubs the head on waking and before leaving the house in order to move the blood. Exercising the head, neck, and arms also helps.

Relations With Other Medical Models

- In occidental medicine this syndrome would correspond to a migraine headache.
- In Chinese traditional medicine a headache in the forehead and temples would signal excess liver *yang*. This type of illness is often brought on by anger repressing the *chi* in the liver which in turn converts to fire and runs through the liver meridian, affecting the throat and the eyes. The liver meridian runs over the forehead to the top of the head.

Dizziness is one of the effects of excess liver *yang*. Another cause of pain in the forehead is heat penetrating the stomach meridian, whether external heat or heat originating in the stomach; the stomach channel passes through the forehead, and this excess heat would bring pain to this region. When the kidney *yin* (water) does not balance the *yang* (fire) of the liver and gall bladder, this heat runs up the liver and gall bladder channels into the head.

KINAN POOL

This is a pain over the entire head and neck. For the Maya it is related to *"corrimiento."*

It is caused by emotional stimuli; the temperature of the bile rises when one becomes angered. It is also brought on by:

- High temperature.
- Anger and lack of emotional care.
- Wind in the night.
- When one looks upward, the brain becomes dizzy.

Kinan pool is a pain in the entire head caused by a weakness of the blood. There may be vomiting, teary eyes, pain in the eyes, and loss of vision. When one goes out in the sun the light hurts the eyes. The pain is greatest in the morning; at noon the pain begins to diminish, and when the sun goes down the pain passes. The patient prefers to stay in the dark and has no appetite. There may be partial deafness accompanied by physical exhaustion.

Diagnosis is made according to signs and symptoms. The patient is asked questions about what she or he has or hasn't done in recent days. Upon palpating the veins in the forehead and temples the blood pressure will be lower than normal.

Kinan pool is most common in adults and elderly people, appearing in any season. It can become chronic or aggravated.

Treatments
- As *kinan pool* is characterized by weakness in the blood, *tok* is not performed.
- The plant known as *corrimiento* (with blue flowers) is mashed in water along with *xbolontibil* (with round leaves) *(Cissus trifoliata,* M.*)* and *xbeskan.* The preparation is left outside in the sun. At twelve noon the head and entire body are bathed in the tea. The preparation has a cool nature and refreshes the body, curing the illness.

Relations With Other Medical Models
- For Western medicine this syndrome would correspond to migraine headache.
- For Chinese traditional medicine, this syndrome might be due to weakness in the bladder channel *(taiyangjing)* brought on by wind. A headache that covers the entire head including the occipital region is characteristic of a stagnation in this meridian.

The wind causes *chi* and blood to stagnate in the meridians, not arriving in the head and thus producing pain. The bladder channel runs up the back and the back of the neck; it is born behind the eyes, which explains the tearing and painful vision. As it is a syndrome of deficiency, the pain passes with rest.

KINAN PACH KA OR JIT A JOOL

This is a headache in the occipital region, also known as pain of *"el celebro"* [a slight mispronunciation of the Spanish *"cerebro,"* meaning "brain"—translator.].

This illness can be described as a nervous condition characterized by anger, pensiveness, tiredness, and overwork. It can be caused by bruises to the back and shoulder blade. If one works too much one gets over tired, and this exhaustion rises to the brain. It can also be brought on when a person bathes but does not wet the hair (causing the head and brain to become hot). Pain in the head may descend to affect the neck and back, as well as the throat. There is general discomfort, sleepiness in the eyes, and exhaustion. Sometimes the pain appears first in the back, then the shoulders and the neck until it arrives in the head. The diagnosis consists of palpation of the tendons in the back of the neck looking for inflammation or hardness.

It can appear at any time of year and is most common in adults and elderly people.

It is not grave or chronic, but it is an illness which returns commonly when there is tension and tiredness.

Treatments
- A massage *(jet)* is given on the back, the neck and the back of the head.

Prevention
- Prevention is difficult as the cause is excess work and worry.

Relations With Other Medical Models
- In occidental medicine pain in the back of the neck would correspond to muscular tension in the neck as a consequence of emotional stress. It might also be a symptom of arterial hypertension.
- For traditional Chinese medicine this type of headache might be caused by excess in the bladder meridian, similar to that described previously in *kinan pach ka*.

JOLON AL

This type of headache, also known as *al jool* or *jolon xale'*, often appears when a woman exposes herself to the wind after giving birth. In the first two days after the birth she is hot from the labor and weak from loss of blood; therefore she is easily susceptible to damage by cold winds. The patient exhibits headache, weakness in the body, dizziness, vomiting, lack of appetite, swollen eyes and eyelids, general swelling of the body, hair loss, dry skin, and fever. There may be anemia and loss of skin coloration.

The diagnosis is carried out according to the symptoms exhibited after labor.

The illness can be grave; if it is not attended, the patient may remain weak and pale.

Treatments
A tea is prepared from the plant known as *xmulix (Tillandsia caput-medusae, E. Morr.)*, a type of epiphytic bromeliad which grows in trees.

Prevention
Do not leave the house for two days after giving birth.

Relations With Other Medical Models
- For occidental medicine postpartum headache might correspond to various illnesses, among them a temporary disorder caused by secondary hormonal imbalance or an ischemia (blood deficit) in the glandular tissues. It might correspond, as well, to Sheehan's syndrome due to cardiac weakness from loss of blood and an acute pyelonephritis brought on by blood loss.
- For Chinese traditional medicine postpartum headache is due to a great loss of *chi* and blood; the *chi* and blood, being insufficient, do not rise to the head, causing dizziness, anemia, palor, weakness, and lack of appetite. Similarly, the loss of hair would be due to the lack of blood and *chi,* or generalized *yin* deficiency. If there is fever it is due to the predominance of *yang* and deficiency of *yin.* When there is weakness of blood and *chi,* the meridians are "empty" and it is easy for the wind to penetrate them, arriving at the head and producing generalized pain; the wind causes lung *chi* to stagnate; the lungs fail in their function of distributing fluids, causing a generalized edema.

K'IL KAB

This is a night sweat which principally attacks children between one and eight years of age when they are asleep. It can be caused by the following:

- The mother sleeps with the child and passes to her an excess of heat accompanied by perspiration.
- Rocking the baby just after a bath.
- Sweeping below the hammock while the child is asleep.
- Changing clothes in the open air.
- Allowing the child to be attacked by evil winds.

Children ill with *k'il kab* sweat at night when they sleep. The skin takes on a yellowish tint, the feet and the hands are cold and weak, and there is red coloration around the ears.

The diagnosis is simple as this illness is very specific and is rarely confused with other illnesses.

K'il kab can appear at any time of year in children under eight years old. If the child is not properly cared for she becomes weak and rickety and lacks appetite. It can be fatal if the child loses an excessive amount of fluid and becomes dehydrated. If the treatment is succesful the illness will not reappear.

Treatments
- Talcum powder is applied for several days until the illness stops.
- The child is bathed with honey in the evening for nine days.
- For nine days the child is bathed in water in which beeswax has been boiled.
- Before sunrise leaves of *tz'utz'uk (Cissampelos pareira, L.)*, basil, *sinan ik*, and *tuxtache'* are soaked in a bucket of water. This bucket is placed in the sun. The child is bathed in this water from noon until one o'clock, daily for nine days. If the water has gotten cold it should be reheated by adding warm water. The medicine should not be put over the fire.

Prevention
- The child should not be rocked at night or after bathing.
- The child should not sleep all night with her or his mother.

Relations With Other Medical Models
- In Western medicine nocturnal sweating might be due to a problem in the autonomic nervous system. In adults it can signal the onset of grave illnesses like lymphoma and diabetes mellitus.
- In Chinese traditional medicine, night sweat caused by external heat arises due to heat entering the gall bladder or triple heater channel *(shaoyang)*. This heat stagnates between the external and internal aspects of the body. This causes the surface of the body to fail in its dispersing function, causing a struggle between the protective *chi* and the pathogenic *chi*, bringing about an exodus of liquids through the pores. This occasions sweating accompanied by chills, bitterness in the mouth (gall bladder fluids rising), and the sensation of distention in the hypochondriac and pericardial regions.

MESANKIL

These are various problems in the menstrual cycle, such as spotting, failure to menstruate, and interruptions in the cycle. There are several variations of *mesankil* such as skipping the period and *"pasmo blanco"* ("white chill").
   Mesankil is caused by:

- Bathing in cold water or drinking cold water in the days before or during menstruation.
- Eating limes in the days before or during menstruation.
- Having excess body heat.
- Anemic women and women who do heavy work have a predisposition towards *mesankil;* twisting or hurting the hips and back, as well as going through abortions can increase the chances of contracting *mesankil.* Some midwives refer to *mesankil* as the failure of the ovules to mature due to *pasmo*—a cramp or ache—produced by body heat or weakness.

Symptoms of *mesankil* include:

- Menstrual irregularities such as interruption of the flow, failure to menstruate on time, or spotting.
- There may be pain in the abdomen, head, back, feet, and hands; the lips become dry and black; there is swelling in the stomach, nausea, lack of appetite, laziness, weakness, dejection, crying, yellow discharge, and leaking breast milk even in young women who have not given birth.

The diagnosis takes the form of questioning: is there pain, excess blood, lack of blood, irregular timing? The abdomen is palpated for pain and the lips are examined for signs of dryness and discoloration. The pulse may be read and *sastún* may be performed.

Mesankil can be confused with internal bleeding from the spleen, and with illnesses of the kidneys and bladder.

It is a common illness attended by midwives and is subject to appear at any time of year in women over fourteen years old.

Not receiving adequate treatment, a women with *mesankil* may experience bleeding from the mouth and nose and runs the risk of becoming sterile. Complications may bring about uterine cancer, and intestinal worms may appear due to the stagnancy of blood. There may be very strong pain, and the dejection experienced may become grave.

Treatments
- Boil a bit of the bark of *te'may (Zuelani quidonia,* Schwartz), two pieces of *yebek,* a bit of the blade of *maguey* (agave), half a quart of honey and a pinch of salt in a half-liter of water. Press out the juice, boil again, rub cooking oil on the abdomen, and administer the medicine to the patient still warm. It is recommended to avoid sour or cold food.
- In a liter of water parboil: four leaves of *chalche '(Pluchea odorata),* nine

leaves of *payche' (Petiveria alliacea)*, a bit of the bark of *chak muk (Rauvolfia hirsuta,* Jacq.) (a white-flowering vine), a quart of honey, a piece of the root of *chelén, (Agave silvestris,* D'utra), a piece of *guaco (Aristolochia pentandra)*, two leaves of bitter orange *(Citrus aurantium,* L.), a pinch of *alucema*, and nine grains of allspice. Take it warm, ideally in one sitting. It is recommended to stay home for three days and to avoid cold or sour foods.

- Boil 30 grams of *altanisa (Ambrosia artemisiaefolia)* in a half-liter of water. Take it three times a day. It is recommended to take vitamins.
- Toast and grind *kep a'í ("pene de lagarto"),* and add a bit to any tea the patient is taking. Once is enough.
- Parboil and eat the testicles of a bull and drink the stock. This remedy assures that the woman will be able to give birth after the illness is cured.
- In a half-liter of water, boil a branch of *chalche' (Pluchea odorata)*, a bit of maguey, two sections of *elel (Oxalis latifolia,* H.B. et K.), five leaves of lime, a young palm of *mulix xaan (Tillandsia caput-medusae,* E. Morr.), a branch of rosemary, and a pinch of salt. Take one cup before breakfast and dinner for three days.
- Soak a branch of *chalche'* in a glass of rum and drink at the onset of menstruation. This is recommended to women who are particularly susceptible to menstrual irregularities and have difficulty conceiving.
- Boil 20 leaves of oregano and one leaf of *chiople' (Eupatorium hemipteropodum,* R.) with a pinch of salt. If there is considerable pain add a slice of sweet orange rind and a young plant of *altaniza (Ambrosia artemisiaefolia,* L.). Allow to cool and take three times a day.
- Mix a cup of anis with a pinch of salt, heat, and take. Avoid ingesting cold foods.
- Boil eight leaves of *chalche'* in a liter of water to be taken over the course of a day for three days. Avoid drinking cold water from the onset of menstruation.
- Parboil one leaf of *chiople' (Hepatorium hemipteropodum)* in a liter of water.
- Parboil one stalk of *chichan p'op'ox (Urera baccifera,* L.) in a liter of water for the bath.
- Parboil five grams of cinnamon in half a liter of water and take over the course of one day.

All of the above remedies are warm-natured, so the patient should avoid drinking cold water for two days after treatment.

Medicinal Plants Indicated for Premenstrual Tension

- *Kanaantzín (Lonchocarpus rugosus, B.).* Infusion of a handful in a quarter of a liter of water to be taken on an empty stomach.
- *Kambalhau* or *contrayerba (Dorstenia contrayerva, L.).* Toast a 15 cm. bit of the root; grind and dissolve in a quarter of a liter of water, to be taken on an empty stomach.
- *Pasmoxiu, chocuil xiu* or *claudiosa (Capraria biflora, L.).* Infusion of nine leaves in 500 ml. of water, to be taken several times.

Prevention

- Make sure young girls eat well, and educate them so that, when they reach the age they take proper measures around menstruation: that they do not eat limes, do not drink cold soft drinks, do not wash their hair or bathe in cold water, and generally stay warm and dry during these days.

Relations With Other Medical Models

- For occidental medicine, this syndrome corresponds to a wide range of menstrual irregularities including menorrhagia, secondary amenorrhea, anemia, premenstrual tension, and vaginal infection.
- For Chinese medicine this syndrome corresponds to an organic weakness affecting the spleen/stomach. This weakness causes the source of blood to dry up, giving rise to symptoms of paleness, dizziness, weakness, and so on.

In the case of older, married women the failure to menstruate could be due to weakness in the kidney, causing the liver to experience an inability to manage the blood; blood does not arrive at the uterus, and there is amenorrhea.

External causes might include cold acquired from wind, or ingestion of cold-natured foods. This causes blood to stagnate in the uterus.

Another cause is the blockage of liver *chi* preventing the blood from circulating well in the collaterals and resulting in amenorrhea.

This is the absence of mother's milk during lactation. It is provoked by:

- Not breastfeeding a newborn baby.
- Weakness and bad diet.
- Fright and pernicious winds.

A mother has no milk in her breasts and is unable to feed her child. The breasts shrink and revert to their pre-pregnant state. Women in this condition are frequently chastised by their husbands out of ignorance for not feeding the child.

This condition may appear at any time of year, after a woman has given birth. A woman with this condition can die if the milk enters the lungs for lack of attention.

Treatments

- Drink a cup of *chocolomo*—a sauce similar to *molé*—of iguana, cooked, and lie face down. If the milk still fails to come, drink a dark beer at room temperature.
- The raceme of the fruit *x'etel* is boiled in a liter of water. Drink at room temperature for three days. Do not leave the house or expose yourself to the wind during these days.
- Drink an *atole* of sesame seeds sweetened with honey four times a day for three days and rest to maintain a normal body temperature.
- When the *nixtamal* (corn being cooked down for tortillas) is being prepared, lean over the pot to receive the vapors. Avoid eating cold foods.
- Make an *atole* from corn and drink warm.

Prevention

- Attention and care during pregnancy.
- Give the woman support and sympathy during pregnancy.

Relations With Other Medical Models

- For occidental medicine the description might correspond to a lack of pituitary stimulus due to emotional stress. The possibility of the milk rising to the lungs and causing death might correspond to postpartum sepsis, currently very rare but still present in memory and in the tradition of the *curanderos*.
- For traditional Chinese medicine, this syndrome is one of deficiency. Mother's milk is a product of the transformation of *chi* and blood. If,

in labor, there was a great loss of blood and *chi,* there is no substrate to be turned into milk. Similarly, this loss of *chi* and blood weakens the body; the spleen and stomach lose their ability to draw nutrients from food, thus failing to produce *chi* and blood and establishing a cycle of weakness.

CHU'U CHUN

These are tumors of the skin which can be caused by:

- Insect bites *("cucaracha natzul").*
- The night air.
- When the body is weak and is scratched or pricked by a thorn.

The patient exhibits a reddish welt on the skin with a whitish tip which is where the "microbe" enters to leave pus. They appear in groups of no more than four on any part of the body. The patient experiences strong pain and fever. The sun aggravates the pain. There is dejection, sadness, and exhaustion. When *chu'u chun* is caused by the night wind it appears as a rash which grows infected when scratched.

The diagnosis consists of an examination of the body to identify the rash, and questioning to determine how long it has been developing. The tumors can grow up to the size of a small lime.

This illness can attack anyone, regardless of age and sex, but is considered rare. It is very painful, and if it goes untreated can develop complications. If the illness is not cured it can result in death, blindness, or loss of physical functions like walking.

Treatments
- The rash or tumor is washed with Princess Soap and salt is spread around the tumor without covering the center.
- To control the illness nine thorns of *"pochote"* are ground and boiled in a half-liter of water to be taken three times after eating. This is taken until the tumors dry up. After this the skin of the *"pochote"* is boiled in a bucket of water and added to the bath regularly until the wounds have healed.
- *Jumpetskín (Tillandsia,* spp.). Infusion of 20 leaves; the tumors are washed and the cooked leaves are placed over the area.
- *Chiké (Chrysophyllum mexicanum,* T.S.) and *saksit (Lasciacis divaricata,* L.).* A handful of each is ground and applied to the area.

- *Boktún (Anthurium, spp.)*. Infusion of a handful of the plant for bathing.
- *Tzunyá (Pereskia, spp.)* and *x'kukemba (Phoradendro)*. Wash, grind, and locally apply a handful of each plant.
- *Popox (Tragia nepetaefolia, Cav.)*. Cook the leaves and apply them to the area affected.
- *Jobonk'ak* or *jobonté (Euphorbia heterophylla, L.)*. Wash a handful of the plant, grind and apply locally.
- *Xikín* or *xikinpek (Calea zacatechichii, Sch.)*. Wash and grind the leaves for local application.
- *X'pujuc, maseual puhuc* or *tuubtok' (Passiflora foethida, L.)*. Wash the area, cook the plant and apply hot to the tumors.
- *Kanán (Hamelia patens, J.)*. Wash a handful of the plant, chop and apply locally to help the scarring of the wounds.
- *Kabalhau (Dorstenia contrayerva, L.)*. Cook ten cm. of the root and apply to the lesions.
- *Pichí (Psidium guajava, L.)*. Cook a handful and apply to the lesions.
- *Ek'k'ixil (Bignonia unguis, Cati, L.)*. Wash the heart of the plant, chop, and apply to the wounds. Functions as a homeostatic.
- *Yaak k'iix (Buetnaria aculeata, Jacq.)*. Infusion of two handfuls in the bath.
- *Xaché xtabay* or *netelok' (Pitecoctenium echinatum, Jacq.)*. Wash and chop a handful of the plant and apply as a poultice.
- *K'uum*, Squash *(Cucurbita moschata, Duch.)*. The endocarp (inside rind) applied locally to abscesses helps in scarring.
- *Utsupek' (Tabernaemontana amygdalifolia, J.)*. The leaves and stems, washed and ground, are applied locally; the resin acts to tame the infection.
- *Boxchechem* or *chechem (Metopium brownei, Jacq.)*. A bit of the bark is washed, ground and applied to the lesions to aid in scarring.
- *Kakaltún* (basil). A handful of the plant is washed, ground, and applied to the infected area.
- *Xanabmucuy (Euphorbia hirta, L.)*. Infusion of the whole plant for bathing.
- *Altaniza (Ambrosia artemisiaefolia, L.)*. A handful of the plant is washed, ground, and applied as a poultice to the lesions.

Prevention
- When one has a flesh wound of any sort, avoid leaving the house uncovered or going to the cemetery.

Disease Classification

Relations With Other Medical Models

- In Western medicine this syndrome might correspond to infectious illnesses of the skin or deeper structures with the formation of abscesses. Tropical *piomiositosis,* of the bacillus staphylococcus, generally forms one or two abscesses accompanied by generalized discomfort and fever.

REUMA IK'

This is a cold-natured illness characterized by generalized discomfort and pain in the bones and joints.

This illness is grouped into two basic categories: in the first, the pain appears at night or in moments of cold—cold *reuma*— while in the second, the joints ache during the day—hot *reuma.*

There are seven types of *reuma:* "renitis," "tapa camino," "grión," "la mariposa," "xist lambe," "cruzacamino," and "culebrilla." The *reuma* can be black or white and can be classified according to what part of the body it attacks. *Reuma* can affect not only the back, ankles, knees, etc., but also the eyes, ears, etcetera.

This illness may come about:

- When it is hot and one becomes exposed to cold and damp.
- When one is barefoot and walks on cold, damp ground, especially when one is hot and steps out of the bath.
- When one is in a hot state and steps out into the night air.
- When one goes to the bathroom in the cold morning air.

The patient experiences pain and inflammation in the bones and joints that make working difficult. Sometimes there is a yellowish skin-tone and hair loss.

If the *reuma* is from a nervous disorder, the painful area feels cold to the touch.

Reuma comes on slowly, little by little. At first there is fatigue; later the patient is unable to walk. This pain and inability to walk are the main diagnostic indications of *reuma.* There may be, as well, a ringing in the ears. Additional diagnostics may include pulse-taking and divination with cards or *sastún.*

White rheumatism causes swelling and little pain; it affects the knees and the blood; when the area is punctured, water escapes.

In black rheumatism the feet turn black because of blood that stagnates there; the foot is "dominated" and can't walk. This rheumatism begins with back pain and is caused by microbes in the skin; the patient should avoid beef, soft drinks, and ice.

If air has penetrated the skin the *reuma* is weaker than if air has penetrated between the bones. The wind can enter the body easily when the body is hot and exposed to wind. The blood becomes thick and dark when wind enters the body, and it must be removed.

This illness is more common in the cold months, most notably November, and during changes in climate. The pain increases just before it rains. It is common in people of all ages. *Reuma* is not a grave illness, but if it goes unattended the patient will be forced to stay in the hammock and rest until the illness passes.

Treatments

- Many Mayan masseuses work the body using the same plants: *tzipche' (Bunchosia swartziana, Gr.), sinanché (Zanthoxylum cuneata, L.),* belladonna, garlic, balsam, *guaco (Aristolochia pentandra), chamico,* and *guarumbo (Cecropia peltata).* In cold-natured rheumatism the plants are cooked in Vaseline to prepare a balm, and for hot-natured *reuma* a tincture is prepared with alcohol. Alcohol is cold-natured, and there is no heat used in the preparation of the tincture.
- A handful of *nabamche' (Bursera graveolens),* a handful of *ko'kobche' (Philocarpus racemosus, Vahl.)* and a pinch of salt are soaked together in alcohol and applied to the patient in a bath.
- White rheumatism is treated with a plant called *chooch (Lucuma hipoglauca,* Standley*);* nine leaves and the seeds are parboiled and taken for nine days until the blood is normalized. The legs of the patient are bathed, and then covered with honey and leaves of cherimoya *(Anona cherimola).*
- The black *reuma* is treated with *tok.* "The stagnant blood is the rheumatism, the bleeding of the wind is to get rid of it."
- *Xoltexnu (Hyptis pectinata, L.).* Infusion of two handfuls in a liter of water for bathing; the hot leaves are applied locally as a poultice.
- With the following plants, an infusion of two handfuls in a liter of water is prepared for bathing; the hot leaves are applied locally as a poultice: *popox, laal,* or *hortiga (Tragia nepetaefolia,* Cav.*), sinanché (Zanthoxylum cuneata, L.),* elder *(Sambucus mexicanus, Presl.)* and *pasmo xiu (Capraria biflora, L.).*
- *Nabanché* or sassafras *(Bursera graveolens,* H.B. et K.*).* Two handfuls are soaked in hot water and applied as a poultice.
- *Tunkusché (Zanthoxylum fagara, L.).* The leaves are heated over a fire and applied hot to the painful area.

Disease Classification

- With the following plants, the leaves are washed, chopped, soaked in alcohol, and then applied as a poultice: *x'mak'ulán (Piper auritum,* H.B. et K.*), chioplé (Eupatorium hemipteropodum,* Rob.*), chokob kat (Ipomea carnea,* J.*), tzipché (Bunchosia swartziana,* Griseb.*), mejen x'tohkú (Datura stramonium,* L.*).*
- *Xtabentún (Turbina corymbosa,* L.*). No description of its preparation is given.*
- *On,* or avocado *(Persea americana,* M.*).* Infusion of a handful of leaves and two seeds in a half-liter of water to be taken at discretion.
- *Teresita.* A handful of leaves and small bits of the root are mashed and applied as a poultice.
- *Op* (cherimoya) *(Annona cherimola,* Mill.*).* Toast a 30 cm. bit of the bark; grind while hot and apply as a poultice with animal feed and a pinch of salt. Cover the region.
- *X'nemis* or *cola de tejón (Cercus gaumeri,* St.*).* Infusion of 30 cm. of the bark in a half-liter of water; strain and leave the liquid to cool in the night air; take in small quantities in the morning. This is a dose for several days.
- Garlic *(Allium sativum).* Cook and mash two bulbs of garlic; spread on bread and eat.
- In one type of rheumatism that attacks the back, *tok* is performed at the level of the *bobox* (coccyx), and in the upper back at the level of the first or second thoracic vertebrae, bleeding the area to release the wind. In the following sessions the puncture moves closer to the center of the back, bringing all of the pain to one point in the spinal column and then removing it.
- For rheumatism in the ear, *tok* is performed in the posterior part of the ear over the mastoid process and in front of the ear at the level of the Chinese point *tinggon* (Palace of Hearing). These points are also used in cases of deafness.
- When the hips hurt because of rheumatism in the knee, *tok* should be performed where there is pain.
- One *curandero,* Máximo Tum, of Camino Real, treats this illness with a subcutaneous injection (with a hypodermic needle) of a substance which he did not reveal to us, but which appeared to have come from a pharmacy. He uses different disposable syringes, depending on the age of the patient, although it looked as if he used the same needle on different patients. Basically he injects in the area where the pain is. In one case he made the injection at the level of the femoral articulation, introducing the needle in the direction of the head of the femur in the lateral part of the hip, subcutaneous to a depth of 1.5 cm. He did the same in

the supra-external part of the knee and in the calf three centimeters below the popliteal hollow. The number of injections applied depends on "the quality of the body, of the blood, and of the wind." He continued applying injections on the medial aspect of the leg two *tsun* beneath the Chinese point *yinlingquan,* and at the level of the vertebral column, two *tsun* above the coccyx. He also prescribed a wine called *Gerian Elci.* He requested of us certain medications that he wanted to use in this treatment as well. These medications are (in Spanish): *Isodalina, Eucaliptol,* and *Alcanfor de aceite.*
- Don Pedro Tzulub Ortega of Santa Cruz Ex Hacienda cures rheumatism, as he says, with the heat of his hands.

Prevention
- Boil drinking water.
- Do not walk barefoot.
- Avoid dampness and cold winds.

Relations With Other Medical Models
- Western medicine gives a wide description to what the Maya call *reuma ik',* bridging a variety of rheumatic and arthritic conditions: cramps from fatigue, heat cramps, lumbago, sciatica, tendonitis, muscular contractions, rheumatoid arthritis, osteo-arthritis, and bursitis.

TREATMENTS FOR OTHER CONDITIONS

Plants Indicated for Intestinal Worms
- *Lukum xiu* (epazote) *(Chenopodium ambrosioides,* L.). Infusion of 5 grams of epazote leaf and 10 cm. of the root in a liter of water to be taken repeatedly in the day; this is one daily dose.
- Coconut *(Cocos nucifera,* L.). Milk and pulp; take repeatedly for several days.
- *Kuché (Cedrella mexicana,* M.). Infusion of a handful of bark in a quarter-liter of water to be taken on an empty stomach for three days.
- *Yakunaax, yakunak* or *cundeamor (Momordica charantia,* L.). Infusion of a handful in a half liter of water to be taken throughout the day for three days.
- *Xukul (Portulaca oleracea,* L.). Infusion of a handful in a half-liter of water, taken during the day for three days.

- *Tzitzin* (Mugwort) (*Artemisa vulgaris,* L.). Infusion of a handful in a half-liter of water, taken during the day for three days.
- *Kuum* or squash *(Cucurbita moschata,* Duch.). Make a drink of 50 grams of seeds to be taken on an empty stomach throughout the week.
- *Piñuela, chakchom* or *chan ch'om (Bromelia karatas,* L.). Prepare a drink with the pulp of ten fruits; take daily on an empty stomach for ten days.

Plants Indicated for Xxej (Nausea)
- Infusion of two stems of *poleo (Mentha pulegium,* L.) and one stem of rue *(Ruta graveolens,* L.) in a half-liter of water; take with sugar repeatedly.
- Infusion of a handful of *toronjil (Cedronella mexicana,* B.) in a half-liter of water; take with a pinch of baking soda.
- *Nabá, bálsamo xiu (Mycroxylon balsamum,* Var. Pareira). Infusion of a handful in a half-liter of water; take with or without bicarbonate.
- *K'uum* or squash *(Cucurbita mosch,* D.). Infusion of a handful of leaves with the flower in a half-liter of water; take with or without bicarbonate.
- Lemon grass *(Cymbopogon nardus,* R.). Infusion of twelve leaves in a half-glass of water.
- *Tsudspakal* or orange *(Citrus aurantium,* L.). Infusion of a handful and a bit of the rind in a half-liter of water.

Plants Indicated for Ele'naak (Gastritis)
- Boil two stems of cilantro *(Coriandrum sativum,* L.) and ten fruits of *abal* (plum) *(Spondias,* spp.) in 300 ml. of water; strain and take daily on an empty stomach.

Plants Indicated for Sasak kal (Cough)
- *Sakmuul* or *amor seco, (Althernathera ramossima,* M.). Infusion of a handful plus eight red flowers in a half-liter of water; take a half glass, warm, several times a day.
- A handful of *chump* or *kanchunup (Clusia flava,* Jacq.) and 20 cm. of bark of *kopté (Cordia dodecandra,* DC.). Infusion of both in 300 ml. of water; take two spoonfuls several times a day.
- *Chocuil xiu, pasmo xiu* or *claudiosa (Capraria biflora,* L.). Infusion of nine leaves in a half-liter of water; take small quantities with discretion. Large doses can be toxic.
- *Tsulutok* or *tsaktsulubtok (Bauhinia divaricata,* L.). Infusion of a handful in a half-liter of water; take warm repeatedly.
- *Jumpetskín (Tillandsia,* spp.). Infusion of a handful in a half-liter of water. Take warm repeatedly.

- *Putxiu, putkán* or *lentejilla (Lepidium virginicum, L.)*. Infusion of a handful with stems in a half-liter of water; take warm repeatedly.
- *Son* or *guayacán (Guaiacum sanctum, L.)*. Infusion of 40 grams of the trunk in 400 ml. of water to be taken as needed.
- A handful of avocado leaves, some branches of *poleo (Mentha pulegium, L.)*, eight leaves of *kuyché* or *amapola (Cedrella odorata, L.)*, eight leaves of *té de china (Micromeria browmei,* Benth.), eight leaves and eight flowers or fruits of *ciricote* or *kopté (Cordia dodecandra, DC.)* are infused in 350 ml. of water. Take two spoonfuls at regular intervals.
- Infusion of oregano leaves *(Lippia graveolens,* H.B. et K.), nine leaves of *jabín (Piscidia piscipula, L.)*, and nine leaves of *beek (Erethia tinifolia, L.)* in 400 ml. of water. Take two spoonfuls repeatedly.
- Infusion of a handful of *kalxilxkooch, koolché* or *guarumbo (Cecropia obtusifolia,* Bert.) in 300 ml. of water; take three times a day; or 15 grams of bark in 250 ml. of water; take fresh.

It is recommended to sweeten these infusions with honey.

Plants Indicated for Sasak ka (Bronchitis) and Jeesbal se'en (Asthma)
- *X'koché, tayché,* or *bokanché (Capparis indica,* H.B. et K.). Infusion of 10 cm. of bark and six leaves in a half-liter of water. Take a half-glass twice a day.
- *X'tujuy xiu (Lippia dulcis,* T.). Infusion of the young leaves in a half-liter of water, to be taken as needed.
- *Chioplé (Eupatorium hemipteropodium,* R.). Squeeze the juice from a handful of the plant and apply as a poultice on the chest.
- *Kuyché* or *amapola blanca (Cedrella odorata, L.)*. Infusion with two flowers in a quarter of a liter of water; sweeten with honey; take three spoonfuls twice a day.
- *Xiu* (oregano) *(Lippia graveolens,* H.B. et K.). Infusion of a handful in a half-liter of water; sweeten with honey and take warm as needed.
- *Tusik xiu.* Infusion of 10 cm. of the root and three leaves in 300 ml. of water; sweeten with honey.
- *Much k'ok, doradilla,* or *flor de piedra (Orobanche,* spp.). Infusion of 10 cm. of the root and three leaves in a half-liter of water; sweeten with honey to be taken as needed.
- *Tsulubtok* or *sak-tsulubtok (Bauhinia divaricata, L.)*. Infusion of one flowering branch in a quarter of a liter of water; add honey and lime-juice and take as needed.
- *Put xiu, putkán, lentejilla* or *mastuerzo (Lepidium virginicum, L.)*. Infusion

Disease Classification

of twenty leaves in a half-liter of water; sweeten with honey and take as needed.

- *Kokché (Croton glabellus, L.).* Heat one branch and apply as a poultice to the chest.
- *X'mak'ulán* or *mak'ulán (Pipper auritum, H.B. et K.).* Heat one branch and apply as a poultice to the chest.
- *Tstutup (Calonyetion aculeatum, L).* Infusion of 10 cm. of root and three leaves in a half-liter of water; sweeten with honey and divide into four doses.
- *Xolte x'nuc (Lippia yucatanna, Loes.).* Infusion of a handful of the plant in a half-liter of water; sweeten with honey and take as needed.
- *Orozús* (Licorice) *(Glycyrrhiza glabra, L.).* Infusion of 20 leaves in 300 ml. of water to be taken repeatedly with honey.
- Infusion in one liter of water of a handful of *bakalché (Bourreria pulchra, M.)*, nine hearts of *jabín (Piscidia piscipula, L.)*, 150 grams of *sakatzín (Mimosa hemiendyta, R.)*, 100 grams of the flowers of *x'tokabán (Calea urticifolia, M.)*, nine seeds of avocado *(Persea americana)*, nine hearts of *chocuil xiu, vasak xiu* or *malva (Boerhavia erecta, L.)*, 150 grams of the bark of *kuché* or cedar *(Cedrela mexicana, M.)*, and one white rose *(Macrosiphonia hypolenca)*. Sweeten with honey and take three cups a day.
- Garlic *(Allium sativum).* For children cook two to four cloves and mash them together with banana; adults should increase the garlic to two bulbs twice a day.
- *Sisal xiu (Pilea microphylla).* Infusion of three leaves in 250 ml. of water; repeat the dose three times a day.
- Bougainvillea. Infusion of a handful of red flowers in 200 ml. of water sweetened with honey; repeat three times a day.

Plants Indicated for Chokuil (Fever)

- With the following plants, mash two handfuls in a liter of warm water for bathing: *chakchaká (Bursera simaruba, L.), siit (Lasiasis divaricata, L.), chalche' (Pluchea odorata, L.), xk'ambalkán (Dorstenia contrayerva, L.), oox, ramón (Brosimum alicastrum, Schwartz),* and *guaco (Aristolochia pentandra, Jacq.).*
- *Tzitzil xiu (Erigeron pusillus, Nutt.).* Crush two handfuls in a liter of warm water for bathing in the sun.
- *Sakbalbelkan* or *pitaya (Hybantus yucatanensis, Mill.).* Soak the flower with a branch of rue in alcohol for a moment and rub on the abdomen, arms, and legs.

- *Xkoché, tayché* or *bokanché (Capparia indica,* H.B. et K.). Soak in alcohol for a moment and apply as a poultice to the abdomen, arms, and legs.
- *Luch* or *jícara (Crescentia cujete,* L.). Infusion of 8 leaves in 150 ml. of water to be taken warm.
- *Achiote* or *kuxub (Bixa orellana,* L.). Crush the leaves with animal feed and apply as a hot poultice to the abdomen.
- *Sakmul (amor seco) (Alternathera ramossima,* Mart.). Infusion of nine flowers in a quarter of a liter of water to be taken warm repeatedly.
- *Arnica (Thitonia diversifolia,* Hemsl.). Infusion of four leaves in 300 ml. of water. Take a teaspoonful every four hours.
- *Jolol,* Yucatec Oak *(Bellotia campbelli,* S.). Soak a handful of the leaves in hot water, let cool, and apply the fresh leaves to the abdomen.
- *Tzulutok* or *sak tzulubtok (Bahuhinia divaricata,* L.). Infusion of a handful of flowers in a quarter of a liter of water to be taken warm; keep covered.
- *Kooch* or *higuerilla* (Castor) *(Ricinus communis,* L.). Parboil the leaves and apply warm to the body.
- *Beek (Erethia tinifolia,* L.). Infusion of a handful of the plant and a bunch of flowers in a liter of water in a hot bath.
- *Xbakenuo (Peperomia pellucida,* L.). Infusion of a handful of the plant and a bunch of flowers in a liter of water in a hot bath.

Plants Indicated for Vaginal Hygeine (Sak mancha)
- *Pasmoxiu, chokuil xiu,* or *claudiosa (Capraria biflora,* L.). Infusion of a handful of leaves in 300 ml. of water for bathing; repeat this dose for several days.
- *Chalche' (Pluchea odorata,* L.). Infusion of a handful of the plant in 300 ml. of water as a vaginal wash; repeat this dose for several days.
- *Yakunaax* or *cundeamor (Mormodica charantia,* L.) boiled for a vaginal wash; repeat this dose for several days.
- With the following plants, wash, grind, and soak a handful of the plant in 300 ml. of water for a vaginal wash: *chichibé (Sida acuta,* Burn.), *chioplé (Eupatorium hemipteropodium,* R.), *kukut* (Onion) *(Allium ceppa,* L.), and *vicaria* (Periwinkle) *(Vinca rosea).*

Plant Tranquilizers Indicated to Calm the Nerves
- *Nabanché (Bursera graveolens,* Jacq.). Soak eight leaves in alcohol for an hour, and then infuse them in a quarter of a liter of water to be taken as needed.
- *Pakal* (Orange) *(Citrus sinensis,* Osb.). Infusion of a handful of blossoms in a quarter of a liter of water to be taken as needed.

Disease Classification

- *Tzipche' (Bunchosia swartziana,* Griseb.*).* Infusion of a handful in a quarter of a liter of water to be taken as needed.
- *Mentha* (Mint) *(Mentha piperita,* L.*).* Infusion of several stems with leaves in a quarter of a liter of water to be taken as needed.
- *Tulub-balam (Hippocratea celastroides,* H.B. et K.*).* Infusion of several stems in a quarter of a liter of water to be taken as needed.
- A handful of *chichibé (Sida actua,* Burm.*),* several stalks of *kaltún* (basil), a handful of *payché (Petiveria alliacea,* L.*),* and a handful of *yaaxhalalché (Pedillantus itzaeus,* M.*).* Soak together for two hours in a liter of water for bathing.
- Four leaves of *chaktzitz* or one of *caballo (Salvia coccinea,* L.*),* three leaves of *muts* or *dormilona,* nine small leaves of epazote *(Chenopodium ambrosioides,* L.*),* and three leaves of rue *(Ruta graveolens,* L.*).* Infusion in a quarter of a liter of water to be taken as needed.
- Infuse a handful of *tankasché, (Zanthoxylum fagara,* L.*),* three leaves of *chioplé (Eupatorium hemipteropodum,* R.*),* and a handful of *kanak (Alchornea latifolia,* S.) in two liters of water for bathing.

Plants Indicated for Mycosis and Erysipelas
- *Yak'unak', yak, unax* or *cundeamor (Momordica charantia,* L.*).* Press the juice from the leaves and apply to lesions on the feet.
- *Xput balam (Solanum hispidum).* Dry, ground, and powder the leaf and apply to the infected area. Prepare an infusion by boiling 10 grams of dry leaves in a half-liter of water for 10 minutes. Wash the lesions. This remedy is used for infected wounds and epidermal fungus.
- *Sak xiu (Boerhaavia erect,* L.*).* Squeeze two handfuls of leaves and apply as a poultice to erysipela lesions.

Plants Indicated for Dermatitis in Lactating Women
- 20 leaves of verbena *(Verbena officianalis,* L.*),* 20 leaves of mint *(Mentha piperita,* L.*),* 20 leaves of *pasmoxiu, chocuilxiu* or *claudiosa (Capraria biflora,* L.*),* 20 leaves of *vicaria (Vinca roseae* or *Catharanthus roseus).* Infuse the mix, allow to cool, add a pinch of salt, six leaves of lime, and six of orange, washed and crushed; apply the infusion as a wash twice a day.

Plants Indicated for Pellagra
- *Box ak' (Nissolia fruticosa,* J.*), chikee' (Chrysophyllum mexicanum,* T.S.*),* and *saksit (Lasciacis divaricata,* L.*).* Wash a handful of each, mix fresh, crush, and apply as a poultice to lesions.

- *X'kulimsiis (Trichilia hirta,* L.*).*Wash a handful of the plant, crush and apply as a poultice to lesions.
- *Xaché x'tabay* or *netolok (Pithecoctenium echinatum,* Jacq.*).* Wash a handful, crush fresh, and apply as a poultice to lesions.

Plants Indicated for Sak Wech (Scabies)
- *K'uinché (Astronium graveolens,* H.B. et K.*).* Crush the leaves and apply locally.
- *Xahauché (Tabebuia chrysantha,* Jacq.*).* Crush the leaves and apply locally.
- *Belsinik'ché (Alvaradoa amorphoides,* Liebm.*).* Squeeze a handful of leaves with 30 cm. of chopped bark; wash the lesions and leave the solids as a poultice.
- *Gobernadora (Larea divaricata,* M.*).* Soak the flowers in alcohol for an hour and apply to the lesions.

Plants Indicated For Burns
- Ten cm. of the root of *op (cherimoya) (Anona cherimola),* 10 cm. of the root and 100 grams of leaf of *ki (hennequen) (Agave,* spp.*),* one clove of garlic *(Allium sativum,* L.*),* 100 grams of aloe leaf *(Aloe vulgaris,* L.*),* and 10 leaves of *kantuul (Nissolia fruticosa,* J.*).* Wash together, toast, grind, and apply to burns.

Plants Indicated for Hemorrhoids
- *Belladona xiu (Bryophyllum pinnatum,* Kurz.*).* Infusion of a handful in 300 ml. of water as a hot enema.
- *Yakunaax, yakunak'* or *cundeamor (Momordica charantia,* L.*).* Infusion of two handfuls with stem in 300 ml. of water as a hot enema; the same dose for several days.
- *Pahalkam* or *yerba mora (Solana niggrum,* L.*).* Infusion of a handful in 300 ml. of water as a hot enema; the same dose for several days.

Plants Indicated for Cholesterol
- *Ya* or *zapote* (Sapodilla) *(Manilkara zapota,* L.*).* Infusion of 12 leaves in 250 ml. of water; take the same dose twice a day.
- *Elemuy* or *yumel (Malmea depressa,* Baillon.*).* Infusion of 30 grams of the root and bark in 400 ml. of water. Take at night on an empty stomach.

Plants Indicated for High Blood Pressure (Arterial Hypertension)
- *Ya* or *zapote* (Sapodilla) *(Manilkara zapota,* L.*).* Infusion of 12 leaves in 250 ml. of water; take the same dose twice a day.

Spiritual Illnesses
JAK'OLAL, JAK'IOOL, ZAK OLAL
(SUSTO, OR FRIGHT)

Fright attacks children as well as adults, though the name generally refers to fright in young children. It is a disease resulting from a strong impression that affects a person's *ool* and alters their will and emotions. There are various kinds of fright:

Jak'iool or Fright in the Maternal Womb is produced when a pregnant woman receives a fright. The less developed the fetus, the stronger the illness; fear enters the fetus and develops with it. Fright can also affect newborns and young children by way of the mother. Fright can attack a pregnant woman in the course of domestic conflicts, because of anger, or simply if it is in her nature to be frightened easily. Sometimes there is nausea and vomiting. When the child is born with fright it is called *"uk'il kel mal"* (Fright Carried in the Blood).

Jasaool is a fright that affects lactating mothers, and which is passed to the infant in the milk. *Xpak'i* is a fright received directly by newborns and children. This fright is brought by the bird *coos,* also known as "the witch bird." The bird shrieks for several hours at a time. It attacks and eats chickens, cutting their throats with its claws so they don't make any noise.

Weakness makes a child more susceptible to fright. Fright affects the *ool,* the emotions and the will. Children are more susceptible to fright because the *ool* is less developed, and therefore weaker. Fright can be passed from mothers to children from pregnancy through the first years of development, because of the strong bond between the *ool* of mother and child.

In *jaki'ool* the child is ill from birth, suffering from fits, weak heart, and muteness or constant crying. Generally a strong mother infected with fright will give birth to a child who later dies in infancy; if the woman is weak, the fright will cause the fetus to be aborted.

Common signs of fright in children are coughing, weeping, and fits.

- In *jasaool* the child suffers cramps and vomiting.
- In *xpak'i* the child does not die but is continually in fear.
- In *paak'il* (chronic fear), one symptom is that the child's hands hang open.
- In other cases of *jaki ool* in children and adults there may be cough, worry, fever, headache, diarrhea, shock, weakness, dreams of death, insomnia, *tuk'ul* (pensiveness), *sakaj* (withdrawal), and *chuputki* (somnambulism).
- When the child is frightened he may wake in the night crying.

The diagnosis of fright is normally carried out by the family according to known signs and symptoms, though occasionally the child may be taken to an herbalist or *j'meen* for diagnosis. In newborns the common signs are opening of the hands, crying, and changes in skin color. An older child will be withdrawn *(sakaj)* and will cry at night.

Fright can be easily confused with nervous illnesses and weakness.

Fright is most common in children under three, although it might attack at any age and at any time of year. In good weather it is less frequent. When there are difficulties like disagreements and deaths in the family, the chance of contracting fright is increased.

In newborns it is very serious. The older the person, the less grave the illness. If it goes unattended in young children they will stay weak and grow up to be easily frightened, or may die. If a child's fright is not cured *(paak'il)*, it becomes somnambulism later in life *(chukut kib)*. If fear in adults is not attended, many nervous illnesses may result: they remain worried, cannot sleep well, grow weak, and die.

Treatments

- For *xa'ak'ool*, parboil *jak'ool xiu (dormilona) (Mimosa pudica,* L.) and use it to massage the child. The herb is applied to sensitive regions: the forehead, the jaw, and the soles of the feet.
- Scrape flakes from the stone *"santa ara"* (a sacred marine stone) and let them sit in holy water; this is for drinking. Baths can be taken as well, with rue and blessed water.
- For adults gather *xkabach'o, kanacho', chalche', tu juchul,* and rue *(Ruta chalapensis)*. Grind to a paste and apply in the form of a cross to the "keys" of the body—elbows, knees, and feet—pointing in the four directions. These "keypoints" are also called *"venas"* (veins) or *uwuatzi*.
- Boil orange leaves and drink the tea.
- Tap the patient nine times with the wick of a beeswax candle or a blessed candle. This is called *chuputki'*.
- Perform *tok* on Good Friday, to cleanse the "cross of blood."
- Burn one feather from the *coos* bird and nine little balls of goat manure beneath the hammock of the sick child.

Prevention

- Make sure that the child stays strong.
- Do not frighten, worry, or disgust pregnant women or small children.

Relations With Other Medical Models

In traditional Chinese medicine it is understood that if the mother is emotionally perturbed, weak, or malnourished during pregnancy, or if the birth is abnormal, prolonged, or difficult, the child may be born ill or predisposed towards illness. This predisposition might be due to general weakness, particular types of mental or emotional imbalance, or weakness in a particular organ or area of the body. It is understood that childhood is the time of major growth and development when certain pressures on the body and mind can have stronger and longer-lasting effects; the mind of the child is especially susceptible to all sorts of influences.

The kidney is the organ associated with fear; if there is fear over a long period of time, it can provoke changes in the action of the kidney meridian, producing incontinence in acute cases and a sense of permanent anxiety in chronic cases.[47]

When there is a *chi* deficiency in the kidney, there may be sudden panic or worry accompanied by other sensations like fatigue and weakness in the knees and hips, lack of will, tension, perspiration, restlessness, and insomnia; the tongue will be reddish with scant fur and the pulse will be thin and weak. These signs should be differentiated from other causes of fear such as weakness of *chi* and blood (weak body, difficult breathing, perspiration, pale face, palpitations, weak, thin pulse, and thin tongue coating).

Another cause of a predisposition to fear is weakness of the liver and gall bladder (discomfort in the ribs, indecisiveness, pale tongue with thin coating, weak pulse).

In sum, it can be said that fright or panic is a symptom of general weakness, and of a deficiency of *chi* and blood. It is said that when there is deficiency of blood there is fear, and when there is an excess of blood there is anger.

EE'K ICH TABI, TU MENTA OJO (EVIL EYE)

This is a series of illnesses which affect small children between two months and one year old—especially those who are weak and malnourished—when they are gazed upon with affection. Along with diseases brought on by material beings—people and animals—*curanderos* often include the diseases known as "eyes of the wind" in the category of *ojo* or evil eye. Evil wind and evil eye comprise a series of illnesses with many common causes and symptoms. The reason for considering "eye of the wind" here is that certain winds are seen as living beings or representatives of the gods and spirits of nature; when passing over a child they may hug him or her admiringly, and they don't want to let go unless they are "paid" and given food.

There are various types of evil eye:

- Evil eye produced by humans and animals.
- Evil eye produced by supernatural beings manifested as wind.

The evil eye is a disease that affects a child most commonly when he is weak and malnourished, when a person or other being gazes upon him admiringly "with a desire to hug the child." The effect of the gaze is heightened if the person is hungry or if it is a woman who is pregnant or menstruating—that is to say, in a state of excess heat.

It can also be caused by a person with a stigmatism in their eye, a drunk, an animal, and by the spirits of the *milpa:* an *alux,* a *balam,* or by the wind of water, the wind of earth, by the water itself, as well as by the sun and the moon. Looked upon by someone with a very strong gaze even the healthiest child may be affected by the evil eye. Animals and small birds are also susceptible.

The action, as it has been described to us, works something like this: the child by her or his actions might attract someone's attention. The attraction becomes mutual. The person looks at the child with a strong gaze, the child loses her or his defenses and falls subject to *ojo,* the eye. It is something like the first sensation of falling in love. If the adult has a desire to hug and hold the child but does not carry through with the desire, this can provoke evil eye in the child.

Evil eye results in an imbalance in the normal thermal state of the child. If the child is fragile, the blood is weak and cannot resist changes in temperature. This depends in large part on whether or not the child is well-nourished. When the person looking at the child is extremely hungry or has a stigmatism in the eye, it can damage the child's *"hiel,"* or gall bladder, and is fatal. It is called "evil eye" because it enters through the gaze of the child when looking at the other person or at the sun, the moon, or any given natural phenomenon whose spirit is attracted to the child.

The first symptoms of evil eye are the presence of a greenish, thick diarrhea and the shrinking of one eye, becoming smaller than the other. The child is dejected, withdrawn and weepy, and shows little desire to suckle. In some cases there is fever, nausea, gas, and inflammation of the stomach.

In the Drunken Evil Eye the child becomes very restless with intense vomiting and diarrhea, sometimes with blood present; the head falls to

Disease Classification

one side, the child is dehydrated with cramps, the right eye becomes smaller than the left, and he or she walks and acts as if drunk.

When the person who caused the evil eye has a stigmatism, the patient's left eye becomes smaller than the right.

- In *ojoy maak* there is vomiting with white phlegm and diarrhea.
- In Evil Eye of Hunger the stomach contracts even though the child eats.
- In Evil Eye of a Breastfeeding Woman there is rapid breathing and pale-colored stool. The child suckling immediately regurgitates the milk. The mother, feeling palpitations in her breast, knows that her child will fall ill; even when she is not feeding the child she feels a pressure on the breasts.
- In Eye of the Whirlwind the mouth or the eyes become pursed or grow small.
- In Evil Eye of the Bird the child exhibits head movements like a bird.
- In *ojoy yi ka ja'* (Eye of the Wind of Water), the child exhibits *chokuil* (fever), the stomach is bloated and the stool may be blueish or white if there was thunder or white clouds with the wind.
- In *ojoy kiin* (Eye of the Sun) the stool becomes yellowish and later greenish.
- In *ojoy uuj* (Eye of the Moon), the child's skin develops a blueish tint.

Generally the child may suffer from diarrhea for several days without any sign of dehydration; if it is not treated it will become worse. In many cases the mother of a sick child will visit medics and professionals to treat the child; when the child remains ill, it is understood that this is not treatable by a doctor and the child is brought to a *j'meen, curandero,* or herbalist for curing.

When the child has taken medicine with no result, when there are changes in the eyes accompanied by diarrhea, and if there has been recent contact with a stranger or peculiar wind or natural phenomena, the illness is diagnosed as evil eye.

Other elements that are useful in diagnosis are:

- In Eye of the Sun in boys the right eye will be smaller than the left.
- In Eye of the Moon in girls the left eye will be the small one.
- The pulse is slower than usual.
- The lungs are palpated for fever or high temperature.

Some *curanderos* use cards to divine what class of evil eye is present.

Evil eye can be confused with *tzan nu yaal* (fall of the crown), or with diarrhea caused by bad hygiene or bad eating habits.

The evil eye will not go away by itself. If the child is not cured, after eight days he may die.

Evil eye may appear at any time of year, in boys or girls, often under one year of age. There are known cases of older children contracting the evil eye.

There are *curanderos* who attend between four and ten cases of evil eye per month in an average-sized village (between 400 and 1000 inhabitants).

Treatments

- The same person who brought about the illness can cure it by carrying the child and blowing into the palm of the hands and the temples. A *curandero* can also cure it by performing a blessing and a cleansing.
- The blessing is done in the name of the Father, the Son, and the Holy Ghost. The *curandero* then asks for help from the four *bacabob*—who hold up the four pillars of the world—and the four cardinal points.
- To perform the cleansing the *curandero* uses basil, *tzipche' (Bunchosia swartziana,* Gr.), *rue (Ruta chalapensis), analche'* and/or *chalche' (Pluchea odorata).* The arms and the forehead are swept from high to low towards the four cardinal points and God the Father, the Son, and the Holy Ghost are invoked, as well as *Santiago Caballero* and the sacred heart of Jesus.
- *Jup* is performed between the eyebrows (the Chinese point *yintang,* or Seal Hall), at the level of the hairline *(shen ting,* or Spirit's Hall), at the middle of the back of the head, and behind the ears in the form of a cross. This causes the child to sweat, dilating the pores and restoring the breathing to normal. This is done only when the child is very sick. As it may not be known where the illness came from, the points punctured open to the four directions so that the disease will leave the body.
- Nineteen leaves of the vine *ojo ak* are mixed with *te chaak* (an algae that appears after rain) in a half-liter of water and given to the patient by the spoonful every hour until the preparation is finished. The *curandero* covers the crown of the child's head with a kerchief and applies a sucking action with his mouth, as described in fall of the crown. Afterwards an incantation is performed.
- *Kakaltún* (basil) is infused in 500 ml. of water and sweetened with honey to be taken repeatedly throughout the day.
- *Luch* or *jícara (Crescentia cujete,* L.) is infused in 500 ml. of water and sweetened with honey to be taken repeatedly throughout the day.
- *Tsutsuk'* or *peteltún (Cissampelos pareira,* L.) is infused in 500 ml. of water and sweetened with honey to be taken repeatedly throughout the day. An equal quantity is used in the bath.

237

- A handful of leaves of *yaax che* (ceiba) *(Ceiba pentandra*, L.) a handful of *kibix (Dalbergia glabra*, M.), a handful of *tsutsuk'* or *peteltún (Cissampelos pareira*, L.), and a handful of *tzitzín* (mugwort), are infused together in a half-liter of water and sweetened with honey to be taken repeatedly.
- With the following plants, a handful is infused in water for bathing: *tzipche (Bunchosia swartziana*, Gr.), *x'tanlum (Ageratum gaumeri*, R.), *kabalyaxn (Ruella nudiflora*, E et G.), *chichibé (Sida acuta*, B.), *payché (Petiveria alliacea*, L.), rue *(Ruta chalapensis*, L.).
- *Kanibinché, chi*, or *nance (Malpighia glabra*, L.). Infusion of 20 cm. of bark in half-liter of water; sweeten with honey and take repeatedly.
- *Yaax-kiix-kanal* or *toxob (Caesalpinia vesicaria*, L.). Toast and crush a 30 cm. bit of bark; add to a half-liter of water, boiled and cooled. Sweeten with honey and take repeatedly.
- For Eye of the Drunk crush two leaves of rue. Lift the child nine times into the air, and on the last time hug the child and apply the crushed leaves to the forehead, followed by a bath in *aguardiente* (sugar cane liquor). Blow into the palms and make the sign of a cross.
- For Eye of a Pregnant Woman, the pregnant woman generally doesn't want to treat the patient herself for fear that her baby will die. Burn the feathers of a vulture or parakeet beneath the child's hammock. This may cause the pregnant woman to lose her hair.
- For Eye of a Breastfeeding Woman heat or parboil leaves of bitter orange, crush them and apply them to the temples.
- For diarrhea associated with evil eye a drink is made from a tuber called *cha'ak* and a peeled young banana. These are ground in water and strained and the drink is administered by the spoonful every two hours. This drink "binds up the insides" and gives nutrition.
- Also for the diarrhea, dry and grind a green banana, mix with corn and water and drink as a rehydration formula.

Prevention
- It is recommended that *yaax jalaalché (Pedilantus itzaeus*, L.) be planted in each corner of the patio of the house.
- When the baby is born, make a bracelet of nine bits of red yarn. Make eight knots, and with the ninth make a knot around the wrist of one hand. The color red has a warm nature. It is said that when the child comes in contact with someone's strong gaze, the yarn will be affected, losing its color.
- When dressing the child, put the underclothes on backwards.

- Turn the father's clothes backwards and massage the child's face and head.
- The child should wear street clothes for going out and change into house clothes at home.
- A protection amulet *(oxo ak)* is made with the seed known as *ojo de venado* or "deer's eye."
- The umbilical cord is dried and sewn into the clothes, or hung and tied with nine knots, the ninth bearing the amulet.
- Draw milk nine times from the mother's breast and throw the milk on the roof.
- Brush the child's face and head nine times with rue and the child will not be susceptible to the evil eye. However, when the child becomes an adult, he will bear a strong gaze, and the evil eye that he may provoke cannot be cured.
- Nine leaves of rue and a pink rose are crushed in a half-liter of boiled water, to be taken three times a day for nine days. Adding a bit more rue, this preparation can be used for washing the head. It is important to make the sign of the cross to get rid of bad air around the patient. Make a reliquary of *Santa Ara Negra* (a black stone particular to the area) and wear it as a necklace.

Relations With Other Medical Models
- The diarrhea that accompanies evil eye is similar to that recognized by occidental medicine as caused by *Escherichia coli,* a normal part of the intestinal flora which only acts up in particular cases related to the body's lowered defenses. In the case of evil eye, the diarrhea remains for several days until the person who caused the illness effects the cure, carrying the child and blowing into the palms of the hands and the temples (at the pressure points), or until the child is healed by a *curandero* performing a cleansing. The general interpretation is that the evil eye involves an imbalance in the body's temperature.
- In Chinese traditional medicine it is understood that *chi* can be passed from one person to another. In these terms it may be possible that the protaganist causes a change in the child's *chi* that is manifested in the large intestine meridian making the child more susceptible to an attack of *E coli* or other illness. For this reason the cure involves a cleansing or treatment by the person who originally caused the illness, reestablishing the balanced *chi,* and the use of specific plants which might have bioenergetic healing properties.

Disease Classification

This is evil eye caused by one of the three variants of the Watery Wind. The three different varieties are: a wind accompanied by thunder, a wind accompanied by white clouds, and a wind which comes alone, unaccompanied.

Eye of the Watery Wind can be caused by a mother's lack of care, taking the child out into bad weather after a bath or making the child hot when it is cloudy or windy, and allowing the child to go out into the wind. This illness is more likely if the child is weak or malnourished. It can also be caused by weakness and malnutrition of the mother, giving birth to a fragile infant.

The events causing Eye of the Watery Wind are related as follows: The child is hot and there is a sudden change in temperature. The child is embraced by the air. Upon embracing the child, the spirit of the wind looks at the child with a strong gaze.

The child with *ojoi yi ka ja'* presents signs of *chokuil* (fever) and stays as if sleeping, eyes closed, but is not asleep. There is greenish diarrhea and bloated belly. The child does not eat or take milk, and may experience nausea. Other illnesses may accompany this, like flu or collapse of the crown.

When the wind that embraces the child is accompanied by thunder, the stool will have a blueish tint; when the wind is accompanied by white clouds, the stool will be whitish. When the wind is unaccompanied, the stool will be greenish.

The diagnosis is carried out by looking at the excrement, as well as by looking at the other symptoms and talking to the family about the child's recent history.

Some *curanderos* diagnose this illness using cards, *sastún,* grains of corn, or an egg.

Evil Eye of the Watery Wind is easily confused with infectious diarrhea, diarrhea caused by teething, amebas, or simple indigestion.

It is more common in the rainy season, in children from one month to two years of age, and it is equally common in both sexes. A child infected as an infant can suffer a relapse at ten years of age. If not attended properly, this illness can lead to chronic weakness, dehydration, and death.

Treatments
- Take two handfuls of *ojoi xiu* (a vine that runs along the ground), and soak in a liter of water. Bathe the child making sure to make nine passes

around the head. The child can drink from one to four swallows of the liquid. This is done once a day for two days.

- Soak two handfuls of *ojoi ak'* in two liters of water, bathe the child, and then put the child to bed, well-covered.
- Give similar baths in water of *nabanché (Bursera graveolens)*.
- Make a necklace of *contraojo* with its fruit.
- Soak a handful of *pi'chi'che' (Psidium yucatanense)* and another of the herb *ojoi kim* in two liters of water. Drink and use as a wash, making sure to make nine passes around the child's head. It is good for inflammation.
- *Uta chaak* is "the excrement of the god *chak;*" it is green and collects on rocks after rain *(chal tun)*. Collect and dry the *uta chaak*, mash in water and use to wash the child's head.
- In a quart of boiling water infuse nine leaves of the tree *tz'utz'uk (Cissampelos pareira, L.)* a small bit of *uta chaak*, some *tak cha*, three petals from a pink rose, and a bit of rue. Give a spoonful to the child before or after each meal for eight days. This preparation should be made daily. What is left over can be used for bathing the child.
- Boil ground squash seed, star anis, half a teaspoon of anis seed, and half a teaspoon of chamomile in a half-liter of water. Administer a spoonful an hour for one day.
- At twelve noon give the child a sponge bath, making nine passes with well water in a little tub; cover the child with a towel. After a half-hour dress the child, light incense, and wave the smoke at his bottomside.
- Wash a handful of the vine *oxolak* in two liters of water and wash the child's head in nine passes. Give the child a bit of the liquid to drink.
- For the evil eye caused by a wind with white clouds, wash and boil a handful of *x'bolenti*. Bathe the child in this and give the child a little drink of it every day for ten days.
- Bathe the child in *aguardiente* (palm alcohol and rum).
- Rub down the child with *agua de cananga, agua florida* and *agua de azahar*—medicinal ointments available in pharmacies throughout rural Mexico.
- Prepare baths with valerian *(Valeriana officinalis, L.)*, rue *(Ruta chalapensis)*, basil, *ojoi che'*, and *ojoi xi*.
- Blow on the soles of the feet and the palm of the hands.

Prevention
- Three days after birth, the child is brought into the sunlight and swept with a branch of rue. If the child is born in the day, the ritual is per-

formed on the fourth day after birth, but if the birth occurs at night, or before dawn, the count is three days. On entering the house, the rue is tossed onto the roof. This ritual is known as "presentation of the child to the sun."

- A month after birth the child is presented to the winds. When the wind of water arrives (the wind that picks up just before rain), the child is stripped of clothes or swaddling and is held up to each of the four directions.

OJOI ALUX

This is Eye of the *Alux,* a type of evil eye. It is caused by walking in the country or in the fields without a shirt; an *alux* takes a liking to a person and its spirit affects the body.

The disease is characterized by sleepiness in the day and restlessness at night; one often talks between waking and dreaming. Restlessness and headache are sometimes accompanied by fever and nausea.

The diagnosis is done by way of orations, invocations of saints, cards, and *sastún.*

It is easily confused with Eye of the Wind.

It can happen in any season and is most common in children.

This is not generally a fatal illness, but if it goes untreated it can develop complications leading to death.

Treatments
- Baths in rue, *tzipche'* (*Bunchosia swartziana,* Gr.) and *ojoiché.*
- Orations.
- When the patient is not cured by other means, a *curandero* performs *ke'j* with a piece of fabric, a chicken, and an egg.

Prevention
- It is very difficult to prevent this illness.

JO' K'O K'IIK TU TUCH

This is when there is bleeding from the umbilicus or *tuch* of a newborn.

This illness comes about when a newborn baby comes into contact with a woman who is menstruating or pregnant, or a pregnant animal.

It is caused by an exchange of energy between the woman or girl whose blood is very strong and the infant whose blood is still weak. It rarely affects strong children. It can also be caused when a woman who has just had intercourse and has not bathed comes in contact with the baby. The affect is produced by the semen that the woman carries within her; in this sense it is caused by the man by way of the woman.

The child affected has gas, swollen belly, frequent bowel movements, and bleeding from the *tuch*.

The diagnosis is simple, based on observing blood in the navel region.

This illness can occur at any time of year, in newborns of both sexes. It is most common in weak babies and is very serious, sometimes leading to death within three days.

Treatments

- Burn the menstrual cloth used by the woman who caused the illness and rub the ashes on the belly of the baby.
- Heat stems of *yerba buena* (mint) and whip the child with it nine times.
- Burn the excrement of a dove and rub the ashes on the umbilical cord of the newborn.
- Burn the excrement and the beard of a black goat and rub it on the baby's belly. The color black has a strong effect.
- Collect nine young leaves of *jabín (Piscidia piscipula),* roast, ground and strain them, and put the fine strained powder on the belly.
- Rub the resin of *ak'an* over the navel, place the plant's leaves over the navel in the form of cross, and tie them in place.
- Put nine leaves of a rubber tree beneath the hammock, wait until they dry and then burn them.
- Roast *alucema*; when it is hot, wrap it in a towel and pass it over the umbilicus.
- In the trunk of the tree *chaká* make a mark like the child's foot, carve out a hole in the tree and put the child's foot in it. When the tree heals, so will the child's *tuch.*
- For *a k'an,* a closely related illness, the mother swings the child up and down nine times. The number nine is strongly associated with the term of pregnancy, and this practice serves to memorialize the pregnancy, reinforcing the bond of the mother with her infant.

Prevention

- Put lime leaves beneath the child's hammock.
- Place a red button over the navel and put tape over it in the form of a cross.

- When the baby is born, put a bracelet of nine red threads on its wrist. Make eight knots and tie it tight with the ninth.
- Make a necklace with black thread and 18 spines of *cazón*, a small shark found in the waters off the Yucatán peninsula.

Relations with Other Medical Models

- In Chinese traditional medicine bleeding from the umbilicus of a newborn might happen if the umbilical cord is badly cut, or it may be a condition of excessive internal heat in the womb which damages the blood causing it to circulate irregularly. In this case the bleeding will be accompanied by phlegm or blood in the urine. The child will exhibit a red tongue and face, irritability, insomnia, and restlessness.

It can also originate because the prenatal *chi* and blood are weak causing an inability of the *chi* to control the blood, and allowing the blood to escape its normal course. The child exhibits a pale face, lips, and tongue, low weeping, and possible symptoms of cold from deficiency (cold limbs, inflexibility, pale tongue).

CHUP YO'LAL DZIBOLAL

This is an illness known in Spanish as *"deseo,"* or desire, which manifests in the skin due to unsatisfied desire. It is apparently also known by the names *ku ben ba', pul baj, tzibola'* and *ku'u benba'*.

There are two kinds of *dzibolal*:

- *Chupul yo'ola poch*—desire for food.
- *Chupul yo'ola xi wach koole*—desire for a man or a woman.

Chupul yo'ola poch, commonly known as *dzibolal* (desire for food), appears when a person with a strong *ool* and a strong gaze experiences an unsatisfied craving for a certain food, and this person comes in contact with another, weaker person—generally a child or younger relative. This disease manifests as skin lesions which, it is said, take the form of the food in question. If the cause was to go without eating the meat of *tuza* (a large rodent native to the area), the skin will break out in lesions bearing "hollows and holes;" if the cause is armadillo meat the skin will develop tough spots; if the cause is candied squash seeds the lesions will resemble wax and honey, and if the cause is beer the lesions will appear like foam around the corners of the mouth. The skin lesions brought on by *chupul yo'ola poch* appear suddenly. It generally rejects medical treatment and can manifest in a variety of forms. While the lesions can appear like the food in question, they can also appear as ordinary welts, thus evading diagnosis.

The standard diagnostic practice to detect *dzibolal* is simple observation and questioning of the family to detect if someone, usually older than the patient, has recently experienced an unsatisfied desire for food. There are some *curanderos* who can identify *dzibolal* and the food that caused it simply by examining the skin lesions. Others find it easily confused with other illnesses of the skin.

Dzibolal can appear at any time of year in both sexes. It is very common, and considerably painful, but not fatal.

Chupul yo'ola xi wak koole appears when one (generally a man) feels a desire for someone of the opposite sex, desiring to "pinch their belly" *("pellizcarle el tuch"),* and remains with the desire unsatisfied. It should be noted again that in Mayan culture the *"tuch,"* or navel, is considered an erotic zone of the body, similar to the breasts for occidental culture.

The lesion generally appears as an infection on the thumb. It is understood that the thumb is the finger where the desire would find its expression—thus the denial of desire manifests in the thumb.

Treatments

- In the case of *dzibolal* from desire for food, the first step is to identify the person responsible. Once this is established, one of two things can be done: get the food that provoked the desire and give it to the person, or ask for a bit of the person's saliva and rub it on the skin lesions.
- In the case of *dzibolal* from sexual desire, the following recommendation is made: go outside in the night and defecate; make nine passes around the excrement with the thumb, and on the ninth abruptly thrust the thumb into the excrement saying an oration in Maya.

K'AK AS IIK (ILLNESS FROM THE EVIL WIND)

This illness comes from the harmful influence of the wind; it is said that "it came from the air, thus it came from the heavens." Many diseases come on the wind, including negative influences from other people, from animals, and from sacred places.

There are two phenomena or categories within the conception of "wind." The first is the wind as a physical phenomena that causes illness through its cold, heat or dampness by causing a thermal imbalance in the body. The illnesses associated with these winds are classified as natural illnesses and are described in the beginning of the appendix.

The other class of wind refers to an influence that can be positive or negative and which comes from the air or wind generated by a material or supernatural being. "Evil wind" or "bad air" is the negative force that is borne on this wind. The wind is thus a vehicle for the transmission of beneficial or harmful forces. This force is not seen as separate from the wind itself; generally the two are expressed in the same terms. For this reason the physical wind is closely related to the "evil wind," making any sharp distinction impossible. Some physical winds, like the west and north winds, are understood to be possessed of malevolent spirits.

Many winds have "owners" or spirits, which might be the principal gods or their helpers. The gods produce these winds and these winds are their earthly manifestations. Thus it is said that the winds have life and can provoke evil eye. The winds are an expression and manifestation of the various phenomena of nature which are related to supernatural forces.

Eye of the Wind is an illness brought on when the spirit of a wind hugs a small child and refuses to let go unless it is paid in food. *"Kumekik' winkili"*—it hugs your body.

Some *curanderos* say that the principal beneficial winds are: *nojoch bil,* God the father; *mejen bil,* the Son, he who produces the holy water; and the Holy Spirit, the wind saint *"el santo iik." Yumi kax,* the god of wild places, is a good wind which dominates the other winds and watches over the wilderness. The people of the Yucatán Peninsula always have the name of this wind on their tongues.

Other names of the evil wind are: *chikin iik'* and *maktzil* (punishment of souls).

The wind is life. *"If a candle is enclosed in a place out of the wind, it will go out."* It is what gives life to people, animals, and plants. *"When we die the breath is choked, the lungs close, and the blood stops."* The wind is not seen, but it is felt and known. There are thousands of kinds of wind, some harmful and others beneficial. Some *curanderos* say that each *j'meen* might have relations with 15 or so wind spirits. *"We are between bad and good,"* they say.

The evil wind is the root of a variety of diseases. As there are a variety of evil winds and ways of being affected by them, and as each one takes a different form, there exists as well a series of causes and manifestations. The winds are produced by the sun, *"k'in,"* the father of everything. The rays of the sun produce various illnesses: *jalch k'in, yokso kin,* and *xui ol'a* (asphyxia). Each color in the sun has a particular effect and an illness that corresponds to it. The most damaging is the color violet or indigo, the main color which heats the body. The sun is the cause of whirlwinds in the dry season, which explains the absence of whirlwinds in the rainy season. The sun can also cause a species of evil eye *(ojoy k'in).*

In the case of *xlu muk* or *xk'amuk ool,* a wind arrives as a punishment when a promise is not fulfilled. Commonly it occurs when one offers a meal to the *pixánob* (the souls of the dead), the saints, or the *balamob* (spirits of the wilderness) and then fails to prepare it; similarly it may occur if one receives an inheritance and fails to offer prayers.

Another cause is the evil wind related with the cardinal directions, like *chikin iik'* or *k'an chik'in,* west wind, "red cloud," and *xaman iik'* or *xam-ankan,* wind from the north. Its most well-known causes are the following:

- Not "curing" the earth before planting. Older generations were accustomed to performing rituals at important times in the agricultural cycle. The evil wind of the wilderness, of the hills and their spirits *(kakab),* and of the *cuyos* will be caused by the failure to perform certain rituals.
- For not feeding the spirits of the wilderness and of the pastures with the offering of an animal and its blood in the ceremony *wahikol* or *lo' corral,* in which an animal is sacrificed. If this is not done the spirits will take revenge, killing animals and causing disease in people.
- For breaking certain agreements with the spirits of the wilderness, like taking things from the woods without asking permission. This happens generally with the four *balamob* protecting the four cardinal points.
- The *cuyos,* stone burial mounds, produce many illnesses (among them *k'ojani kakab iik'*) because the bones of the dead are gathered there, and because the *aluxob* live there protecting the remains. This wind comes most commonly at 12 o'clock noon, 6 o'clock in the afternoon, and 5 o'clock in the morning.
- In the species of evil wind resulting from the work of a *j'meen,* a traditional cane liquor called *xjool ja'* is used to perform a cure and what is

left over is tossed out, or an animal, plant, or object that was used to perform *k'ej* is discarded afterwards, having been infected with the evil wind (which was expelled from the patient). A person passing by the place where these things have been left can be infected by the evil wind and become ill.

- People who don't understand or don't have faith in these spirits and these winds are most susceptible to damage by them.
- It is said that when the owl hoots it is pulling out the fingernails of one who is going to die. When someone's time has come, the owl flies looking up to alert the spirits.
- If an abortion is performed and the fetus is carelessly disposed of, this can produce an evil wind.

The person infected with evil wind might exhibit signs of asthma or bronchitis, aching bones, or back pain. There may be swelling in the arms, fever, and various other illnesses, such as headache, nausea, vomiting, diarrhea, and indigestion. Children become agitated and depressed and shows signs of fever.

A partial description of various distinct winds:

- In the case of *xlu muk* or *xk'amuk ool*, a person's will becomes exhausted. When a promise is fulfilled, the state of will and energy is restored.
- *Jik'al janli kol*—Wind of the Food of the *Milpa*—is produced by not fulfilling a promise. It causes headache, fever and dejection. One has the sense of being bombarded with bits of sugarcane or pumpkin seeds. Sometimes there is vomiting and the vomit bears the ingredients of *sakab*—the ritual offerings.
- *K'ojani kakab iik'*—the wind produced by *aluxob* that live in the stone mounds—causes insomnia, vomiting, and hallucinations.
- *Juntul wakax ik'*—air produced by cattle—causes chills.
- *Iik'al keej*—Wind of the Deer—consists of high fevers leading to death.
- *Xtus (alkab) iik'*—Evil Wind from the Grave—produces asphyxia.
- *Xpap (chi, ximbal) iik'* is caused by a wind which, circulating through the body, stings like chili pepper.
- *(Alkab) k'ok'ppb iik'* causes dejection and chill and results from the shock of seeing an iguana or a green snake which speaks.
- *Chikin iik'* or *k'an chik'in* (west wind or "red cloud") causes asthma. It is also known as the Wind of Bile, and it affects the will.
- *Xaman iik'* or *xamankan* (north wind) causes or complicates asthma, eye problems, *chokuil* (fever), and *chiba pool* (headache).

The diagnosis involves:

- Seeing if a particular wind is blowing or has blown.
- Noting that the illness has been attended by doctors but cannot be cured.
- Divination. This can be done with kernels of corn, observing the patterns in burning charcoal, observing an egg that has been passed over the patient, observing the entrails of an animal or reading a deck of cards or the shadows in the *sastún*.
- Seeing the results of the treatment offered by a *j'meen*.

The various illnesses caused by the different winds are easily confused.

The Wind of the Earth and the Wind of Rain only pass at five o'clock in the afternoon. Some winds occur all year round while others are season-specific, like the Wind of Rain and the whirlwind *("mozón")*, which occur in the rainy season and the dry season, respectively. Wind of the Owl happens only in the rainy season, while there are certain winds that are more frequent on particular days of the week, specifically Tuesdays and Fridays.

The evil wind can affect anyone, but is more common in children, both because they are weaker and because they don't yet know how to obey the rules of nature and society. Although there are many kinds of wind and many illnesses involved, these illnesses are not extremely frequent. Illness due to wind is not grave at first, but can become very serious, especially if it goes unidentified. If it doesn't receive adequate treatment the patient might come down with *xmaol ximbal iik' (xme'ol)*—wind exhaustion—and if an oration is not done, death may follow.

Treatments

The winds can be cured by an herbalist or *j'meen* but not by a doctor. Depending on the kind of wind and its gravity, the treatment may be any of the following:

- It is treated basically with prayers and cleansings. An incantation is sung in Maya while an herbal preparation—*tzipche' (Bunchiosa swartziana,* Gr.) or *chalche'*—is prescribed. *Tzipche'* smells of *caoba* (mahogany) and has yellow flowers and red fruit, while *chalche'* smells of anis. These aromas have the property of chasing away evil winds, while the colors red and blue, being hot, attract cold airs which draw the wind from the body. Other commonly used herbs are basil and rue, although they are not native to the region.
- By performing orations and cleansings *(lu'usa' k'eebaan)* the *curandero* brings the evil wind to the surface of the body, and from there brushes

Disease Classification

it away. This is done using aromatic plants of the colors red and blue which are later burned and thrown away.

- By performing *k'ej*. The patient brings an animal, plant, egg, or other object and the evil wind is channeled into it, leaving the person healthy. The animal dies, the plant dries out and changes color, and the egg cooks and goes bad.
- To treat *k'ojani kakab iik*—a wind produced by the *aluxob* that live in the mounds—it is necessary to offer *saká*—a wild plant (whose name is untranslated)—as food for the *aluxob*.
- In some places the rites of the *j'meen* are done in the shade of the ceiba *(Ceiba pentandra)*. It is one of the few trees that harbors a spirit. Many *curanderos* have their own secrets about how to harness the strength of the ceiba.

The treatment of wind can be completed with:

- Temperate herbal baths.
- Infusions of *kantemok, makulis, chiople' (Epitorium hemipteropodum,* R.), and flowers of *lo'l katzin*.
- A syrup of the fruit of young *jicara* or *luuch (Crescentia cujete)* with sugar and raisins.
- Iodine.
- The completion of a promise.

Prevention
- Stay out of the wind, do not leave the house at the times when specific winds blow.
- Fulfill promises and respect traditional practices. Give thanks for the harvest and perform the various rituals—*janikol, hakab, wahikol, cham, chan, pib*—for the spirits of the *milpa*, the corral, and so on.
- *Wahikol* and *lo'corral* consist of a ceremony in which an animal is sacrificed and its blood offered to the earth; the performer spins 13 times to the right and then 13 to the left. This ceremony should be performed every year to ensure the happiness of the spirits so that they won't bring disease and death to the animals or their owners.
- Kill an owl, remove its claws, disinfect them in boiling water, and keep them.

Meyak'as

This is a form of witchcraft or spell cast with malicious intent. There are many forms of *meyak'as*. This illness is caused by spells cast in envy, anger, hate, or vengeance. These spells are cast at night, generally on Tuesdays and Fridays.

- The protagonist may put a harmful substance in the food.
- The protagonist may toss something in the yard or in the house, for example dirt from the cemetery over which a spell has been cast.

The victim of witchcraft may show various symptoms, among them:

- Disassociation, paleness, lack of will, exhaustion, swollen belly, dryness in the body.
- Generalized pain, swelling, fever, asthma, blurred vision, vomiting.
- He or she loses money easily.
- Constant illness.
- When a massage is given to cure body aches but there is no effect, this is a sign that there is witchcraft involved.

A Western diagnosis using laboratory exams or x-rays will reveal nothing; diagnosis involves questioning the patient and performing divination. Apart from the above-mentioned indications, diseases caused by witchcraft can be easily confused with more common illnesses.

Illnesses associated with witchcraft seem to be fairly common, especially in adults. The gravity depends on the spell. If it is not adequately treated, the victim may experience great suffering, loss of will, ruin, and death.

Treatments
- The treatment depends on the spell. "Changes" are performed using totems, seven-colored ribbons, and candles.
- Other types of changes *(k'exob)* are performed using eggs or animals like black or calico hens.
- The treatment can be done through the medium of a family member using the victim's name or photo.
- Take a half-cup of olive oil with lime-juice and salt, accompanied by a blessing, to induce vomiting.
- If a man leaves his wife for another woman, a spell can be cast on a photograph and the photograph hidden in the man's clothes. With

Disease Classification

this spell he will no longer be attracted to the other woman and will return to his wife.

Prevention

- Clean the house and grounds. Protect the house with the marine stone known as *"la santa Ara negra,"* placing it at the four corners of the house, and burning something to smoke out the house.
- Carry a talisman—an amulet or relic—at all times.

A NOTE ON PRONUNCIATION

THE LANGUAGE SPOKEN IN THIS REGION of the state of Campeche is generally referred to by scholars as Yucatec or Yucatecan Maya, while its native speakers refer to the language simply as Maya. This can cause some confusion, as there are many distinct Mayan languages spoken in the different regions of the Mayan zone: Tzotzil, Tzeltal, Ch'ol, Tojolobal, Mam, Quiché, to name a few. All Mayan terms from the original text have been left in their original form, as have words from Chinese.

The pronunciation of all Maya words is as in Spanish, with the following exceptions: **c** is always hard; **x** is sounded like *sh* in English (xiu is pronounced "shu"). The letter **k** and the consonants **p, t, ch,** and **tz,** when marked by an apostrophe (**p', t', ch',** and **tz'**), are preceded by a muscular contraction of the mouth and then sounded suddenly, as glottal stops. Thus **tz'** sounds to the English speaker as if it were **dz,** as it is often written (as in *dzibolal*). The Mayan languages lack the English speech sounds **d,** hard **g, j, z,** and **f;** Yucatec Maya also lacks the **r.** As pronunciation is similar to Spanish, the **j** is pronounced as an aspirated **h,** so *j'meen* is pronounced *"h-meen."*

The plural suffix in Yucatec Maya (the equivalent of the English "s") is "ob." In keeping with recent Mayan scholarship, this standard is observed here; thus more than one *alux* is written *aluxob*, more than one *chak* is written *chakob*, and so on.

253

GLOSSARY OF MAYAN TERMS

Alux—a dwarf-like being or spirit (equivalent to a *chaneke* and *achene* of other Mesoamerican cultures). According to some Mayan people, the *aluxob* are leftover men of clay from the third creation, remaining on earth as helpers of the underworld gods. The *aluxob* guard the woods, jungles, springs, and stone mounds know by earlier Maya as *cuyos*.

Balam—meaning "jaguar" in everyday use, balam also refers to the guardian spirits of the woods, towns, and particular places.

Chak—a rain god. There are four *chakob,* one for each of the cardinal directions.

Haab—the Mayan calendar of 365 days, comprised of eighteen twenty-day months and one additional "month" of five days.

Jet—a form of massage imparted by midwives to pregnant women to insure a healthy birth.

J'meen—a shaman or healer whose role involves cleansings, incantations, herbal treatments, massage, *jup* and *tok.*

Jup—a therapy in which points on the body are pricked with a spine, without drawing blood, to move stagnant blood and air.

K'ak'as iik'—evil wind.

Kantis—denotes the sacred geography—veneration of the four directions and their manifestation in all aspects of life.

K'ej—meaning "change," denotes a type of spirit cleansing or cure for evil wind.

Lu'usa' k'eebaan—a spirit cleansing or treatment of evil wind in which a j'meen uses oration, laying on of hands and plant remedies to expel the wind from the body, and pass it into an inanimate object.

Ool—*"the wind of life,"* the animating spirit of the body, the vital impulse governing health, strength and emotional balance.

Causality and Illness

Pixán—"that which leaves me when I die." The body's vital force which exists from before birth, and at death leaves the body to be reincarnated in another form.

Sastún—a glass ball used in divination. Every *j'meen* has a *sastún* which is used in divining and diagnosing illnesses.

Sakáb—an offering of ritual food given to *aluxob, balamob,* or divinities.

Tipté—an organ or seat of energy, known in Spanish as *cirro*, located in the *tuch*.

Tok—a therapy in which points on the body are opened with a serrated spine to draw out stagnant blood and cure illnesses associated with evil wind.

Tu menta ojo—evil eye.

Tuch—the umbilical region of the body, center of the body's sacred geometry, equivalent to the *dan tian* in Chinese thought.

Tzak xiu—"plant medicine." Refers both to herbalists and to the practice of herbology.

U muuk'nak—one of the principal energies of the body, which palpitates with life and resides in the region of the of the *tuch*.

COMMENTS
ON THE TRANSLATION

THE BOOK YOU HOLD IS A DIRECT translation, from the Spanish, of the original *Medicina Maya Tradicional: Confrontacion con el Sistema Conceptual Chino* (Merida, Yucatán, EDUCE, 1996). I have stayed as close to the original as possible, while making small changes to bring the text before a North American audience, and I have reduced certain sections where I felt that streamlining the text would contribute to its cohesiveness and coherence. I have not added annotation, though I have included a short bibliography of books in English that have been useful to the translation and might be useful to the reader as well.

Although the emphasis of *Wind in the Blood* is on the present state of indigenous medical practice, it should provide an entrance into various fields of scholarship, looking at once to the ancient past and to the near future. The bibliographic notes presented here reflect a small fragment of the available scholarship. As mentioned in the text, very little scholarly work has been done on Mesoamerican forms of massage and acupuncture; however, a vast literature covers areas such as the ethnobotany of the Mayan regions, Mesoamerican shamanism, the calendric systems, Precolumbian mythology, religious syncretism and, of course, the ruins and the hieroglyphic writing system. To begin to create a bibliography covering every aspect of Mayan scholarship would be a work larger than can be undertaken here; rather, I would lead the reader to the bibliographies presented in some of my source materials. The ethnographic works by Barbara and Dennis Tedlock cover detailed and intimate aspects of Mayan timekeeping, myth, history, and religious practice in highland Guatemala; the seminal ethnobotanical research of Dennis Breedlove and Brent Berlin gives extensive treatment to the plants used in the Mayan world; Douglas Gillettes's tract on the resurrection teachings of the ancient Maya may provide a useful complement to the information on Mayan spiritual healing; and the extensive archeological work of Linda Schele, David Freidel and their collaborators uncovers facets of the ancient and contemporary Mayan worldview that may give greater depth to the vistas opened here.

Similarly, extensive resources are available in the field of Chinese medicine. Three books that give direct and simple treatment to complement and expand on the information presented here are *The Web That Has No Weaver*, by Ted Kaptchuk, *Between Heaven and Earth: A Guide To Chinese Medicine* by Harriet Beinfield and Efrem Korngold, and *The Way of Qigong* by Kenneth S. Cohen.

Certain words in the text have been left in the original Spanish, for a variety of reasons. Some terms, like *campesino* and *curandero,* have no direct translation which would reveal their social dimension; others, like the names of a few plants—*alucema, incienso maravilloso*—lack a Latin binomial in the original text, so no English equivalent could be found. One hopes that further editions of this work will alleviate these omissions, or that the work of other researchers will make this information available. In many cases, the villagers themselves may not know the name of a given plant, though they will be quite familiar with its uses.

I am not a scholar nor a speaker of Yucatec Maya; where English equivalents are given for Mayan words, these terms have not been translated directly from Maya, but rather from the Spanish; any inconsistencies or irregularities in the translation of Mayan terms may be due to the two-step removal of the English version from the Mayan original. One hopes that such variations and inconsistencies are slight and do no harm to the original sense.

BIBLIOGRAPHY

THIS IS THE BIBLIOGRAPHY EXACTLY as it appears in the original, published version of *Medicina Maya Tradicional: Confrontación con el sistema conceptual chino,* Mérida, Yucatán: EDUCE, 1996. These references have not been researched by the translator. Where an edition of the book is available in English I have listed these references in the Translator's Bibliography.

Aguilar Cerón: *La medicina empírica yucateca en el siglo XVII a través de sus fuentes.* Talleres Gráficos del Sureste. Mérida, Yucatán, México, 1987.

Aguirre Beltrán, Gonzalo: *Antropología médica.* CIESAS, SEP/Cultura. México, D.F., 1986.

Aparicio Alegría, Bertha: "El Susto y sus distintas modalidades en una comunidad totonaca." Ponencia presentada en el IV Congreseo Internacional de Medicina Tradicional y Folklórica, San Cristóbal de Las Casas, Chiapas, diciembre de 1990.

Arnold, Paul: *El libro maya de los muertos.* Editorial Diana, México, D.F., 1983.

Arsovska, Liljana: "Breve historia de la filosofia china." Primer Encuentro Académico de Acupuntura de la Asociacíon Mexican de Asociaciones y Sociedades de Acupuntura (AMASA A.C.A) Guadelajara, Jalisco, enero 23 y 24 de 1993.

Arzápalo Marín, Ramón: *El ritual de los Bacabes.* Edicíon facsimilar con traducción rítmica, traducción, notas, índice, glosario y cómputos estadísticos. UNAM. México, D.F., 1987.

Balam P., Gilberto: "Del origen, desarollo, y actualidad social del conocimineto médico de los mayas de Yucatán." Tesis presentada para obtener el grado de doctor en sociología. UNAM. México, D.F.,1990.

Balam P., Gilberto: "Medicina indígena en la península yucateca," México indígena, núm. 9, marzo-abril de 1986. INI, México.

Barrera Marín, A., et al: *Nomenclatura etnobotánica maya. Una interpretación taxonómica.* Editorial Centro Regional del Sureste, INAH, México, D.F., 1976.

Barrera Vázquez, Alfredo: *Las fuentes para el estudio de la medicina nativa de Yucatán.* Mérida, Yucatán, 1963.

Bello, M.A.G., y Pérez, A.: "El papel de los hueseros en la medicina tradicional en Xochipala, Guerrero." Ponencia presentada en el IV Congreso Internacional de Medicina Tradicional y Folklórica. San Cristóbal de las Casas, Chiapas, diciembre de 1990.

Bonfil Batalla, Guillermo: *México profundo: Una civilización negada.* Editorial Grijalbo, México, D.F., 1990.

Bossy, J: *Bases neurobiológicas de las reflexoterapias.* Monografías de Reflexoterapia Aplicada. Masson, S.A. Barcelona, España, 1985.

Brailowski, Simón, Stein, Donald G., y Bruno, Will: *El cerebro averiado: Plasticidad cerebral y recuperación funcional.* Fondo de cultura económica. Sección de obras de ciencia y tecnología, México, D.F., 1992.

Cardeña, V.: *El judío.* ECAUDY. Mérida, Yucatán, 1984.

Códice Pérez. Traducción del original por E. Solis A. Editorial de la Liga de Acción Social. Mérida, Yucatán, 1949.

Colección de artículos de acupuntura y moxibustión. de 1978 a 1983. Primera parte, Instituto de Medicina Tradicional China de Tianjin y la Clínica de Acupuntura del Hospital Anexo 1 de Tianjin, República Popular China, 1983.

Cuevas, Benjamín: *Plantas medicanales de Yucatán. Guía médica práctica doméstica.* Imprenta de la Lotería de Yucatán. México, D.F., 1913.

Chen Jing: *Anatomical Atlas of Chinese Points.* Shandong Science and Technology Press. Jinan, Republica Popular China, 1982.

De Landa, Diego: *Relación de las cosas de Yucatán.* Editorial Porrúa. México, D.F., 1982.

Devereux, George: *De la ansiedad al método en las ciencias del comportamiento.* Siglo XXI Editores, México, 1989.

Dian Cong et al: *Coleccíon de moxibustion china.* Ediciones Científicas de Lioning, Yucatán, 1930.

Diccionario de Motul. Maya-español. Edición particular de Juan Martínez, Mérida, Yucatán, 1930.

Dondé, J. y J.: *Apuntes sobre las plantas de Yucatán.* S/Ed. Mérida, Yucatán, 1876.

Estudio de Acupuntura. Instituto de Medicina Tradicional de Shanghai, Editorial Salud del Pueblo, República Popular China, 1986.

Florescano, Enrique: "Muerte y resurrección del dios del maíz." *Nexos.* México, D.F., abril, 1993.

García López, Marcelina: "Concepcíon indígena de las patologías, acciones terapéuticas y análisis de algunos métodos de curación." Ponencia presentada en el IV Congreso Internacional de Medicina Tradicional y Folklórica, San Cristóbal de las Casas, Chiapas, diciembre de 1990.

García Ramírez, Hernán: *Salud, conciencia y organización.* CRT y Fomento Cultural Educativo, México, 1990.

Gómez, A., M. Gispert y A. Ramírez: "El ramo de limpias; su composición botánica e importancia en la medicina tradicional," Ponencia presentada en el IV Congreso Internacional de Medicina Tradicional y Folklórica, San Cristóbal de las Casas, Chiapas, diciembre, 1990.

González, Roberto: "Historia de la medicina tradicional china." Primer encuentro académico de acupuntura de la Asociación, Mexicana de Asociaciones y Sociedades de Acupuntura (AMASA A.C.) Guadalajara, Jalisco, enero 23 y 24 de 1993.

Gui Yong Fan, Chen Qi, Li Yin Fa y Jiang Shan: "Características fisicas del *qi'* emitido." Instituto Aeronáutico de Nanjing. Artículo publicado en el *Compendio de la Primera Conferencia de Intercambio Académico de* qi gong *Médico.* Beijing, China 1988.

Gutiérrez, Enrique: *Tomar conciencia,* Fomento Cultural Educativo, México, 1985.

Guzmán, Eulalia: "La lengua maya y la lengua china." *Magisterio,* número 242, enero de 1987. Sindicato Nacional de Trabajadores de la Educación.

Lévi-Strauss, Claude: *Antropología estructural.* EUDEBA. Buenos Aires, 1977.

Liu Bing Quan: *Optimum time for acupuncture: A Collection of Traditional Chinese Chronotherapeutics.* Shandong Science and Technology. Beijing, Peoples' Republic of China, 1988, pp. 1 á 20.

López Austin, Alfredo: *Cuerpo humano e ideología.* UNAM, México, D.F., 1980.

Locke, Steven y Douglas Colligan: *El médico interior. La nueva medicina que revela la incidencia de la mente en nuestra salud y en el tratamiento de las enfermedades.* Editorial Sudamericana-Hermes. México, D.F., 1991.

Lovelock, James: *Gaia, una nueva visión de la vida.* Editorial Orbis, Biblioteca de divulgacíon científica. Barcelona, España, 1986.

Lozano, Francisco: "Etiologia en medicina tradicional china." En: Primer Encuentro Académico de Acupuntura de la Asociación Mexicana de

Bibliography

Asociaciones y Sociedades de Acupuntura (AMASA, AC.) Guadelajara, Jalisco, enero 23 y 24 de 1993.

Lu Zu Yin y Wang Yao Lan: *Un método para detectar el campo de* qi. Instituto de Alta Energía Física. Academia Sinica Yan Xin. Instituto Municipal de Medicina Tradicional China de Chong Quing, Provincia de Sichuan. Artículo publicado en el *Compendio de la Primera Conferencia de Intercambio Académico de* qi gong *Médico.* Beijing, Republica Popular China, 1988.

Memorias del Primer Congreso de Medicina Tradicional y Herbolaria. San Cristóbal de las Casas, Chiapas, noviembre de 1983.

Memorias del Primer Encuentro de Médicos Indígenas del Estado de Chiapas. OMIECH, San Cristóbal de las Casas, Chiapas, noviembre de 1986.

Memorias del Cuarto Encuentro de Médicos Indígenas del Estado de Chiapas. OMIECH, San Cristóbal de las Casas, Chiapas, agosto de 1989.

Menéndez, Eduardo L.: *Poder, estratificación y salud. Análisis de las condiciones sociales y económicas de la enfermedad en Yucatán.* Ediciones de la Casa Chata 13. México, D.F., 1981.

Montulio Villar, María: "Cosmovisión y salud entre los mayas de Yucatán," del libro *Plantas medicinales de México.* Erik Estrada, compilador. Universidad Autónoma de Chapingo. Departamento de Fitotecnia, Unidad de Estudios Etnobotánicos, México, D.F., 1990.

Montulio Villar, María: *"La medicina maya."* Del libro *Plantas medicinales de México.* Erik Estrada, Compilador. Universidad Autónoma de Chapingo. Departamento de Fitotecnia, Unidad de Estudios Etnobotánicas. México, D.F., 1990, pp. 102 á 110.

Negrete, G., y A. Gómez: *"La herbolaria tradicional aplicada a enfermedades de la piel en Xochipala, Guerrero."* Ponencia presentada en el IV Congreso Internacional de Medicina Tradicional y Folklórica. San Cristóbal de las Casas, Chiapas, diciembre de 1990.

Ordoñez, Crisóforo y Roberto González: *"Historia Clínica."* Segundo Encuentro Académico de Acupuntura de la Asociación Mexican de Asociaciones y Sociedaded de Acupuntura (AMASA A.C.) Puebla, Puebla. Marzo 27 y 28 de 1993. Pp. 9 á 43.

Oropeza Gutiérrez, Alejandro: *"Tui na Masaje Chino."* Segundo Encuentro Académico de Acupuntura de la Asociaciónes y Sociedades de Acupuntura (AMASA A.C.). Puebla, Puebla. Marzo 27 y 28 de 1993. Pp. 136–154.

Pérez Tamayo, Ruy: *El concepto de enfermedad, su evolución a través de la historia.* Tomo II. UNAM, CONACYT, FCE. México, D.F., 1989.

Principios básicos de medicina tradicional. Primer Tomo. Ediciones de Medicina Tradicional Escritas en Lengua Antigua China. Beijing, China.

Redfield, R. y Villa Rojas, A.: *Chan Kom: A Maya Village*. The University of Chicago Press. Chicago, 1934.

Rejón, Pastor: *Manual para encargados de fincas*. Ed. de la Facultad de Mérida, Yucatán, México, 1905.

Riojas Horacio: *Una aproximacíon a tres nosolgías de la medicina tradicional en el suroccidente de Puebla y límites con el estado de Morelos*. Mimeo, 1991.

Rodríguez Rivera, Luis: "La entidad nosológica: un paradigma," *Revista cubana de administración de la salud*, Número 8. Julio–septiembre de 1988. La Habana, Cuba, pp. 253 á 257.

Rogers, Fred B.: *Compendio de historia de la salud pública*. Siglo XXI Editores, México, D.F., 1981.

Roys, Ralph: *Mayan Ethnobotany*. New Orleans, LA. Tulane University Press, 1931.

Sagan, Carl: *Cosmos*. Editorial Planeta. Barcelona, España, Séptima edición, 1983, pp. 46 y 48.

Sanginés, Agustín: *Medicina liberadora, teoría, método y práctica*. Praxis, México, 1989.

Sasoon Lombardo, Yolanda: *El alma y los síndromes patológicos populares actuales*. Dirección General de Culturas Populares. Unidad regional Michoacán, SEP, Cuadernos 41, mayo de 1983.

Shi Xue Ming: *Acupuntura práctica*. Instituto de Medicina Tradicional China de Tianjin. Clínica de Acupunctura del Hospital Anexo 1 de Tianjin. Editorial Científica de Tianjin, 1980.

Técnica de sangrado por punción. Ci xue liao fa. Editorial Científica de la Provincia de Anhui, República Popular China, 1988.

The Chinese-English Medical Dictionary. Ediciones Salud del pueblo, Beijing, República Popular China, 1987.

Tompkins, Peter, y Bird, Christopher: *La vida secreta de las planta*. Editorial Diana, México, D.F., 1985.

Thompson, Eric S.: *Historia y religión de los mayas*. Siglos XXI. México, D.F., 1979.

Tratado de Acupuntura. Colección de Publicaciones de Medicina Tradicional China, primera parte. Editorial de Libros Antiguos. Instituto de Medicina Tradicional China de Beijing, China, 1985.

Villa Rojas, A.: *Los elegidos de Dios. Etnografía de los mayas de Quintana Roo*. INI, México, D.F., 1978.

Yuan Ke: *Chugoku kodai Shinwa.* (Mitología antigua de la China). Shanghai, China, 1957.

Yuan Zhu, et al.: *Atlas de puntos acupunturales.* Editorial Científica de Sahnghai, República Popular China, 1988.

Zhang Jun y Zheng Jing: *Fundamentos de acupuntura y moxibustión de China.* Ediciones en Lenguas Extranjeras, Beijing, República Popular China, 1984.

Zhang Mingwu y Sun Xingyuan: *Chinese* quigong *therapy.* Shandong Science and Technology Press. Jinan, China, 1985.

Zolla, Carlos, Sofía del Bosque, Antonio Tascón y Virginia Mellado: *Medicina tradicional y enfermedad.* Centro Interamericano de Estudios de Seguridad Social (CIESS), México, 1988.

TRANSLATOR'S BIBLIOGRAPHY

NOTE: LATIN PLANT NAMES ARE notated according to *The Plant Book, A Portable Dictionary of the Vascular Plants,* by D.J. Mabberley (see below). English translations of the names of Chinese acupuncture points are translated in accordance with *Acupuncture, A Comprehensive Text,* by John O'Connor and Dan Bensky (see below).

Barrera Vásquez, Alfredo and Redon, Silvia. *El libro de los libros de Chilam Balam.* México, D.F.: Fondo de Cultura Economica, 1948.

Beinfield, Harriet and Korngold, Efrem. *Between Heaven and Earth: A Guide To Chinese Medicine.* New York: Ballantine Books, 1991.

Bensky, Dan, and Gamble, Andrew, with Kaptchuk, Ted. *Chinese Herbal Medicine: Materia Medica.* Seattle, WA: Eastland Press, 1986.

Berlin, Brent. *Principles of Tzeltal Plant Classification, An Introduction to the Botanical Ethnography of a Mayan-Speaking People of Highland Chiapas.* New York, NY: Academic Press, 1974.

Breedlove, Dennis E. and Laughlin, Robert M. *The Flowering of Man: a Tzotzil Botany of Zinacantan.* Washington, D.C.: Smithsonian Institution Press, 1993.

Brotherston, Gordon and Dorn, Edward (translators). *The Sun Unwound: Original Texts from Occupied America.* Berkeley, CA: North Atlantic Books, 1999

Cohen, Kenneth S. *The Way of Quigong: The Art and Science of Chinese Energy Healing.* New York, NY: Ballantine Books, 1997.

Connelly, Dianne M. *Traditional Acupuncture: The Law of the Five Elements.* Columbia, MD: Centre for Traditional Acupuncture Inc., 1989.

De Landa, Friar Diego (Translated by William Gates). *Yucatán Before and After the Conquest.* New York, NY: Dover Press, 1978.

Gillete, Douglas. *The Shaman's Secret: The Lost Resurrection Teachings of the Ancient Maya.* New York, NY: Bantam Books, 1997.

Kaptchuk, Ted J. *The Web That Has No Weaver: Understanding Chinese Medicine.* Chicago, IL: Congdon and Weed, 1983.

Lévi-Strauss, Claude. *Structural Anthropology.* New York, NY: HarperCollins, 1963.

Lovelock, James. *Gaia: A New Look at Life on Earth.* Oxford, England: Oxford University Press, 1979.

Mabberley, D.J. *The Plant Book: A Portable Dictionary of the Vascular Plants.* Cambridge, England: Cambridge University Press, 1997.

Maoshing Ni, (translator). *The Yellow Emperor's Classic of Medicine.* Boston and London: Shambhala, 1995.

Markman, Roberta H. and Markman, Peter T. *The Flayed God, The Mythology of Mesoamerica.* San Francisco: Harper San Francisco, 1992.

O'Connor, John, and Bensky, Dan, (translators). *Acupuncture, A Comprehensive Text—Shanghai College of Traditional Medicine.* Seattle: Eastland Press, 1981

Pitchford, Paul. *Healing With Whole Foods: Oriental Tradition and Modern Nutrition.* Berkeley, CA: North Atlantic Books, 1993.

Porter, Roy. *The Greatest Benefit to Mankind: A Medical History of Humanity.* New York, NY: W.W. Norton & Company, 1998.

Schele Linda, and Freidel, David. *A Forest of Kings: The Untold Story of the Ancient Maya.* New York, NY: William Morrow and Company, 1990.

Schele, Linda, Frediel, David, and Parker, Joy. *Maya Cosmos: Three Thousand Years on the Shaman's Path.* New York, NY: William Morrow and Company, 1993.

Tedlock, Barbara. *Time and the Highland Maya.* Albuquerque, NM: University of New Mexico Press, 1982.

Tedlock, Dennis (translator). *Popul Vuh.* New York, NY: Simon and Schuster, 1985.

Tedlock, Dennis. *Breath On The Mirror.* New York, NY: HarperCollins, 1993.

Thompson, Eric S. *Maya History and Religion.* Norman, OK and London, England: University of Oklahoma Press, 1970.

Tompkins, Peter, and Bird, Christopher. *The Secret Life of Plants.* New York, NY: Harper & Row, 1973.

NOTES

1. De Landa, Diego, *Relación de las cosas de Yucatán*, 1982
2. Barrera Vásquez, Alfredo, *El libro de los libros de Chilam Balam*, 1948
3. Roys, Ralph, *Mayan Ethnobotany*, 1931
4. Arzápalo, Marín Ramón, *El ritual de los Bacabes*, 1987
5. Barrera Vásquez, Alfredo, *Las fuentes para el estudio de la medicina nativa de Yucatán*, 1963
6. Cardeña, V., *El Judio*, 1984
7. Donde, J. y J., *Apuntes sobre las plantas de Yucatán*, 1876
8. Cuevas, Benjamín, *Plantas Medicinales de Yucatán*, 1913
9. Rejón, Pastor, *Manual para encargados de fincas*, 1905
10. Sangines, Agustín, *Medicina liberadora, teoria, metodo y practica*, 1989
11. Tedlock, Dennis (translator), *Popul Vuh*, 1985
12. Yuan Ke, *Chugoku kodai Shinwa*, 1957
13. Montulio Villar, María, "La medicina maya"
14. Thompson, Eric S., *Historia y Religion de los mayas*, 1975. This is the version referred to by the authors. See also the original English version: Thompson, Eric S., *Maya History and Religion*, 1970
15. Arnold, Paul, *El libro maya de los muertos*, 1983
16. Arzapalo R., *El ritual de los bacabes*, 1987
17. Tedlock, Dennis (translator), *Popul Vuh*, 1985
18. Montulio Villar, María, "*Cosmovisión y salud entre los mayas de Yucatán*"
19. Ni, Maoshing (translator), *Yellow Emperor's Classic of Medicine*, 1995, pg. 27
20. Balám, Gilberto, *Del origen, desarollo, y actualidad social del conocimiento médico de los mayas de Yucatán*, 1991
21. Florescano, Enrique, *Muerte y resurrección del dios de maíz*, 1993
22. ibid.
23. Ni, Maoshing (translator), *Yellow Emperor's Classic of Medicine*, 1995, pg. 8
24. ibid., pg. 39
25. Liu Bing Quan, *Optimum Time for Acupuncture*, 1988, pp. 1-20
26. Ni, Maoshing (translator), *Yellow Emperor's Classic of Medicine*, 1995, pg. 23
27. ibid., pg. 11
28. ibid., pg. 19

29. ibid., pg. 11
30. ibid., pg. 58
31. ibid., pg. 243
32. ibid., pg. 27
33. García López, Marcelina, *"Concepción indígena de las patologías, acciones terapéuticas y análisis de algunos métodos de curación,"* 1990
34. González, Roberto, *"Historia de la medicina tradicional china,"* 1993
35. Arzapalo R., *El ritual de los Bacabes,* 1987
36. Bossy, J., *Bases neurobiologicas de las reflexoterapias,* 1985
37. Ni, Maoshing (translator), *Yellow Emperor's Classic of Medicine,* 1995, pg.172
38. Mingwu, Zhang, *Chinese Quigong Therapy,* 1985
39. Lu Zuyin, *Un metodo para dectectar un campo de qi* 1988
40. González, Roberto, *Historia de la medicina tradicional china,* 1993
41. Oropeza Gutiérrez, Alejandro, *Tui na Masaje Chino,* 1993, pp. 136–154
42. Sagan, Carl, *Cosmos,* 1983, pp. 4–48
43. Brailowsky, Símon, *El cerebro averiado,* 1992
44. Riojas, Horacio, *Una aproximacíon,* 1991
45. Pérez Tamayo, Ruy, *El concepto de enfermedad,* 1989
46. Rodríguez Rivera, Luis, *"La entidad nosologica: un paradigma,"* 1988, pp. 253–257
47. Lozano, Francisco, *Etiología en medicina tradicional china,* 1993

INDEX

Index

Sa'p u k'aab u yim, 219–20
Sasak ka, 227–28
Sasak kal, 226–27
Sastún
    appearance of, 69
    diagnosis by, 69
    importance of, to *j'meen*, 143
Sauco, 88
Scabies, 231
Scarlet sage, 81
Seasons, 59–61
Se'en, 208–9
Sensitive plant, 84
Sesame, 80
Sesamum orientale, 80
Seven Emotions, 56–58
Sexual activity, excessive, 58–59
Sexual desire, 245
Shamans, 147
Shang Hai Jing, 147
Shang Han Lun, 76
Shaoyang, 8
Shaoyin, 8
Shen, 32, 33, 162
Shencang, 114
Shenfeng, 114
Shenmai, 122
Shensu, 130–31
Shenting, 116
Shufu, 114
Shuigou, 115
Shuoyuan, 147
Sida acuta, 82
Sidu, 117
Siit, 88
Simarouba glauca, 92
Sinanche', 88
Sinan ik, 89
Sisal xiu, 89
Sisín, 90
Sizhukong, 117
Skin disease, 220–22

Small intestine
    fire element and, 36
    summer and, 24
Solanum hispidum, 92
Solanum niggrum, L., 87
Son, 89
Sotuta, xxvii
Soul, concepts of, 30, 162. *See also*
    Vital principles
Sour orange, 86
Soursop, 83
Spirits, 52–53
Spleen
    earth element and, 19, 36
    function of, 37, 38
    late summer and, 24
Spondias purpurea, 82
Squash, winter, 85
Star-apple, 81
Stars, influence of, 15
Stomach
    ache, 198–99
    cold in, 181
    earth element and, 36
    late summer and, 24
    sour, 199–201
Subín, 89
Suciedad, 27
Suction treatment, 104–5
Summer heat, 64. *See also* Heat and
    cold
Sun
    chi and, 8
    influence of, 15
    winds and, 52, 247
Susto, 232–34

Taa chak, 89
Tabebuia chrysantha, 90
Tabernaemontana amygdalifolia, 90
Tagetes patula, L., 92
Taiyang, 129

About North Atlantic Books